This is the first volume to look in depth at the functioning of the vascular endothelium, and at the diseases and tissue injury that arise as a result of inflammation and immunological responses. The vascular endothelium is a metabolically highly active layer of cells lining all blood vessel walls. Through its interactions with leukocytes and other mediators, it is central to the development of inflammatory foci and to lymphocyte trafficking around the body. Tissue injury may arise here as a result of abnormal inflammatory or immune responses. The potential for such injury to contribute to autoimmune disease is discussed in this book, particularly in relation to autoimmune vascular disease of the renal, rheumatological and neurological systems, as well as in organ transplantation.

Immunological aspects of the vascular endothelium

CAMBRIDGE REVIEWS IN CLINICAL IMMUNOLOGY

Recent advances in immunology, particularly at the molecular level, have led to a much clearer understanding of the causes and consequences of autoimmunity. The aim of this series is to make these developments accessible to clinicians who feel daunted by such advances and require a clear exposition of the scientific and clinical issues. The various clinical specialities will be covered in separate volumes, which will follow a fixed format: a brief introduction to basic immunology followed by a comprehensive review of recent findings in the autoimmune conditions which, in particular, will compare animal models with their human counterparts. Sufficient clinical detail, especially regarding treatment, will also be included to provide basic scientists with a better understanding of these aspects of autoimmunity. Thus each volume will be self-contained and comprehensible to a wide audience. Taken as a whole the series will provide an overview of all the important autoimmune disorders.

Autoimmune endocrine disease A. P. Weetman
Immunological aspects of renal disease D. B. G. Oliveira
Gastrointestinal and hepatic immunology R. V. Heatley

Immunological aspects of the vascular endothelium

EDITED BY

CAROLINE O. S. SAVAGE
Senior Lecturer in Medicine, Department of Medicine,
The Medical School, University of Birmingham, UK

AND

JEREMY D. PEARSON
Professor of Vascular Biology, King's College, London, UK

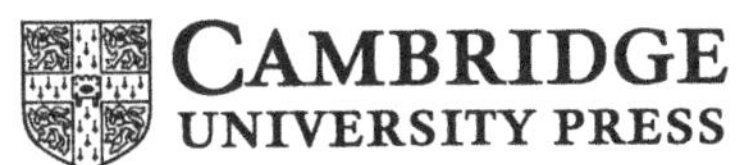
CAMBRIDGE
UNIVERSITY PRESS

CAMBRIDGE UNIVERSITY PRESS
Cambridge, New York, Melbourne, Madrid, Cape Town, Singapore,
São Paulo, Delhi, Dubai, Tokyo, Mexico City

Cambridge University Press
The Edinburgh Building, Cambridge CB2 8RU, UK

Published in the United States of America by Cambridge University Press, New York

www.cambridge.org
Information on this title: www.cambridge.org/9780521184311

First published 1995
First paperback edition 2010

A catalogue record for this publication is available from the British Library

Library of Congress Cataloguing in Publication data

Immunological aspects of the vascular endothelium/edited by Caroline O.
Savage and Jeremy D. Pearson.
p. cm.—(Cambridge reviews in clinical immunology)
Includes index.
ISBN 0-521-45249-X (hc)
1. Vascular endothelium—Immunology. 2. Inflammation.
3. Vascular endothelium—Pathophysiology. I. Savage, Caroline O. S.
II. Pearson, Jeremy D. III. Series.
[DNLM: 1. Endothelium, Vascular—Immunology. WG 500 133
1995]
RC694.5.I53I48 1995
616.13′079—dc20
DNLM/DLC
for Library of Congress 94–48324 CIP

ISBN 978-0-521-45249-6 Hardback
ISBN 978-0-521-18431-1 Paperback

Contents

List of contributors

ANN AGER
Laboratory of Cellular Immunology
National Institute for Medical Research
The Ridgeway
Mill Hill
London NW7 1AA, UK

DANIEL M. ALTMANN
Transplantation Biology Section
Clinical Sciences Centre
Royal Postgraduate Medical School
Du Cane Road
London W12 0NN, UK

P. ATHANASSIOU
Rheumatology Unit
Hammersmith Hospital
Du Cane Road
London W12 0NN, UK

HUW BEYNON
Rheumatology Research Unit
Royal Free Hospital
Pond Street
London NW3 2QG, UK

JOHN R. BRADLEY
Department of Medicine
Addenbrooke's Hospital
Cambridge CB2 2QQ, UK

VIRGINIA CALDER
Institute of Ophthalmology
Bath Street
London EC1V 9EL, UK

K. A. DAVIES
Rheumatology Unit
Hammersmith Hospital
Du Cane Road
London W12 0NN, UK

M. J. DILLON
Department of Nephrology
Hospital for Sick Children
Great Ormond Street
London WC1N 3JH, UK

P. EMERY
Department of Rheumatology
The Medical School
University of Birmingham
Edgbaston
Birmingham B15 2TT, UK

JOHN GREENWOOD
Institute of Ophthalmology
Bath Street
London EC1V 9EL, UK

MICHAEL J. MAY
Vascular Biology Research Centre
Biomedical Sciences Division
King's College
Campden Hill Road
London W8 7AH, UK

R. J. MOOTS
Department of Rheumatology
The Medical School
University of Birmingham
Edgbaston
Birmingham B15 2TT, UK

SUSSAN NOURSHARGH
Department of Applied Pharmacology
National Heart & Lung Institute
Dovehouse Street
London SW3 6LY, UK

ABEED A. PALL
CCRIS
The Medical School
University of Birmingham
Edgbaston
Birmingham B15 2TT, UK

JEREMY D. PEARSON
Vascular Biology Research Centre
Biomedical Sciences Division
King's College
Campden Hill Road
London W8 7AH, UK

GIUSEPPE REMUZZI
Mario Negri Institute for Pharmacological Research
Via Gavazzeni 11
24125 Bergamo
Italy
and
Division of Nephrology and Dialysis
Ospedali Riuniti di Bergamo
24100 Bergamo
Italy

CAROLINE O. S. SAVAGE
Renal Immunobiology Laboratory
The Medical School
University of Birmingham
Edgbaston
Birmingham B15 2TT, UK

CARLA ZOJA
Mario Negri Institute for Pharmacological Research
Via Gavazzeni 11
24125 Bergamo
Italy

Preface

Endothelial cells form the interface between blood and tissues throughout the body. They are thus the first barrier between cellular or humoral components of the immune system and any challenging extravascular antigen. In recent years it has become apparent that this barrier is far from being metabolically inert, that the properties of endothelial cells contribute critically to the physiological and pathological extravasation of leukocytes, and that these properties can be modulated substantially by inflammatory and immune mediator molecules. In addition, in a subset of autoimmune diseases, vascular damage is prominent, suggesting that immunological effector processes are being targeted inappropriately to the cells of the vessel wall. Similar processes may also underlie rejection of transplanted organs, where donor blood vessels are prominently and primarily affected.

In this volume we have gathered a series of expert authors to describe in more detail the immunological aspects of vascular endothelial cell function summarized above, introduced by a chapter that updates current general concepts of autoimmunity as a framework for what follows. The next three chapters review the ways in which the endothelial phenotype can be modulated by inflammatory and immune cytokines, particularly surveying the recent enormous increase in our understanding of how endothelial cells control leukocyte adhesion and emigration, and of the molecular families implicated in this control. These fall into overlapping but distinct patterns directing the selective emigration of different leukocyte classes in acute or chronic inflammation, and the recirculation of lymphocytes through the lymphyoid tissue.

The next five chapters cover what is known (or suspected) of the role of endothelial cells in individual autoimmune diseases where there is a greater or lesser degree of vascular involvement. These include diseases where specific organ involvement is prominent, ranging from the brain or eye to the kidney, joints or skin, and also the primary systemic vasculitic diseases. The final chapter emphasizes the under-appreciated ability of endothelial cells, when stimulated, to present antigens with the correct co-stimulatory signals to lymphocytes, and hence to trigger the immunological process of graft rejection. Taken together, we hope that the second half of the book provides a persuasive argument as to why understanding normal endothelial cell function and its dysregulation is vital if we are to succeed in designing effective therapies for the treatment of these diseases.

Caroline Savage and Jeremy Pearson
March 1995

–1–
New concepts of mechanisms in autoimmunity

DANIEL M. ALTMANN

Introduction

Autoimmune diseases are, by definition, ones in which pathology results directly or indirectly from specific immune recognition of self-tissues. Although the ultimate mediators of destruction may include T cells, antibody and complement or activated macrophages, attention has focused on the central interaction of antigenic peptide, major histocompatibility complex (MHC) molecule and T cell receptor (TCR) needed to trigger recognition. The paradigm for analysis of these events has come largely from studies in a small number of mouse and rat models. In particular, experimental allergic encephalomyelitis (EAE), an experimentally induced disease where animals show CNS inflammation sometimes including demyelination, is a model for some aspects of multiple sclerosis (MS), while the non-obese diabetic (NOD) mouse offers a good model for the spontaneous, autoimmune destruction of pancreatic beta cells in insulin dependent, type I diabetes (IDDM).

Experiments in such models have raised the hope that characterization of the molecular components involved in the activation of autoreactive T cells will pave the way for the design of highly selective immunosuppressive therapies. Since the stimulation of specific T cells to kill targets or secrete cytokines depends on signals which follow precise binding of the TCR to a complex formed by antigenic peptide lodged in the 'cleft' of a specific MHC molecule, therapeutic intervention may be offered by competition with, or blocking of, any of these compounds. Indeed, many major pharmaceutical companies currently base much of their research and development for diseases such as rheumatoid arthritis and diabetes on this premise.

The aim of this chapter is to summarize and evaluate what is known about the molecular mechanisms underlying autoimmune disease in animal models and in man and thus to appraise the potential for specific immunotherapies. It also provides a framework for understanding the possible pathogenic process involved in the autoimmune vascular diseases described in Chapters 5 to 10. The following pages review current work on each of the three central components in the stimulation of autoreactive T cells: MHC, antigenic peptide and TCR. However, in considering these questions it is germane to start by considering some of the current views on the nature of self-tolerance and how autoimmune diseases could nevertheless emerge.

Current concept of self-tolerance

Older textbooks often introduce immunology as the science of discrimination between self and non-self, a view rooted in Ehrlich and Burnet, whereby 'forbidden clones' recognizing any self components are tolerized or deleted during development, and clonal selection then operates on the remaining T cell repertoire. Autoreactivity would thus be viewed as a pathological accident resulting from a failure or bypassing of tolerance. Data accrued in recent years imply that the question must be more complex than this view suggests. Many laboratories which have set out to clone T cells against human self-antigens such as myelin basic protein (MBP) and acetylcholine receptor (AChR) have found this fairly easy to do using blood from healthy laboratory personnel (Burns *et al.*, 1983; Ota *et al.*, 1990; Zhang *et al.*, 1990). Autoreactive cells may exist in all individuals at a low precursor frequency and/or under some form of control such that they do not necessarily trigger disease. Network theories of immune regulation have long been debated by immunologists, and there is currently one school of thought which maintains that recognition of some self-antigens is a necessary and physiological part of the shaping of the immune repertoire (Cohen, 1992; Coutinho, 1993).

However, there clearly also exists a form of self-tolerance to some self-antigens which is absolute and presumably results from deletion of the responsive T cells. For example, from studies on elution of endogenous peptides from MHC class II molecules, transferrin receptor peptides constitute one of the self components which quite commonly occupy the cleft of MHC molecules, but we know of no diseases resulting from autoreactivity to this molecule and no T cells which recognize it.

It has long been appreciated that the thymus is the black box where there is some selection from among the random repertoire of antigen receptors on developing T cells. The current concept of T cell deletion or 'negative selection' dates from experiments conducted largely in the late 1980s. In one series of experiments, Kappler and Marrack's laboratories first generated a monoclonal antibody specific for mouse T cell receptors encoded by TCR genes which include the variable region gene segment, Vβ17a. They noted that many of their T cell clones which were reactive against the mouse MHC class II molecule, H-2E (formerly termed I-E), used this Vβ17a gene rather than the 23 other possible variable regions in the germline repertoire (Kappler *et al.*, 1987). It was then possible to track Vβ17a$^+$ cells by flow cytometry, asking what became of these cells in a mouse which actually carried the H-2E target molecule. Cells bearing the autoreactive receptor were found equally in the thymuses of E$^+$ or E$^-$ mice when the immature, CD4$^+$8$^+$ double positive TCR^{lo} thymocytes were analysed (Kappler, Roehm & Marrack, 1987). Among mature cells in the thymus or those which had emerged into the periphery (CD4$^+$ TCR^{hi} or CD8$^+$ TCR^{hi}), mice expressing H-2E had totally deleted the population of cells bearing the autoreactive receptor. This was one of the first experiments which allowed the nature of thymic or central tolerance by clonal deletion to be described at the level of ligand/receptor interactions. Since that time it has become clear that the self-antigen recognized by the Vβ17a clones was, in fact, H-2E complexed with so-called endogenous superantigen encoded by the endogenous mouse mammary tumour virus integrants carried in the mouse germline (for review see Simpson *et al.*, 1993). Nevertheless, this principle of tolerance through thymic elimination of T cells bearing a particular, autoreactive repertoire has since been confirmed in numerous experimental models and a wide range of self-antigens.

If this central tolerance is one of the consequences of TCR engagement of ligand during thymic development, the question that arises is how this tolerance could be achieved for self-antigens which are never encountered in the thymus. A number of laboratories addressed this question by constructing transgenic mice in which the transgene-encoded self-antigen was under the control of a promoter such that gene expression would be limited to a particular, extra-thymic tissue. In one example, the MHC class I antigen H-2K^b (which would normally be expressed by the majority of tissues) was expressed in a very restricted fashion by juxtaposing the coding region of the gene with the regulatory sequence of the insulin gene, so permitting expression of the MHC gene only in pancreatic beta cells (Miller & Morahan, 1992). Despite the lack of H-2K^b expression in the thymus, mice became tolerant to this antigen since H-2K^b skin grafts were not rejected. When thymocytes were extracted from these mice for study in culture, however, *in vivo* tests readily detected T cells which could respond to K^b. When T cells from the periphery were tested in the same assay, they too could respond, provided they received the 'kick-start' of some exogenously supplemented interleukin-2 (IL-2) as growth factor. Experiments of this type were interpreted as showing another form of tolerance, acquired not in the thymus but in the periphery, and involving not deletion of cells but, rather, some alternative form of programming to become inactive or anergic. It may be this type of tolerance in the form of anergy (rather than deletion) which is overcome when experimental mice are manipulated by immunization in powerful adjuvants to respond to self-myelin or when similar reactivities are elicited from human peripheral blood by culture in IL-2 and IL-4.

Disease genes

HLA class II genes

The dominant theme in the search for susceptibility factors in autoimmune disease has been the importance of HLA genes and particularly genes mapping to the class II region. In the HLA region on chromosome 6, the class I and class II regions are separated by a large genetic distance (some 1100 Kb), the main functional gene products from the class II region being HLA-DP, -DQ and -DR. Although the pattern of expression and general function of these molecules, i.e. peptide presentation is the same, it remains unclear whether they have differential roles in development of immune responses. Most attention has focused on -DR since it is expressed at the highest level on most cells and therefore accounts for the HLA restriction of the majority of $CD4^+$ T cells.

It has been noted for many years that, in a number of autoimmune diseases, particular HLA alleles are found at a higher frequency than in control populations and these alleles are thus deemed to confer a raised relative risk. As technologies for characterizing the products of the different HLA loci and distinguishing polymorphism have improved, the assignment of disease-associated genes has become more precise and the relative risks observed have become higher. However, until there is both a continuous map of the HLA region, all the genes within it cloned, and functional proof that any candidate gene has some role in disease susceptibility, the possibility will always remain that associations found are identifying a locus which is in linkage disequilibrium with the actual susceptibility gene. Linkage disequilibrium is a serious consideration in some parts of the HLA region where genes are relatively close together and, for example, particular DR alleles invariably occur with particular DQ alleles.

The problem can be illustrated by the progress of IDDM immunogenetics over the past 20 years. In the early 1970s when only typing for HLA class I was possible, an association was picked up with HLA-B15 and -B8. By the early 1980s, when reagents were available for HLA-DR typing, it became clear that the earlier reports probably reflected linkage disequilibrium between these class I alleles and alleles at the DR locus, particularly DR3 and DR4. In IDDM there is a very high relative risk associated with DR3,4 heterozygosity, rising as high as 23 among the young onset group (Caillat-Zucman *et al.*, 1992). When DQA and DQB alleles were analysed, initially by restriction fragment length polymorphism (RFLP) and subsequently by polymerase chain reaction (PCR), it became evident that the DR association may, in turn, simply have been a marker for a stronger association with the nearby HLA-DQ locus (Bohme *et al.*, 1986). This has now been confirmed in many studies. There were several reasons for reaching this conclusion:

1. Across ethnic groups, the increase in DQA1*0301/DQB1*0302 was found on haplotypes involving various different DRB1 products.
2. Although DR4 also occurs with DQA1*0301/DQB1*0301, this combination is under-represented in diabetics.
3. There was an increase in DQA1*0301/DQB1*0201 again associated with various different DRB1 haplotypes.
4. Disease implicated DQA/DQB pairs which were increased in the disease group could be encoded either *cis* or *trans* (that is, whether from the same or different chromosomes).
5. When the DQB alleles associated with susceptibility or resistance were sequenced and aligned by Todd, Bell & McDevitt (1987), they pointed out an underlying motif, in which alleles associated with susceptibility had a serine or valine at position 57 in the DQβ product, whereas alleles associated with protection had an aspartic acid.
6. The DQA1*0102/DQB1*0602 combination was protective irrespective of whether the chains were encoded in *cis* or *trans* and irrespective of ethnic group or the DR haplotype on which it was carried.

Even these findings, which are among the most compelling for any HLA association with autoimmune disease, fall short of proof that a primary association has been found, and no experiments to establish a causal relationship between MHC type and susceptibility have been possible. The case is supported by the fact that, in the NOD mouse, which spontaneously develops T cell dependent diabetes, the trend with respect to position 57 motif is continued since NOD mice have serine while most diabetes-resistant strains have aspartic acid. Nevertheless, the search for other linked genes which may offer stronger associations has continued (see below).

Meanwhile, many other diseases were analysed in this way, and coeliac disease and pemphigus vulgaris both appear more strongly associated with alleles of DQ than DR (for reviews see Nepom & Erlich 1991; Altmann, 1992). Rheumatoid arthritis and Goodpasture's syndrome, on the other hand, are both associated with the DR; the former with the DR4 alleles *0401, *0404, *0405 as well as DR1, and Goodpasture's with DRw15.

The assignment of a DR or DQ risk factor in MS has been somewhat confounded by the problem of linkage disequilibrium of DR and DQ in DRw15 individuals, a situation not helped by sometimes poor and over-interpreted serological and RFLP HLA-typing studies. In general, studies of North European and American Caucasians show an increase in DRw15 and DQw6, although in Jordanians and Sardinians the association is with DR4, and in Japanese with DR6. It seems likely that in these cases again the association is really with the DQ locus. For example, among the Southern Chinese there are novel DR/DQ haplotypes such that DQw6 (0602) can occur on various different DR haplotypes, not just DRw15. Among the relatively small patient group studied, the association is with DQA1*0102/DQB1*0602 and not with DRw15 (Serjeantson *et al.*, 1992). Furthermore, among the $DR4^+$ Sardinian patients there is deviation from the normal proportions having DQB1*0302 and DQB1*0301, giving an excess in the disease group of $DR4^+$ DQB1*0302^+ (Marrosu *et al.*, 1992). This again implies a stronger association with DQ than with DR.

There are many theories as to the mechanisms underpinning these genetic associations but few facts. The simplest working hypothesis is that HLA genes act as immune response genes (Ir), as defined originally in rodents with respect to the regulation of the magnitude of responsiveness to particular antigens. Thus particular HLA products predispose to disease in an appropriate genetic and environmental setting because they allow large responses to be generated to a given self-antigen. It should thus be possible to show, for example, that in MS patients who are DRw15 DQw6 on one chromosome and some other haplotype, X, on the other, T cells recognizing myelin peptides are more likely to be restricted by the disease-related haplotype than by X. Evidence of this type has been remarkably hard to come by. There is, however, one example, where gliadin-specific T cells isolated from the small intestinal mucosa of coeliac disease patients were predominantly restricted via HLA DQA1*0501/B1*0201, the pair implicated by the disease-gene associations (Lundin *et al.*, 1993).

Another possibility is that particular genes are associated with disease because their expression skews T cell receptor development, favouring the emergence of those cells with appropriate TCR expression to recognize the self-antigen. This can be illustrated by considering T cell receptor positive selection in inbred mice, where all mice which express an intact H-2E molecule have an increased proportion of TCR $V\beta10^+$ T cells in the periphery, and there is a hierarchy with some alleles of H-2E exerting a stronger effect than others (Tomonari, Hederer & Hengartner, 1992). If there were an autoimmune disease where recognition of the self-antigen depended especially on $V\beta10^+$ T cells, the mice with the strongest H-2E-mediated $V\beta10$ positive selection might be expected to be more disease-prone then H-$2E^-$ mice. Again, there are very few experimental data from humans for or against this model, although there are many studies addressing the issue of TCR skewing among the specific T cells of patients with autoimmune diseases (see below).

A related possibility again involves the influence of particular MHC products on shaping of the TCR repertoire, but this time on the ability or inability of a given MHC allele to negatively select T cells. Drawing again on knowledge of TCR selection in inbred mice, it has become clear in recent years that products of the endogenous mouse mammary tumour virus (MMTV) integrants act as endogenous superantigens, the effect of TCR engagement of MMTV/MHC complexes during thymocyte development being gross deletions in TCR repertoire on the basis of the TCR $V\beta$ product recognized. Thus, large holes accounting for 10–20% of all T cells may be punched in the repertoire, but in a highly TCR-skewed fashion. Most mouse strains which carry Mtv-7 (as well as mice carrying some other Mtv integrants) delete a part or all of their T cells with $V\beta6^+$ receptors. The only exceptions to this are mice where the only expressed class II molecule is H-$2A^q$. One might argue that this would give H-2^q mice a greater risk of developing some hypothetical disease which depends on attack by cells which are $V\beta6^+$.

New genes in the HLA region

As discussed above, since the HLA region still contains uncharted territory, the possibility remains that new genes will be found (for which the old genes were simply neighbouring markers) which are more closely associated with disease and offer a stronger explanation for disease predisposition. This possibility was recently addressed by several groups when a number of new loci were identified in the HLA class II region. Two of the new genes, now termed *TAP1* (transporter associated with antigen processing 1) and *TAP2*, form a heterodimer located in the endoplasmic reticulum and are members of the ATP-binding cassette transporter family (Trowsdale *et al.*, 1990). It is inferred from gene transfection to mutant cell lines as well as from mice with gene-targeted mutations that these gene products function in transport of antigenic peptides from the cytoplasm into the endoplasmic reticulum where they are loaded into the grooves of newly formed class I molecules. Polymorphisms in these genes, leading presumably to variation in the spectrum of peptides presented by class I molecules, can affect T cell recognition since the rat *TAP2* genes were originally tracked through an effect on generation of an allogeneic T cell epitope. Furthermore, although the possible mechanisms are more uncertain, some experiments imply that TAP genes may also affect peptide presentation by class II molecules.

Many diseases are currently under investigation for associations with TAP polymorphisms. Three alleles of *TAP1* have been identified and eight of *TAP2*, and the human alleles show considerably less variability than the rat alleles (Powis *et al.*, 1993*b*). Studies on coeliac patients showed no association with any TAP alleles (Powis *et al.*, 1993*a*). Analysis of IDDM panels also showed no association beyond that which would be expected from linkage disequilibrium between TAP genes and other genes in the class II region (Ronningen *et al.*, 1993), although a more recent study has claimed that there is indeed an association (Caillat-Zucman *et al.*, 1993).

The other new loci which have generated much interest are the low molecular mass polypeptide (LMP) genes, *LMP2* and *LMP7*. These genes encode components of large LMP complexes which are related to proteasomes (for review see Monaco, 1992). Proteasomes are cytoplasmic proteolytic complexes involved in non-lysosomal protein turnover. While it is clear that *LMP2* and *LMP7* can indeed influence protein degradation to generate peptidic fragments, the precise function of these genes in antigen presentation is still unclear. However they do, at least in the mouse, appear to be polymorphic, and it will be important to determine whether variability in LMPs influences disease susceptibility.

Non-HLA genes

The diseases under discussion here have complex aetiologies involving a number of genetic loci as well as environmental factors. In IDDM studies, monozygotic twins show concordance of 36% and in MS the level of concordance is 25%. Environmental factors including infectious agents must therefore play an important part. Furthermore, even in a disease with a relatively strong HLA class II association like IDDM, the MHC contribution to susceptibility is estimated at only 20–60%. Other genes contributing more minor effects to disease susceptibility could presumably be ones encoding anything from products affecting the cell biology or structure of the target cell to products involved in aspects of the immune response. It may be necessary to consider not only polymorphism in products of the target tissue and the cells attacking it but also in products which may influence susceptibility to some disease-triggering environmental pathogen.

There have been great efforts in recent years to collect and analyse large DNA panels from patients for polymorphisms segregating with disease. Aside from the problem of collecting sufficient numbers of families, a major limiting factor in these studies had been the need to find polymorphic markers peppered across each chromosome at a high enough density to make the detection of disease linkages a viable proposition. The situation changed drastically when groups started to analyse polymorphisms by PCR amplification of microsatellite repeats. Examples of these are the $(CA)_n$ repeats, which are scattered throughout the genome in most species, n the number of repeats (and thus the size of the amplifiable PCR product when primers are chosen on each side of the repeat) showing a high degree of polymorphism (Litt and Lutty, 1989).

In the spontaneous IDDM NOD mouse model, microsatellite analysis of backcrosses to follow polymorphisms which segregate with the disease phenotype has allowed the allocation of ten linkages on various chromosomes, termed *Idd*-(1–10). Two of these are the MHC association and a linkage near the insulin locus. Some others map near to loci of immunological interest, for example *Idd-3* may be at or near to the locus for the high affinity Fc receptor, FcγRI (Prins *et al.*, 1993).

There are now national and international initiatives to collect DNA panels for many other diseases, and it is likely that more and more linkages will accrue for complex genetic diseases in the next few years. There has been much interest in a reported linkage of MS to the MBP (myelin basic protein) gene, although studies on different patient groups have produced conflicting results (Tienari *et al.*, 1992).

Pathogenic T cells

The search for disease-related T cells

In the early days of T cell cloning, it was demonstrated that a T cell clone against MBP, when injected into an appropriate rat, was necessary and sufficient to induce EAE in the recipient. Koch's postulates were thus obeyed, and the T cell was seen to be the cause of disease. This scenario differed from anything which could be achieved with human T cells, not just with respect to the opportunity for cell transfer but also because it has been possible to prime the rat T cell donors actively with a defined antigen, rescue newly activated cells during acute disease, and then restimulate the cells with the correct antigen *in vitro*. On the other hand, experiments on T cells from autoimmune patients have often depended on taking lymphocytes from patients at various stages of ongoing disease and screening them for reactivity to the available, candidate autoantigens in the hope that something interesting will show up. The notion that patients would have an obvious 'fault in self-tolerance' so that antigen-reactive T cells would be identifiable in blood from patients but not from healthy controls was soon dispelled. Since T cells recognizing many of the human disease-related antigens which have been studied (such as those implicated in MS and Goodpasture's syndrome) have been readily cultured from healthy individuals, the question has had to be sharpened to ask whether pathogenesis is distinguished by some particular pattern of T cell recognition. Thus there have been efforts to map the HLA restriction, peptide recognition and TCR usage of T cell clones in search of disease-specific patterns. This logic again draws to some extent on the EAE model, where various strains of rat and mouse can mount a T cell response to various peptides from the MBP sequence, but the tendency to develop disease in the susceptible strains is associated with recognition of particular, dominant, encephalitogenic epitopes.

Many thousands of autoreactive human T cell clones from MS patients and controls have been generated against human MBP in several laboratories. On the whole, the search for a dominant, disease-specific pattern of recognition common to the clones from patients is a fairly disheartening experience. Clones restricted via either DRw15 products (DRB1 or DRB5) or DQw6 are not represented at a much higher frequency than other HLA-restrictions. In terms of MBP epitopes, there seems to be dominance of two regions, one around amino acid residues 87–102 (which also encompasses the encephalitogenic epitope in SJL mice) and another in the region 139–154. In one or two studies, recognition of the 87–102 epitope was a particular feature of clones from MS patients, although others found no differences (Ota *et al.*, 1990; Pette *et al.*, 1990). Indeed, some of the studies are noteworthy for the sheer lack of any pattern found with respect to peptide recognition (Olsson *et al.*, 1992) and the incredible diversity of clones against different MBP epitopes which can be cultured. This type of approach has reached something of an impasse which may only be overcome when a new generation of experiments can be devised which offers some evidence of the pathogenic capacity of particular clones. Such experiments may involve cell transfer of human T cell clones to HLA transgenic mice, expression of human TCR and HLA genes in transgenic mice, cell transfer to severe combined immune deficiency mice reconstituted with human cells (Hu-SCID mice), or some combination of these.

In myasthenia gravis the current data give a slightly different picture. The α subunit of the ACLR dominates the T cell response as it does the autoantibody response. However, unlike MS, the ability to generate reactive T cell clones appears somewhat more specific to patients with relatively severe disease (although responses have been obtained from normal donors). The cumulative data from these clones suggest absolutely no dominant peptide epitope and no particular HLA class II restriction molecule (Oshima *et al.*, 1990; Manfredi *et al.*, 1992). Thus, this is an example which, even more than MS, seems to diverge from the paradigm from the mouse EAE autoimmune model of a pathogenic process which is highly focused and homogeneous with respect to the presenting MHC class II molecule, the self-peptide presented and the TCR recognizing the complex.

An interesting exception to this rather confusing picture is the T cell response in coeliac disease (CD) patients. In this case, T cells against the wheat protein, gliadin, could be cultured from biopsies of CD patients but not controls. The disease has a DQ association and the expression of DQ is raised at the site of inflammation. Furthermore, the majority of clones are restricted via the DQA1*0501/DQB1*0201 encoded heterodimer which is strongly associated with disease (Lundin *et al.*, 1993). This may therefore turn out to be an example where the HLA association with disease reflects a simple *Ir* gene mechanism of strong local immune responsiveness in the context of a particular HLA allele. A general lesson to be learnt from this study and others is that more interpretable patterns of immune recognition tend to be obtained when T cells are isolated from the site of the autoimmune lesion than from peripheral blood.

T cell receptor heterogeneity in animal models

When T cell receptors of encephalitogenic clones against MBP1-11 in the PL/J mouse model of EAE were sequenced, it was found that there was remarkable homogeneity. The vast majority of receptors sequenced used the same Vβ gene segment (Vβ8.2), Jβ segment (Jβ2.7) and Vα segment (Vα4 or Vα2) (Acha-Orbea *et al.*, 1988). Antibodies to either Vα2 or Vβ8.2 could block disease when administered *in vivo*, confirming that these specificities, indeed, account for most of the pathogenic response. Such experiments also suggest the hope of developing similar TCR-specific antibody therapy in human disease. Similar findings were obtained in B10.PL mice and in Lewis rats. However, the trend does not extend to all examples of EAE since, in another common model using the SJL strain of mouse (where pathology seems to involve mainly the response to another myelin component, proteolipoprotein (PLP)), TCR heterogeneity was more apparent. Another caveat which confuses the issue is that, even in mice where clones predominantly use Vβ8.2 and disease can be blocked by monoclonals against this product, the actual T cells infiltrating the CNS may express a diverse array of receptors (Bell *et al.*, 1993).

Some of the other experimental models of autoimmune disease were then analysed for heterogeneity of TCR usage. While there have been some hints of fairly limited TCR usage among pathogenic clones, for example, the expansion of Vβ6$^+$ clones in experimental myasthenia gravis and of Vβ6 and Vβ8.2 in collagen-induced arthritis, no models have provided results as clear-cut as in EAE (Infante *et al.*, 1992; Haqqi *et al.*, 1992). Analysis of pancreas infiltrates in the spontaneous NOD mouse model of diabetes has revealed no clear bias in TCR usage.

T cell receptor heterogeneity in clinical disease

The potential for TCR Vβ-specific therapy implied by the initial mouse EAE experiments triggered a flurry of activity with respect to analysis of TCR usage in human diseases. The most extensively studied disease has been MS. There is little consensus with some workers finding marked homogeneity akin to the mouse studies and others, none at all. For example, two studies reported pronounced skewing in favour of MBP-reactive T cell clones using Vβ5.2 (Kotzin *et al.*, 1991; Martin *et al.*, 1991), while others were unable to detect this effect. Indeed, some workers could find no preference for any particular TCR Vα/Vβ combinations in MBP-reactive clones (Giegerich *et al.*, 1992).

Pursuing the idea that the clearest answers will be found by analysing the actual cells that have homed to the site of the lesion rather than just sampling peripheral blood, one group used PCR to analyse TCR transcripts in MS brains (Oksenberg *et al.*, 1993). Interestingly, it was found that rearranged Vβ5.2 genes were present in the brains of all of the patients who were DRw15, DQw6. Furthermore, a V-D-J sequence occurring frequently in the brain T cell samples was similar to a common sequence seen in the TCR from DRw15 restricted T cells against MBP 89-106. The two camps in the ongoing TCR homogeneity debate, the sceptics and the enthusiasts, now have to wait and see whether the brain-derived TCR sequences, when transfected back into a functional T cell, indeed respond to the MBP 89-106 epitope. This would be fairly compelling evidence that, at least for the DRw15 DQw6 patients, recognition of MBP 89-106 is a step in MS pathogenesis and Vβ5.2$^+$ TCRs have an important role in the process. Although some of the most interesting data have been produced by workers analysing T cells at the site of the autoimmune lesion, it is nevertheless worth bearing in mind that many largely irrelevant cells may also home to the site in the course of an inflammatory response.

Among the many diseases where efforts have been made to analyse TCR usage of T cells infiltrating the site of autoimmune attack are rheumatoid arthritis and thyroid diseases such as Graves' and Hashimoto's thyroiditis. In the thyroid diseases, only Vα gene usage has so far been reported in detail, but there does indeed seem to be some bias to infiltration by cells expressing a fairly small range of specificities (Davies *et al.*, 1991). Analysis of synovial infiltrates in rheumatoid arthritis has produced conflicting results, with TCR V gene usage appearing highly homogeneous (Paliard *et al.*, 1991), relatively homogeneous (Stamenkovic *et al.*, 1988) or completely heterogeneous (Uematsu *et al.*, 1991).

Autoantigens

All of the work on HLA restriction and TCR usage of T cell clones described above is meaningless if we are not studying clones directed against the true disease autoantigens. By a slightly precarious form of circular logic, one argument seems to go that we will know when we have found the correct antigen because we will get interpretable patterns of HLA restriction and TCR usage.

A more logical approach to defining an autoantigen would be first to make the correct cellular probes with which to isolate it: these should be T cells cloned (preferably early in disease) from the target site, without imposing any selection on them, for example, by using mitogenic stimulation with anti-CD3 antibody and IL-2. Armed with such cloned T cells, it is possible to screen an expression library. This is simply any DNA library carrying amplified, cloned copies of all of the genes expressed by a given tissue, designed so that they are available not simply as DNA sequences but are also expressed as protein. For T cell screening purposes, this generally means generating a library in a vector which permits expression of the DNA sequences after transfection into a mammalian cell. Thus, the transfectant carrying the autoantigen gene is the one which stimulates the T cell clones to proliferate. This kind of approach has been successfully used by tumour immunologists to identify and clone the genes for melanoma-specific antigens (Van der Bruggen *et al.*, 1991). However, while there are numerous ongoing projects using this approach to autoimmunity, it has as yet yielded no autoantigen T cell epitopes, essentially because each of the steps (generating appropriate T cells, making an appropriate expression library, screening the library) constitute fairly Herculean tasks.

Among this uncertainty, those investigating the diseases of antibody-mediated destruction have been at an advantage. In Goodpasture's syndrome, for example, monoclonal antibodies capable of competing for the binding to renal basement membrane by patients' autoantibodies were generated (Butkowski *et al.*, 1987; Pusey *et al.*, 1987). These monoclonal antibodies could then be used to affinity purify the protein of interest from renal basement membrane for peptide sequencing. The antigen recognized both by autoantibodies and by the T cells supplying the help for those antibodies to be made was thus shown to be a non-collagenous domain (NC1) of type IV collagen present in glomerulus as well as in some other basement membranes such as those of lung alveoli. Similarly, in myasthenia gravis the vast majority of evidence points to recognition of the α chain of the acetylcholine receptor and in pemphigus vulgaris to an epithelial cadherin involved in the junctional adherence of keratinocytes (Amagai, Klaus-Kovtun & Stanley, 1991).

In MS there have been attempts to look at T cell responses to more or less every myelin protein component which can either be purified or expressed as a recombinant molecule. The focus on MBP comes partly from the fact that it was the first of the myelin proteins which could be plentifully isolated and partly from the fact that, in a number of animal models where injection of spinal cord homogenate and adjuvant triggered an acute encephalomyelitis, the major part of the effect could be accounted for by reactivity to MBP. However, this is not the case in EAE of SJL mice where reactivity is primarily against another protein, proteolipid protein (PLP) (Kennedy *et al.*, 1990). T cell responses of MS patients to PLP, myelin-associated glycoprotein (MAG) and myelin oligodendrocyte glycoprotein (MOG) have each been analysed and certainly look no less relevant or interesting than the response to MBP (Sun *et al.*, 1991).

In diabetes research, despite the availability of a mouse model from which infiltrating T cells can be isolated, there is a similar level of confusion. Unlike myasthenia, pemphigus and Goodpasture's where tissue destruction is clearly antibody mediated, and mapping autoantibody recognition was a sure route to the target antigen, this approach has, if anything, caused confusion in diabetes where the pathology is T cell mediated. Thus, early studies looked mainly at the so-called islet cell antigen (ICA) which was defined by recognition with patients' autoantibodies (for review see Harrison, 1992). The antigen(s) localize to islets but not specifically to beta cells, and this antibody response is seen in other polyendocrine disorders, not just IDDM.

Another antigen initially defined by autoantibodies, glutamic acid decarboxylase (GAD), also known as 64K antigen, looks a more promising candidate. The GAD autoantibody is present in the serum of recent onset patients, precipitates a 64K molecular weight band on protein gels and is beta cell specific. More recently, there have been extensive studies on T cell responses to GAD showing that the majority of recent-onset patients make a response (Harrison *et al.*, 1993). However, there are numerous other candidate autoantigens. For example, the so-called 36K antigen was identified by separating the proteins of a rat insulinoma cell line on a protein gel, cutting out the bands and asking which would stimulate specific T cell responses in recent onset diabetics. 36K is the molecular weight of the fraction which stimulated responses in the majority of diabetics but not in controls (Roep *et al.*, 1991). Meanwhile, other workers found that disease could be accelerated in the NOD mouse model by transfer of T cell clones against the stress protein, Hsp60 (Elias *et al.*, 1990). The stress or heat shock proteins are highly conserved in prokaryotic and eukaryotic cells where they act as 'molecular chaperones', guiding cellular proteins to the correct cellular compartments and maintaining functional conformation of proteins during stresses such as heat shock. Much of the current interest in Hsps among immunologists stems from models showing that certain T cells, when activated by Hsps of invading microorganisms such as bacteria or mycobacteria, may cause autoimmunity by a cross-reaction with molecules in autologous tissue. The prototype here was the finding that adjuvant arthritis, a model for rheumatoid arthritis in Lewis rats, was induced in response to a peptide derived from mycobacterial Hsp65 (Van Eden *et al.*, 1988). Hsps are now under investigation as candidate autoantigens, with some interesting results, in various diseases including arthritis, MS and IDDM. As antigens they have the conceptual advantage that they offer a highly plausible explanation for the link between infectious agents and autoimmune disease. On the other hand, autoreactivity to a ubiquitously expressed protein might be expected to cause disseminated disease rather than the tissue-specific and localized lesions associated with these diseases. It may thus be more appropriate to propose that there is some initial tissue-specific target, the response to this causing local stress and elevation of Hsps, with the subsequent anti-Hsp response acting as a general, secondary, mechanism for amplifying autoimmune pathology.

Concluding remarks

It may appear from this brief review of current developments in autoimmune disease that there has been little progress in unravelling the mechanisms underlying pathogenesis. Certainly, there is still no disease where it is possible to make any definitive statement about the specific T cells, peptide and MHC molecule contributing to antigen recognition and tissue damage. While there are many initiatives to intervene therapeutically in specific immune recognition in a highly targeted way (for example, oral tolerance induction with MBP or TCR peptide treatments), the majority of these approaches are still highly speculative and hope to bypass a vast number of unknowns. Nevertheless, the past few years have been a period of great progress, both with respect to the ability to clone great numbers of autoimmune T cells from patients and analyse their TCR usage and specificity and to define HLA associations and exciting linkages with other parts of the genome with far greater precision and speed than previously thought possible. It seems likely that, during the next few years, it will also be possible to look at some of the genes of interest in transgenic and 'knockout' mouse models and arrive at firmer conclusions about mechanisms.

References

Acha-Orbea, H., Mitchell, D. J., Timmerman, L., Wraith, D. C., Tausch, G. S., Waldor, M. K., Zamvil, S., McDevitt, H. O. & Steinman, L. (1988). Limited heterogeneity of T cell receptors from T lymphocytes mediating autoimmune encephalomyelitis allows specific immune intervention. *Cell*, **54**, 263–73.

Altmann, D. M. (1992). HLA-DQ associations with autoimmune disease. *Autoimmunity*, **14**, 79–83.

Amagai, M., Klaus-Kovtun, V. & Stanley, J. R. (1991). Autoantibodies against a novel epithelial cadherin in pemphigus vulgaris, a disease of cell adhesion. *Cell*, **67**, 869–77.

Bell, R. B., Lindsey, J. W., Sobel, R. A., Hodgkinson, S. & Steinman, L. (1993). Diverse T cell receptor Vβ gene usage in the central nervous system in experimental allergic encephalomyelitis. *Journal of Immunology*, **150**, 4085–92.

Bohme, J., Carlsson, B., Wallin, J. Moller, E., Persson, B., Peterson, P. A. & Rask, L. (1986). Only one DQβ restriction fragment pattern of each DR specificity is associated with insulin dependent diabetes. *Journal of Immunology*, **137**, 941–48.

Burns, J., Rosenzweig, A., Zweiman, B. & Lisak, R. P. (1983) Isolation of myelin basic protein reactive T cells from normal human blood. *Cellular Immunology*, **81**, 435–40.

Butkowski, R., Langveld, J., Wieslander, J., Hamilton, J. & Hudson, B. (1987). Localization of the Goodpasture's epitope to a novel chain of basement membrane collagen. *Journal of Biological Chemistry*, **262**, 7874–7.

Caillat-Zucman, S., Garchon, H.-J., Timsit, J., Assan, R., Botard, C., Djilali-Saiah, I., Bougneres, P. & Bach, J. F. (1992). Age-dependent HLA genetic heterogeneity of type 1 insulin dependent diabetes mellitus. *Journal of Clinical Investigation*, **90**, 2242–50.

Caillat-Zucman, S., Bertin, E., Timsit, J., Boitard, C., Assan, R. & Bach, J.-F. (1993) Protection from insulin-dependent diabetes is linked to a peptide transporter gene. *European Journal of Immunology*, **23**, 1784–8.

Cohen, I. R. (1992). The cognitive principle challenges clonal selection. *Immunology Today*, **13**, 441–4.

Coutinho A. (1993). Beyond clonal selection and network. *Immunological Reviews*, **133**, 63–87.

Davies, T. F., Martin, A., Concepcion, E. S., Graves, P., Cohen, L. & Ben-Nun, A. (1991). Evidence of limited variability of antigen receptors on intrathyroidal T cells in autoimmune thyroid disease. *New England Journal of Medicine*, **325**, 238–44.

Elias, D., Markovits, D. Reshef, D., van der Zee, R. & Cohen, I. R. (1990). Induction and therapy of autoimmune diabetes in the non-obese diabetic (NOD/Lt) mouse by a 65-kDa heat shock protein. *Proceedings of the National Academy of Sciences, USA*, **87**, 1567–80.

Giegerich, G., Pette, M., Meinl, E., Epplen, J. T., Wekerle, H. & Hinkkanen, A. (1992). Diversity of T cell receptor α and β chain genes expressed by human T cells specific for similar myelin basic protein/major histocompatibility complexes. *European Journal of Immunology*, **22**, 753–8.

Haqqi, T. M., Anderson, G. D., Banerjee, S. & David, C. (1992). Restricted heterogeneity in T cell antigen receptor Vβ gene usage in the lymph nodes and arthritic joints of mice. *Proceedings of the National Academy of Sciences, USA*, **89**, 1253–5.

Harrison, L. (1992). Islet cell antigens in insulin dependent diabetes: Pandora's box revisited. *Immunology Today*, **13**, 348–52.

Harrison, L. C., Honeyman, M. C., DeAizpurua, H. J., Schmidli, R. S., Colman, P. G., Tait, B. D., Cram, D. S. (1993). Inverse relation between humoral and cellular immunity to glutamic acid decarboxylase in subjects at risk of insulin-dependent diabetes. *Lancet*, **341**, 1365–9.

Infante, A. J., Levcovitz, H., Gordon, V., Wall, K. A., Thompson, P. A. & Krolick, K. A. (1992). Preferential use of a T cell receptor Vβ gene by acetylcholine receptor reactive T cells from myasthenia gravis susceptible mice. *Journal of Immunology*, **148**, 3385–90.

Kappler, J. W., Roehm, N. & Marrack, P. (1987). T cell tolerance by clonal elimination in the thymus. *Cell*, **49**, 273–80.

Kappler, J. W., Wade, T., White J., Kushnir, E., Blackman, M., Bill, J., Roehm, N. & Marrack, P. (1987). A T cell receptor Vβ segment imparts reactivity to a class II major histocompatibility complex product. *Cell*, **49**, 263–71.

Kennedy, M., Tan, L.-J., Dal Canto, M. C., Tuohy, V. K., Lu, Z., Trotter, J. L., Miller, S. D. (1990). Inhibition of murine relapsing experimental autoimmune myelitis by immune tolerance to proteolipid protein and its encephalitogenic peptides. *Journal of Immunology*, **144**, 909–15.

Kotzin, B. L., Karuturi, S., Chou, Y., Lafferty, J., Forrester, J., Better, M., Nedwin, G., Offner, H. & Vandenbark, A. (1991). Preferential T cell receptor β chain variable gene use in myelin basic protein reactive T cell clones from patients with multiple sclerosis. *Proceedings of the National Academy of Sciences, USA*, **88**, 9161–5.

Litt, M. & Luty, J. A. (1989). A hypervariable microsatellite revealed by in vitro amplification of a dinucleotide repeat within the cardiac muscle actin gene. *American Journal of Human Genetics*, **44**, 397–401.

Lundin, K. E. A., Scott, H., Hansen, T. *et al.* (1993). Gliadin specific, HLA-DQ(α1*0501, β1*0201) restricted T cells isolated from the small intestinal mucosa of coeliac disease patients. *Journal of Experimental Medicine*, **178**, 187–96.

Manfredi, A. A., Protti, M. P., Wu, B. S., Howard, J. F. & Conti-Tronconi (1992). $CD4^+$ T epitope repertoire on the human acetylcholine receptor α subunit in severe myasthenia gravis: a study with synthetic peptides. *Neurology*, **42**, 1092–100.

Marrosu, M. G., Muntoni, F., Murru, M., Costa, G., Pischedda, M. P., Pirastu, M., Sotggiu, S., Rosati, G. & Cianchetti, C. (1992) HLA-DQB1 genotype in Sardinian multiple sclerosis: evidence for a key role of BQB1*0201 and *0302 alleles. *Neurology*, **42**, 883–6.

Martin, R., Howell, M. D., Jaraquemada, D., Ferlage, M., Richert, J., Brostoff, S., Long, E. O., McFarlin, D. & McFarland, H. F. (1991). A myelin basic protein peptide is recognized by cytotoxic T cells in the context of four HLA-DR types associated with multiple sclerosis. *Journal of Experimental Medicine*, **248**, 19–24.

Miller, J. F. A. P. & Morahan, J. (1992). Peripheral T cell tolerance. *Annual Review of Immunology*, **10**, 51–69.

Monaco, J. J. (1992). A molecular model of MHC class I-restricted antigen processing. *Immunology Today*, **13**, 173–9.

Nepom, G. T. & Erlich, H. (1991). MHC class II molecules and autoimmunity. *Annual Review of Immunology*, **9**, 493–525.

Oksenberg, J., Panzara, M., Begovich, A., Mitchell, D., Erlich, H., Murray, R., Shimonkevitz, R., Sherrit, M., Rothbard, J., Bernard, C. C. & Steinman, L. (1993). Selection for T cell receptor Vβ-Dβ-Jβ gene rearrangements with specificity for a myelin basic protein peptide in brain lesions of multiple sclerosis. *Nature*, **362**, 68–70.

Olsson, T., Sun, J., Hillert, H., Hojenberg, B., Ekre, H.-P., Andersson, G., Olerup, O. & Link H. (1992). Increased numbers of cells recognizing multiple myelin basic protein epitopes in multiple sclerosis. *European Journal of Immunology*, **122**, 1083–7.

Oshima, M., Ashizawa, T., Pollack, M. S. & Atassi, M. Z. (1990). Autoimmune T cell recognition of human acetylcholine receptor: the sites of T cell recognition in myasthenia gravis on the extracellular part of the α subunit. *European Journal of Immunology*, **20**, 2563–9.

Ota, K., Matsui, M., Milford, E., Mackin, G. A., Weiner, H. L. & Haffler, D. A. (1990). T cell recognition of an immunodominant myelin basic protein epitope in multiple sclerosis. *Nature*, **346**, 183–7.

Paliard, X., West, S., Lafferty, J., Clements, J., Marrack, P. & Kappler, J. (1991). Evidence for the effects of a superantigen in rheumatoid arthritis. *Science*, **253**, 325–9.

Pette, M., Fujita, K., Wilkinson, D., Altmann, D., Trowsdale, J., Giegerich, G., Hinkkanen, A., Epplen J., Kappos, L. & Wekerl, H. (1990). Myelin autoreactivity in multiple sclerosis: recognition of myelin basic protein in the context of HLA-DR2 products by T lymphocytes of multiple sclerosis patients and controls. *Proceedings of the National Academy of Sciences, USA*, **87**, 7968–73.

Powis, S. H., Rosenberg, W., Hall, M., Mockridge, I., Tonks, S., Ivinson, A., Ciclitira, P. J., Jewell, D. P., Lanchbury, J. S., Bell, J. I. & Trowsdale, J. (1993*a*). TAP1 and TAP2 polymorphism in coeliac disease. *Immunogenetics*, **38**, 345–50.

Powis, S. H., Tonks, S., Mockridge, I., Kely, A. P., Bodmer, J. G. & Trowsdale, J. (1993*b*). Alleles and haplotypes of the MHC-encoded ABC transporters TAP1 and TAP2. *Immunogenetics*, **37**, 373–80.

Prins, J.-B., Todd, J. A., Rodrigues, N. R., Ghosh, S., Hogarth, M., Wicker, L. S., Gaffney, E., Podolin, P. L., Fischer, P. A., Sirotina, A. & Peterson, L. B. (1993). Linkage on chromosome 3 of autoimmune diabetes and defective Fc receptor for IgG in NOD mice. *Science*, **260**, 695–8.

Pusey, C., Dash, A., Kershaw, M., Morgan, A., Reilly, A., Rees, A. & Lockwood, C. (1987). A single autoantigen in Goodpasture's syndrome identified by a monoclonal antibody to human glomerular basement membrane. *Laboratory Investigation*, **56**, 23–30.

Roep, B. O., Kallan, A. A. & Hazenbos, W. L. W., Bruining, G. J., Bailyes, E. M., Arden, S. D., Hulton, J. C. & de Vries, R. R. P. (1991). T cell reactivity to 38 kD insulin secretory granule protein isolated from pancreatic granules. *Lancet*, **337**, 1439–41.

Ronningen, K., Undlien, D. E., Ploski, R., Maouni, N., Konrad, R. J., Jensen, E., Hornes, E., Reijonen, H., Colonna, M., Monos, D., Srominger, J. L. & Thorsby, E. (1993) Linkage disequilibrium between TAP2 variants and HLA class II alleles; no primary association between TAP2 variants and insulin dependent diabetes mellitus. *European Journal of Immunology*, **23**, 1050–6.

Serjeantson, S. W., Gao, X., Hawkins, B. R. Higgins, D. A. & Wu, Y. L. (1992). Novel HLA-DR2-related haplotypes in Hong Kong Chinese implicate the DQB1*0602 allele in susceptibility to multiple sclerosis. *European Journal of Immunogenetics*, **19**, 11–19.

Simpson, E., Dyson, P. J., Knight, A. M., Robinson, P. J., Elliott, J. I. & Altmann, D. M. (1993). T cell receptor repertoire selection by mouse mammary tumor viruses and MHC molecules. *Immunological Reviews*, **131**, 93–115.

Spies, T., Cerundolo, V., Colonna, M., Cresswell, P., Townsend, A. & De Mars, R. (1992). Presentation of viral antigen by MHC class I molecules is dependent on putative peptide transporter heterodimer. *Nature*, **355**, 644–6.

Stamenkovic, I., Stegagno, M., Wright, K., Krane, S., Amento E., Colvin, R., Dusquesnoy, R. & Kurnick, J. (1988). Clonal dominance among T lymphocyte infiltrates in arthritis. *Proceedings of the National Academy of Sciences, USA*, **85**, 1179–83.

Sun, J.-B., Link, H. Olsson, T., Xiao, B. G., Andersson, G., Ekre, H.-P., Linnington, C. & Diener, P. (1991). T and B cell responses to myelin-oligodendrocyte glycoprotein in multiple sclerosis. *Journal of Immunology*, **146**, 1490–5.

Tienari, P. J., Wikstrom J., Sajantila, A., Palo, J. & Peltonen, L. (1992). Genetic susceptibility to multiple sclerosis linked to myelin basic protein gene. *Lancet*, **340**, 987–91.

Todd, J. A., Bell, J. I. & McDevitt, H. O. (1987). HLA-DQβ gene contributes to susceptibility and resistance to insulin-dependent diabetes mellitus. *Nature*, **329**, 599–604.

Tomonari, K., Hederer, R. & Hengartner, H., (1992). Positive selection of TCR-V10b$^+$ T cells. *Immunogenetics*, **35**, 9–15.

Trowsdale, J., Hanson, I., Mockridge, I., Beck, S., Townsend, A. & Kelly, A. (1990). Sequences encoded in the class II region of the MHC related to the 'ABC' superfamily of transporters. *Nature*, **348**, 741–4.

Uematsu, Y., Wege, H., Straus, A., Ott, A., Bannwarth, W., Lanchbury, J., Panayi, G. & Steinmetz, M. (1991). The cell receptor repertoire in the synovial fluid of a patient with rheumatoid arthritis is polyclonal. *Proceedings of the National Academy of Sciences, USA*, **88**, 8534–8.

van Eden, W., Thole, J. E., van der Zee, R., Noordzij, A., van Embden, J., Hensen, E. & Cohen, I. R. (1988). Cloning of the myobacterial epitope recognized by T lymphocytes in adjuvant arthritis. *Nature*, **331**, 171–3.

van der Bruggen, P., Traversari, C., Chomiez, P., Lurquin, C., de Plaen, E., van den Eynde, B., Knuth, A. & Boon, T. (1991). A gene encoding an antigen recognized by cytolytic T lymphocytes on a human melanoma. *Science*, 254, 1643–4.

Zhang, Y., Schleup, M., Frutiger, S., Hughes, G. J., Jeannet, M., Steck, A. & Barkas, T. (1990). Immunological heterogeneity of autoreactive lymphocytes against the nicotinic acetylcholine receptor in myasthenic patients. *European Journal of Immunology*, **20**, 2577–83.

–2–

Regulation of endothelial cell function by cytokines

JEREMY D. PEARSON and MICHAEL J. MAY

Introduction

Control of the access of soluble mediators and leukocytes to sites of inflammation and immune reactions is a crucial function of blood vessels, particularly within the microvasculature. Careful *in vivo* studies, especially those employing intravital microscopy, first revealed increases in small vessel permeability, apparently caused by direct action of inflammatory mediators on the endothelial cells, and altered properties of the endothelium provoking leukocyte adhesion and emigration (for review see Ryan & Majno, 1977).

Mainly *in vitro* studies of endothelial cells, starting in the early 1970s, have delineated a rapidly expanding range of properties of endothelium that actively contribute to the maintenance of vascular homeostasis and regulate blood vessel tone and permeability, blood coagulation and fibrinolysis (for review see Pearson, 1994). Following the recognition that communication between different leukocytes to orchestrate their specific functions was due to a variety of secreted polypeptides (the lymphokines) it became pertinent to examine whether endothelial cell properties relevant to the control of inflammatory and immune responses were, in addition, modulated by such molecules. This led, in the 1980s, to the first reports that the adhesive interactions between leukocytes and endothelium could be substantially enhanced by the action of either of two inflammatory cytokines, interleukin 1 (IL-1) and tumour necrosis factor (TNF), or bacterial endotoxins (lipopolysaccharide: LPS) on endothelial cells. Although LPS is not a cytokine, its effects on endothelial cells largely overlap with those of IL-1 and TNF, and it will be discussed in this context in this chapter. As the number of cytokines identified has increased steadily, the breadth of their ability to affect, differentially, a wide variety of endothelial cell functions has also been recognized.

Phenotypic modulation of endothelial cells by cytokines, now often referred to as endothelial activation, a term introduced by Pober (1988), was first reviewed in depth by Pober & Cotran (1990) and aspects have been well summarized in two more recent articles (Libby & Hansson, 1991; Mantovani, Bussolino & Dejana, 1992). It is the purpose of this chapter to survey the effects of specific cytokines on endothelial cells, with the emphasis on updating the information contained in those reviews.

Interleukin 1, tumour necrosis factor and endotoxin

Receptors

Although the two monocyte/macrophage-derived cytokines IL-1 and TNF act on different receptors, with few exceptions (noted below) their effects on endothelial cells are almost identical. The two distinct forms of IL-1 (α and β) were first described as T cell costimulatory molecules, where either can bind to type I or type II receptors (Sims *et al.*, 1988; McMahan *et al.*, 1991). However, endothelial cells possess only the type I receptor (Akeson *et al.*, 1992; Colotta *et al.*, 1993*b*). The multiple biological actions of TNF (for review, see Vassalli, 1992) are mediated by two receptors, p55 and p75, which also bind the related molecule lymphotoxin (Smith *et al.*, 1990; Loetscher *et al.*, 1990; Schall *et al.*, 1990). Both receptors are present on endothelial cells (Shalaby *et al.*, 1990), though p55 is the predominantly active form (Mackay *et al.*, 1993).

In monocytes, the glycosylphosphoinositol-anchored membrane protein CD14 binds LPS complexed with a plasma component, lipopolysaccharide binding protein (LBP), and initiates signalling (Wright *et al.*, 1990). Endothelial cells lack anchored CD14, but the action of LPS on endothelium depends on internalization of LPS that has bound soluble CD14, a process substantially enhanced in the presence of LBP (Pugin *et al.*, 1993; Goldblum *et al.*, 1994).

Responses

IL-1, TNF and LPS induce altered transcription of a large array of endothelial genes, effectively reprogramming the cells' homeostatic properties in terms of: (1) inflammatory mediator secretion; (2) expression of leukocyte adhesion molecules; (3) the balance of pro- and anti-thrombotic functions: (4) the synthesis of matrix molecules and their receptors; (5) secretion of growth factors, secondary cytokines and enzymes related to matrix degradation. Each of these responses is outlined in the following sections.

Details of the signal transduction mechanisms leading to these changes are a subject of intensive current research, though it is clear that early events include activation of the transcription factor NFκB and synthesis of the transcription factor c-fos (e.g. Mantovani *et al.*, 1992; Read *et al.*, 1993;

Muller, Ziegler-Heitbrock & Bauerle, 1993; Larner *et al.*, 1993; Collins, 1993). The effects are typically transient, involving new mRNA and protein synthesis that peak within 12 hours and often return towards basal levels after 24 h, though they can be modified by coincubation with other cytokines. Processes for reversing endothelial activation may be set up concomitantly, since one of the gene products rapidly formed in response to IL-1 or TNF is the specific inhibitor of NFκB (d'Aniello *et al.*, 1993; Read *et al.*, 1994).

Inflammatory mediators

The ability of endothelial cells to synthesize two important inflammatory mediators, the potent vasodilators nitric oxide (NO) and prostacyclin (PGI_2), is enhanced by LPS, TNF or IL-1 treatment. NO is formed in endothelial cells, in response to Ca^{2+}-mobilizing agonists, from the amino acid arginine by the constitutively present Ca^{2+}/calmodulin-sensitive enzyme NO synthase (eNOS). In several cell types, epitomized by macrophages and smooth muscle cells, which lack eNOS, exposure to IL-1, TNF or LPS induces the expression of an alternative, Ca^{2+}-insensitive, isoform of NO synthase (iNOS) leading to substantial generation of NO, which is utilized by activated macrophages as a cytotoxic agent (Knowles & Moncada, 1994). Cytokine-induced expression of iNOS has also been reported in porcine and murine endothelial cells (Kilbourn & Belloni, 1990; Radomski, Palmer & Moncada, 1990; Gross *et al.*, 1991). It has proved more difficult to express iNOS in human cells *in vitro*, and, as yet, there are no reports of human endothelial iNOS. Indeed, recent results have shown in contrast that eNOS mRNA levels are greatly reduced in response to IL-1 or TNF plus interferonγ (IFNγ) (Yoshizumi *et al.*, 1993; Rosenkranz-Weiss *et al.*, 1994). However, the activity of eNOS is actually enhanced because of a concomitant increase in the levels of the essential cofactor, tetrahydrobiopterin (BH_4), owing to cytokine-induced synthesis of the rate limiting enzyme of the BH_4 biosynthetic pathway (Schoedon *et al.*, 1993; Rosenkranz-Weiss *et al.*, 1994). Another element in the upregulation of NO production, demonstrated in macrophages in response to cytokine treatment, is the parallel induction of increased levels of the arginine transporter at the cell membrane (Bogle *et al.*, 1992).

A similarly coordinated set of changes is responsible for the enhanced ability of endothelial cells to synthesize PGI_2 after treatment with IL-1, TNF or LPS. Mobilization of the precursor, arachidonate, from phospholipids is increased owing to increased levels of phospholipase A_2 (Breviario *et al.*, 1990; Jackson *et al.*, 1993). Levels of the rate-limiting enzyme, cyclooxygenase (COX1), are also increased, and there is induction of a second isoform (COX2) (Maier, Hla & Maciag, 1990; Jones *et al.*, 1993). As a consequence, agonist-stimulated PGI_2 synthesis is greatly elevated in pretreated cells (Zavoico *et al.*, 1989). Synthesis of two further endothelium-derived inflammatory mediators, the lipid platelet-activating factor (PAF) and the potent constrictor peptide endothelin-1, and of the recently described C-type natriuretic peptide, are each stimulated by IL-1, TNF and LPS (Bussolino *et al.*, 1986; Yoshizumi *et al.*, 1990, Suga *et al.*, 1993).

It has been reported also that these cytokines lead to the induction of either Cu/Zn or Mn superoxide dismutase in endothelial cells, thus enhancing their oxidant defence mechanisms (Kong & Fanberg, 1992; Visner *et al.*, 1992; Suzuki *et al.*, 1993).

Coagulation, thrombosis and fibrinolysis

Endothelial cells are actively involved in maintaining the fluidity of the blood within healthy vessels, though they are also concerned with reactions to ensure that a haemostatic plug is formed efficiently at the site of damage to a blood vessel (for review see Pearson, 1993). Thus they are the source for the circulating initiator of fibrinolysis, tissue-type plasminogen activator (tPA), and of its inhibitor (PAI-1), which normally circulates in excess of tPA. The luminal endothelial surface presents antithrombin, the primary inactivator of active thrombin, and also thrombomodulin, which binds thrombin and converts it to an anticoagulant enzyme. Endothelial cells also secrete von Willebrand factor: this highly multimerized glycoprotein circulates as the cofactor for Clotting Factor VIII, and is also secreted into the subendothelial matrix where it is a primary ligand for the platelet glycoprotein (Gp) Ib, and is important for trapping platelets from flowing blood when exposed at the site of damage to the vessel wall.

PGI_2 and NO, whose synthesis is enhanced by IL-1, TNF and LPS (as noted above), are inhibitors of platelet aggregation in addition to being vasodilators. However, the predominant effect of IL-1, TNF or LPS is to alter endothelial properties in a procoagulant direction. As discussed in Chapters 9 and 11, these effects may be of clinical importance in early vasculitis and during allograft rejection. Cytokine pretreatment has no effect on basal secretion of von Willebrand factor, but for a period of hours enhances the ability of agonists such as thrombin to induce secretion of von Willebrand factor from its endothelial granular storage site (Paleolog *et al.*, 1990). At the same time, thrombomodulin expression is down-regulated (Nawroth & Stern, 1986) and PAI-1 secretion is up-regulated while tPA release is unaltered or decreased (Bevilacqua *et al.*, 1986; Emeis & Kooistra, 1986; Nachman *et al.*, 1986; Schleef *et al.*, 1988). Finally, endothelial cells, unlike extravascular cells, do not normally express the primary initiator of blood coagulation (Tissue Factor, thromboplastin). However, at least *in vitro* Tissue Factor is efficiently induced at the surface of endothelial cells by

IL-1, TNF or LPS (Bevilacqua *et al.*, 1984; Brox *et al.*, 1984). It has been hard to demonstrate induction of endothelial Tissue Factor *in vivo*, perhaps (reasonably) implying an extra level of control which is lacking *in vitro*, to prevent disseminated intravascular coagulation. This is plausible, because LPS increases the lifespan of Tissue Factor mRNA, rather than inducing transcription (Crossman *et al.*, 1990). *In vitro* studies also suggest that Tissue Factor is mostly expressed at the basal (abluminal) surface of endothelium (Ryan *et al.*, 1992).

Leukocyte adhesion molecules

The demonstration that IL-1, TNF and LPS caused enhanced leukocyte adhesion to endothelial cells (Bevilacqua *et al.*, 1985; Cavender *et al.*, 1986) launched the search for specific adhesion molecules inducible on the endothelial cell surface, which has led to the identification of several classes of such molecules, providing selectivity for the emigration of different classes of leukocyte. Details of the molecules are described in the next two chapters, and are reviewed by Needham, Pearson & Hellewell (1991), Bevilacqua (1992), and Springer (1994).

The first adhesion molecule to be characterized, E-selectin, is not constitutively expressed by endothelial cells, but is rapidly induced and reaches maximal levels after 4–6 hours of IL-1, TNF or LPS treatment. Both *in vitro* and *in vivo* expression is usually transient, returning to zero after about 24 hours, though more recent *in vitro* data, based on observations of prolonged *in vivo* expression in response to certain stimuli, have indicated that longer-lived expression can be achieved (Keelan *et al.*, 1994; Sepp *et al.*, 1994). E-selectin is involved in the binding of neutrophils, monocytes and some T lymphocytes to endothelial cells, and is specifically concerned with the initial stages in which flowing leukocytes are captured to roll on endothelium (Bevilacqua *et al.*, 1987, Graber *et al.*, 1990; Needham *et al.*, 1991; Springer, 1994: also see Chapters 3 and 4).

Within the wide-ranging group of molecules belonging to the immunoglobulin superfamily, at least three members play a role on the endothelial surface in binding leukocytes: ICAM-1, ICAM-2 and VCAM-1. ICAM-1 is expressed at low levels on resting endothelium but is markedly up-regulated by IL-1, TNF or LPS, with maximal expression 24 hours after activation which is maintained for >72 hours (Dustin *et al.*, 1986; Pober *et al.*, 1986*a*). The counterligands for ICAM-1 on leukocytes are in the β_2 integrin (CD11/CD18) family (see Chapter 3). ICAM-2, constitutively present on resting endothelial cells at rather higher levels than ICAM-1, also binds leukocytes via one member of the β_2 integrin family (CD11a/CD18), but its level is not modulated by cytokines (de Fougerolles *et al.*, 1991). VCAM-1 is normally present minimally on nonactivated endothelial cells, but is induced with a similar time course to ICAM-1 (Osborn *et al.*, 1989; Thornhill & Haskard, 1990). The integrin counterligands for VCAM-1 are $\alpha_4\beta_1$ (VLA-4) present on lymphocytes and monocytes but not neutrophils, and $\alpha_4\beta_7$ on lymphocytes (Elices *et al.*, 1990; Chan *et al.*, 1992; Ruegg *et al.*, 1992: also see Chapters 3 and 4).

Not all surface adhesion molecules are increased by IL-1, TNF or LPS: for example, CD34 (which may also have a role in cell adhesion as a ligand for L-selectin expressed by lymphocytes) is reciprocally down-regulated (Delia *et al.*, 1993), and CD31 (PECAM-1: a homotypic endothelial cell adhesion molecule) is redistributed towards cell junctions rather than uniformly expressed as in non-activated cells (Ioffreda *et al.*, 1993).

In addition to these leukocyte adhesion molecules, there is a series of endothelial molecules, known collectively as addressins (which are still being identified) that are expressed at particular sites, especially in the high endothelial venules of lymph nodes, and are responsible for ensuring the correctly directed homing or recirculation of lymphocytes (for review see Picker, 1994; Springer, 1994; and discussed further in Chapter 4). Of these, the levels of several are modulated by cytokines; for example the mucosal addressin MAdCAM is increased on IL-1 treated high endothelial cells (Sikorski *et al.*, 1993).

Matrix growth factors and secondary cytokines

IL-1, TNF or LPS treatment significantly modulates the interactions of endothelial cells with the extracellular matrix, particularly in terms of selective alterations in the levels of cell surface integrins that can bind matrix components and in the secretion of matrix metalloproteinases and their inhibitors. Thus, α_6 integrin mRNA is decreased, leading to reduction of the $\alpha_6\beta_1$ molecule (laminin receptor) at the cell surface, while levels of other integrin α chain mRNAs (α_1, α_2, α_5) are unaltered (Defilippi, Silengo & Tarone, 1992). In contrast, the vitronectin receptor ($\alpha_v\beta_3$) is increased (Lafrenie *et al.*, 1992). The expression of several matrix metalloproteinases is enhanced by IL-1 or TNF, while production of their major inhibitor (TIMP-1) is apparently suppressed (Shingu *et al.*, 1993; Hanemaaijer *et al.*, 1993). A further example of induction of altered cell surface properties, in this case due to activation of a glycolipid metabolic pathway by IL-1, is the appearance of a novel ceramide derivative (Van de Kar *et al.*, 1992). This may be relevant in the pathogenesis of forms of the haemolytic uraemic syndrome associated with bacterial infection, since the ceramide is a specific receptor for verocytotoxin (see Chapter 10).

IL-1, TNF or LPS can inhibit endothelial cell growth, but they also induce the synthesis and secretion of a series of cytokines and haemopoietic growth factors from endothelial cells. It was initially described that exposure to IL-1 for several days strongly stimulated the autocrine secretion of IL-1 from endothelial cells, as detected by its T cell stimulatory activity in bioassays (Stern *et al.*, 1985; Locksley *et al.*, 1987; Warner, Auger & Libby, 1987). However, the mechanism of IL-1 secretion is not understood, since the molecule has no signal sequence for export, and subsequent studies indicate that the majority of endothelial IL-1 (IL-1α) is associated with the membrane (Kurt-Jones, Fiers & Pober, 1987) or is intracellular (Maier *et al.*, 1990). It is likely that at least part of the activity originally attributed to secreted IL-1 was due to IL-6, which is secreted readily from endothelial cells in response to IL-1 (Sironi *et al.*, 1989; Jirik *et al.*, 1989). Maier and coworkers have identified intracellular IL-1α as a critical factor in controlling endothelial cell lifespan, providing evidence that it is targeted to the cell nucleus and initiates senescence (Maier *et al.*, 1990; Maier, Statuto & Ragnotti, 1994).

Endothelial activation with IL-1, TNF or LPS induces the secretion of a large number of defined haemopoietic growth factors, including the colony stimulating factors GM-CSF, G-CSF, and M-CSF (Sieff *et al.*, 1988; Broudy *et al.*, 1988; Zsebo *et al.*, 1988; Clinton *et al.*, 1992) and increases constitutive expression of stem cell factor (Koenig *et al.*, 1994). Activated cells also secrete two growth factors known to be smooth muscle cell mitogens, PDGF and a more recently described heparin-binding growth factor (Libby & Hansson, 1991; Yoshizumi *et al.*, 1992).

Stimulation of endothelial cells with IL-1, TNF or LPS induces the synthesis of at least three members of the chemokine family of leukocyte chemoattractant peptides, IL-8, gro-α and MCP-1 (Strieter *et al.*, 1989*a,b*; Schroder & Christophers, 1989; Sica *et al.*, 1990*a,b*). The first two of these selectively act on neutrophils (and some lymphocytes), whereas the third attracts monocytes. These molecules were detected by screening libraries from IL-1-activated endothelial cells, and this approach has been used to identify several other novel endothelial gene products induced by IL-1 or TNF, particularly by Dixit's group (e.g. Wolf *et al.*, 1992) and Mantovani's group (e.g. Breviario *et al.*, 1992; which describes a new member of the pentaxin family that includes C-reactive protein).

Differential effects of TNF

Although the actions of IL-1, LPS and TNF on endothelial cells are virtually identical, TNF causes a few extra effects that cannot be mimicked by IL-1. There are indications that TNF may prolong the up-regulated expression of leukocyte adhesion molecules or the secretion of IL-6, by comparison with IL-1 (e.g. Hettmannsperger *et al.*, 1992) but there is a qualitative difference in the up-regulation of several proteins, in that TNF, but not IL-1 or LPS, increases the levels of class I major histocompatibility (MHC) molecules

(Wedgewood, Hatam & Bonagura, 1988; Lapierre, Fiers & Pober, 1988). TNF, but not IL-1, has also been shown to up-regulate the expression of endothelial GpIbα (Rajagopalan *et al.*, 1992). In conjunction with the TNF-induced increase in MHC Class I molecules, there is also a (more rapid) increase in the intracellular antigen processing transporter (TAP-1) required to assemble peptide antigen with nascent MHC Class I (Epperson *et al.*, 1992).

It has also been reported that the effects of TNF, but not of IL-1, on adhesion molecule expression are synergistically enhanced by coincubation with IFNγ (Doukas & Pober, 1990), though similar additive effects with either IL-1 or TNF were found by Leeuwenberg *et al.* (1990).

Interferon γ

Originally named, along with the unrelated molecules interferon α and β, because of its potential to inhibit viral replication, IFNγ is a T cell-derived cytokine with immunomodulatory properties, acting at a specific receptor (Aguet, Dembic & Merlin, 1988), which has recently been shown to require an accessory protein in the same family to signal cellular responses (Hemmi *et al.*, 1994; Soh *et al.*, 1994). IFNγ acts on endothelial cells to increase lymphocyte adhesion (Yu *et al.*, 1985) concomitantly with the slow (over a period of days) up-regulation of ICAM-1 and MHC Class I expression on endothelium (Pober *et al.*, 1986*b*).

However, the effects of IFNγ are clearly distinct from, and less pleiotropic than those of IL-1 or TNF. Although, as noted above, it can enhance the effects of TNF or IL-1, IFNγ alone does not induce the expression of early genes such as c-fos or the up-regulation of release of inflammatory mediators such as NO or PGI_2 (e.g. Colotta *et al.*, 1988). Nor does IFNγ up-regulate E-selectin or VCAM-1 expression on umbilical vein endothelial cells (Thornhill & Haskard, 1990), though it has been reported to induce VCAM-1 expression on a murine brain endothelial cell line (Sikorski *et al.*, 1993), and it enhances the levels of VCAM-1 present on cells derived from high endothelial venules (Sikorski *et al.*, 1993; May *et al.*, 1993).

Uniquely, IFNγ induces the expression of MHC Class II molecules on endothelium, allowing the cells to present foreign antigen productively to T cells (Pober *et al.*, 1983; Wagner, Vetto & Burger, 1984; see Chapter 11); it also acts synergistically with TNF in the induction of MHC class I molecules (Doukas & Pober, 1990) and with TNF or IL-1 in stimulating IL-6 production (Leeuwenberg *et al.*, 1990; Hashimoto *et al.*, 1992).

In contrast, IFNγ opposes some of the actions of IL-1 or TNF, for example reducing IL-1 induced PGDF synthesis and the IL-1 induced upregulation of Tissue Factor and urokinase-type plasminogen activator (uPA) (Suzuki *et al.*, 1989; Wojta *et al.*, 1992; Hashimoto *et al.*, 1992). It has also been reported to have varying effects on the expression of addressins, inducing MECA-325 but repressing MAdCAM (Duijvestijn *et al.*, 1986; Sikorski *et al.*, 1993).

Little is known of the effects of IFNα or β on endothelial cells. These interferons, produced by tissue cells (including endothelial cells) act via a distinct receptor from the IFNγ receptor (Merlin, Falcoff & Aguet, 1985). They have, however, been reported, like IFNγ, to augment endothelial MHC Class I expression and to depress uPA production (Pober & Cotran, 1990; Wojta *et al.*, 1994), and to interact with IL-2 to modulate endothelial phenotype (see below).

Interleukin 2

IL-2 is an important T cell-derived T cell growth factor (for review see Arai *et al.*, 1990). Until recently, though there were suggestions that IL-2 could enhance endothelial cell growth (Pober & Cotran, 1990), IL-2 receptors had not been detected on endothelial cells. IL-2 receptors belong to a subgroup of the dimeric class I cytokine receptor family, which binds IL-2, IL-4 and IL-7. They share a common γ chain, but have distinct α chains responsible for ligand binding specificity (Sato & Miyajima, 1994).

IL-2 therapy can cause widespread increases in vascular permeability, but this has been attributed to indirect effects of IL-2 caused by the induction of secondary cytokine release or mast cell activation (Cotran *et al.*, 1988; Edwards, Heniford & Miller, 1992). Recently, though, Cozzolino *et al.* (1993) reported that IL-2 receptors could be induced on IFNα-treated endothelial cells, and that exposure to IFNα followed by IL-2 stimulated basic fibroblast growth factor secretion. Thus, although IL-2 alone has no effect on properties such as adhesion molecule expression, its effects on endothelial cells in combination with other cytokines may need re-evaluation.

Interleukin 4, interleukin 10, interleukin 13

IL-4 is another T cell-derived cytokine (Arai *et al.*, 1990) first shown to act on endothelial cells to increase lymphocyte but not neutrophil binding (Thornhill, Kyan-Aung & Haskard, 1990). It was subsequently demonstrated that this was due to the induction of VCAM-1 (Thornhill & Haskard, 1990). IL-4 also acts synergistically to enhance IL-1- or TNF-induced VCAM-1 and T cell binding, but it concomitantly reduces both stimulated ICAM-1 and E-selectin levels (Thornhill & Haskard, 1990; Thornhill *et al.*, 1991). Recent evidence suggests that IL-4 co-induces another, as yet undefined, adhesion molecule for lymphocytes via a cAMP-dependent pathway (Galéa *et al.*, 1993): this signalling pathway may also be responsible for the inhibitory effects of IL-4 on E-selectin expression (Pober *et al.*, 1994). Interestingly, although monocytes possess VLA-4 (the ligand for VCAM-1), monocyte binding to activated endothelial cells can be reduced by concomitant IL-4 treatment (Elliott *et al.*, 1991) indicating that, at least under the conditions in which those experiments were performed, VCAM-1 is not of primary importance for monocyte adhesion.

IL-4 alone, or in synergy with other cytokines (IL-1, TNF, IFNγ) induces IL-6 and MCP-1 production (Howell *et al.*, 1991; Colotta *et al.*, 1992; Rollins & Pober, 1991). In common with IFNγ, IL-4 induces the production of complement accessory proteins (Ripoche *et al.*, 1988; Brooimans *et al.* 1989; Moutabarrik *et al.*, 1993). It has also been reported that IL-4 is a mitogen for capillary endothelial cells (Toi, Harris & Bicknell, 1991).

As well as antagonizing IL-1- or TNF-induced evaluations of ICAM-1 and E-selectin, IL-4 counteracts the increases in Tissue Factor, BH_4, PAI-1 and GM-CSF, and decreases in thrombomodulin, induced by IL-1, TNF or LPS (Kapiotis *et al.*, 1991; Herbert *et al.*, 1992; Schoedon *et al.*, 1993; Zoellner *et al.*, 1993; Martin, Jamieson & Tuffin, 1993).

IL-10 acts on a receptor in the same family as the IFNγ receptor, and also shares some signalling properties, including the activation of STAT (p91) transcription factors (Larner *et al.*, 1993; Sato & Miyajima, 1994). However, it often antagonizes the actions of IFNγ or other activating cytokines; for example, IL-10 inhibits monocyte production of cytokines and MHC Class II molecules (De Waal Malefyt *et al.*, 1991), and in common with IL-4 (Liew *et al.*, 1991) it inhibits induction of macrophage iNOS (Gazzinelli *et al.*, 1993). The latter effect may be due to inhibition of the autocrine production and action of TNF in macrophages, since IL-10 can, in fact, enhance iNOS production when exogenous TNF is present (Corradin *et al.*, 1993). In endothelial cells, IL-10 has been shown, like IL-4, to enhance IL-6 and MCP-1 synthesis (Sironi *et al.*, 1993), and to block IL-1- or TNF-induced BH_4 synthesis (Schoedon *et al.*, 1993).

Herbert *et al.* (1993) showed that IL-13, a recently characterized cytokine with actions similar to those of IL-10 (Minty *et al.*, 1993), acted on endothelial cells in the same way as IL-4 to oppose the induction of Tissue Factor and down-regulation of thrombomodulin by IL-1, TNF or LPS.

Interleukin 6

As noted above, IL-6 is secreted from IL-1-activated endothelial cells, and it is thought to be a major determinant of the acute phase response (Gauldie *et al.*, 1987; Kishimoto, 1989). The IL-6 receptor is a member of another subgroup of the dimeric class I family, which includes the G-CSF receptor (Sato & Miyajima, 1994). Initial work provided no evidence that IL-6 acted on endothelium: it does not modulate adhesion molecule or class I MHC molecule expression (Pober & Cotran, 1990), nor does it modulate basal or agonist-stimulated von Willebrand factor release (Paleolog & Pearson, 1990). However, it has recently been shown that IL-6 (like IL-1) increases endothelial monolayer permeability reversibly (Maruo *et al.*, 1992*b*) and alone or in synergy with IL-1 increases PDGF-B chain synthesis (Calderon *et al.*, 1992). In contrast to IL-1, IL-6 down-regulates COX1 expression (Maruo *et al.*, 1992*a*). G-CSF, like GM-CSF (see below) has been reported to increase endothelial cell growth and migration (Bussolino *et al.*, 1989).

Interleukin 3 and granulocyte/monocyte colony stimulating factor

The class I receptor subgroup recognizing IL-3, IL-5 and GM-CSF, all haemopoietic growth factors, again shares a common β chain while receptor specificity is imparted by separate α chains (Sato & Miyajima, 1994). Early reports indicated that GM-CSF enhanced endothelial growth and migration (Bussolino *et al.*, 1989) and tPA secretion (Kojima *et al.*, 1989). Subsequently, IL-3 was shown to enhance endothelial cell growth and to induce E-selectin expression (Brizzi *et al.*, 1993): this study also demonstrated the presence of mRNAs for both the β and α chain of the IL-3 receptor. Korpelainen *et al.* (1993) confirmed this and showed that the receptor is up-regulated by TNF, IL-1 or LPS, leading to potentiation of E-selectin expression and IL-8 secretion in the additional presence of IL-3. Colotta *et al.* (1993*a*) showed that the α chains for GM-CSF and IL-3 receptors are present in endothelial cells, but the IL-5-specific α chain was not detectable.

Transforming growth factor β

Although originally described as a mitogen for various cell types, with a widespread range of cell sources (including lymphocytes and endothelial cells) (Massagué, 1990) it is sensible to consider here the actions of TGFβ on endothelial cells, as they complement those of the cytokines described above. TGFβ binds to two related surface receptors, recently shown to act in concert to signal cellular responses (Wrana *et al.*, 1994). *In vitro*, TGFβ is an inhibitor of endothelial cell growth (Takehara, LeRoy & Grotendorst, 1987; Muller *et al.*, 1987). Gamble & Vadas (1988) found that TGFβ antagonized cytokine-up-regulated adhesion of neutrophils to endothelium, and the same group has now shown that TGFβ, additively with IL-4, inhibits E-selectin up-regulation (Gamble, Khew-Goodall & Vadas, 1993). TGFβ also reverses the enhanced BH_4 and GM-CSF production induced by IL-1 or TNF (Schoedon *et al.*, 1993). However, like IL-1, TGFβ can increase superoxide dismutase, and PAI-1 and endothelin-1 secretion (Saksela, Moscatelli & Rifkin, 1987; Kurihara *et al.*, 1989; Kong & Fanberg, 1992).

Conclusions

The multiple and diverse effects of cytokines on the modulation of endothelial cell phenotype are important factors influencing the involvement of endothelial cells in inflammatory and immune processes, where local or systemic production of one or more leukocyte-derived cytokines is occurring.

The most clear-cut example, though the details of the sequential elements of the interactions are still being explored, is the modulation of expression of adhesion molecules at the endothelial cell surface. These molecules are designed to capture and guide emigration of the appropriate leukocyte populations in a controlled manner, so that they can deal with the inflammatory or immune reactions taking place outside the blood vessel. Cytokines also modulate the release of a series of endothelium-derived soluble inflammatory mediators and regulators of haemostasis, to reinforce signals for leukocyte recruitment and to alter the haemostatic balance at the site of potential vessel damage.

However, the wide range of effects of cytokines on endothelial cells described in this chapter supports the concept that these responses are important in a variety of other pathophysiological situations, such as the developing atherosclerotic lesion, where intimal infiltration of monocytes and smooth muscle cells occurs; in rejecting organ grafts, where lymphocyte-mediated damage to endothelial cells is prominent; and in autoimmune diseases with a local or systemic vasculitic component. Several of these processes are discussed in detail in subsequent chapters.

Acknowledgement

J.D. Pearson thanks Ono Pharmaceutical Company for support. M.J. May holds an ARC studentship award.

References

Aguet, M., Dembic, Z. & Merlin, G. (1988). Molecular cloning and expression of the human interferon-γ receptor. *Cell*, **55**, 273–80.

Akeson, A. L., Mosher, L. B., Woods, C. W., Schroeder, K. K. & Bowlin, T. L. (1992). Human aortic endothelial cells express the type I but not the type II receptor for interleukin-1 (IL-1). *Journal of Cellular Physiology*, **153**, 583–8.

Arai, K., Lee, F. Miyajima, A., Miyatake, S., Arai, N. & Yokota, T. (1990). Cytokines: coordinators of immune and inflammatory responses. *Annual Reviews of Biochemistry*, **59**, 783–836.

Bevilacqua, M. P. (1993). Endothelial–leukocyte adhesion molecules. *Annual Reviews of Immunology*, **11**, 767–804.

Bevilacqua, M. P., Schleef, R. R., Gimbrone, M. A. Jr. & Loskutoff, D. J. (1986). Regulation of the fibrinolytic system of cultured human vascular endothelium by interleukin-1. *Journal of Clinical Investigation*, **78**, 587–91.

Bevilacqua, M. P., Pober, J. S., Majeau, G. R., Cotran, R. S. & Gimbrone, M. A. Jr. (1984). Interleukin-1 (IL-1) induces biosynthesis and cell surface expression of procoagulant activity in human vascular endothelial cells. *Journal of Experimental Medicine*, **160**, 618–23.

Bevilacqua, M. P., Pober, J. S., Mendrick, D. L., Cotran, R. S. & Gimbrone, M. A. Jr. (1987). Identification of an inducible endothelial–leukocyte adhesion molecule. *Proceedings of the National Academy of Sciences USA*, **84**, 9238–42.

Bevilacqua, M. P., Pober, J. S., Wheeler, M. E., Cotran, R. S. & Gimbrone, M. A. Jr. (1985). Interleukin 1 (IL-1) activation of vascular endothelium: effects on procoagulant activity and leukocyte adhesion. *American Journal of Pathology*, **121**, 393–403.

Bogle, R. G., Baydoun, A. R., Pearson, J. D. & Mann, G. E. (1992). L-Arginine transport is increased in macrophages generating nitric oxide. *Biochemical Journal*, **284**, 15–18.

Breviario, F., D'Aniello, E. M., Golay, J., Peri, G., Bottazzi, B., Bairoch, A., Saccone, S., Marzella, R., Predazzi, V., Rocchi, M., Della Valle, G., Dejana, E., Mantovani, A. & Introna, M. (1992). Interleukin-1-inducible genes in endothelial cells. Cloning of a new gene related to C-reactive protein and serum amyloid P component. *Journal of Biological Chemistry*, **267**, 22190–7.

Breviario, F., Proserpio, P., Bertocchi, F., Lampugnani, M. G., Mantovani, A. & Dejana, E. (1990). Interleukin-1 stimulates prostacyclin production by cultured human endothelial cells by increasing arachidonic acid mobilization and conversion. *Arteriosclerosis*, **10**, 129–34.

Brizzi, M. F., Garbarino, G., Rossi, P. R., Pagliardi, G. L., Arduino, C., Avanzi, G. C. & Pegoraro, L. (1993). Interleukin 3 stimulates proliferation and triggers endothelial–leukocyte adhesion molecule 1 gene activation of human endothelial cells. *Journal of Clinical Investigation*, **91**, 2887–92.

Brooimans, R. A., Hiemstra, P. S., Van Der Ark, A. A. J., Sim, R. B., Van Es, L. A. & Daha, M. R. (1989). Biosynthesis of complement factor H by human umbilical vein endothelial cells. Regulation by T cell growth factor and IFN-γ. *Journal of Immunology*, **142**, 2024–30.

Broudy, V. C., Kaushansky, K., Harlan, J. M. & Adamson, J. W. (1988). Interleukin 1 stimulates human endothelial cells to produce granulocyte-macrophage colony-stimulating factor and granulocyte colony-stimulating factor. *Journal of Immunology*, **139**, 464–8.

Brox, J. H., Østerud, B., Bjørklid, E. & Fenton, J. W. (1984). Production and availability of thromboplastin in endothelial cells: the effects of thrombin, endotoxin in platelets. *British Journal of Haematology*, **57**, 239–46.

Bussolino, F., Breviario, F., Tetta, C., Aglietta, M., Mantovani, A. & Dejana, E. (1986). Interleukin-1 stimulates platelet activating factor production in cultured human endothelial cells. *Journal of Clinical Investigation*, **77**, 2027–33.

Bussolino, F., Wang, J. M., Defilippi, P., Turrini, F., Sanavio, F., Edgell, C. J., Aglietta, M., Arese, P. & Mantovani, A. (1989). Granulocyte- and granulocyte-macrophage colony stimulating factors induce human endothelial cells to migrate and proliferate. *Nature*, **337**, 471–3.

Calderon, T. M., Sherman, J., Wilkerson, H., Hatcher, V. B. & Berman, J. W. (1992). Interleukin 6 modulates c-sis gene expression in cultured human endothelial cells. *Cellular Immunology*, **143**, 118–26.

Cavender, D. E., Haskard, D. O., Joseph, B. & Ziff, M. (1986) Interleukin 1 increases the binding of B and T lymphocytes to endothelial cell monolayers. *Journal of Immunology*, **136**, 203–7.

Chan, B. M., Elices, J. J., Murphy, E. & Hemler, M. E. (1992). Adhesion to vascular cell adhesion molecule-1 and fibronectin. Comparison of $\alpha_4\beta_1$ (VLA-4) and $\alpha_4\beta_7$ on the human B cell line JY. *Journal of Biological Chemistry*, **267**, 8366–70.

Clinton, S. K., Underwood, R., Hayes, L., Sherman, M. L., Kufe, D. W. & Libby, P. (1992). Macrophage colony-stimulating factor gene expression in vascular cells and in experimental and human atherosclerosis. *American Journal of Pathology*, **140**, 301–16.

Collins, T. (1993). Endothelial nuclear factor-kappa B and the initiation of the atherosclerotic lesion. *Laboratory Investigation*, **68**, 499–508.

Colotta, F., Bussolino, F., Polentarutti, N., Guglielmetti, A., Sironi, M., Bocchietto, E., De Rossi, M. & Mantovani, A. (1993*a*). Differential expression of the common beta and specific alpha chains of the receptors for GM-CSF, IL-3, and IL-5 in endothelial cells. *Experimental Cell Research*, **206**, 311–17.

Colotta, F., Lampugnani, M. G., Polentarutti, N., Dejana, E. & Mantovani, A. (1988). Interleukin-1 induces c-fos protooncogene expression in cultured human endothelial cells. *Biochemical and Biophysical Research Communications*, **152**, 1104–10.

Colotta, F., Sironi, M., Borré, A., Luini, W., Maddalena, F. & Mantovani, A. (1992). Interleukin 4 amplifies monocyte chemotactic protein and interleukin 6 production by endothelial cells. *Cytokine*, **4**, 24–8.

Colotta, F., Sironi, M., Borre, A., Pollicino, T., Bernasconi, S., Boraschi, D. & Mantovani, A. (1993*b*). Type II interleukin-1 receptor is not expressed in cultured endothelial cells and is not involved in endothelial cell activation. *Blood*, **81**, 1347–51.

Corradin, S. B., Fasel, N., Buchmüller-Rouiller, Y., Ransijn, A., Smith, J. & Manuël, J. (1993). Induction of macrophage nitric oxide production by interferon-γ and tumor necrosis factor-α is enhanced by interleukin-10. *European Journal of Immunology*, **23**, 72045–8.

Cotran, R. S., Pober, J. S., Gimbrone, M. A. Jr., Springer, T. A., Wiebke, E. A., Gaspari, A. A., Rosenberg, S. A. & Lotze, M. A. (1988). Endothelial activation during interleukin 2 immunotherapy. A possible mechanism for the vascular leak syndrome. *Journal of Immunology*, **139**, 1883–8.

Cozzolino, F., Torcia, M., Lucibello, M., Morbidelli, L., Ziche, M., Platt, J., Fabian, S., Brett, J. & Stern, D. (1993). Interferon-alpha and interleukin 2 synergistically enhance basic fibroblast growth factor synthesis and induce release, promoting endothelial cell growth. *Journal of Clinical Investigation*, **91**, 2504–12.

Crossman, D. C., Carr, D. P., Tuddenham, E. G. D., Pearson, J. D. & McVey, J. H. (1990). The control of tissue factor mRNA in human endothelial cells in response to endotoxin or phorbol ester. *Journal of Biological Chemistry*, **265**, 9782–7.

D'Aniello, E. M., Breviario, F., Padura, I. M., Lampugnani, M. G., Dejana, E., Mantovani, A. & Introna, M. (1993). Interleukin-1 and tumor necrosis factor induce transient expression of an inhibitor of nuclear factor kB in endothelial cells. *Endothelium*, **1**, 161–5.

De Fougerolles, A. R., Stacker, S. A., Schwarting, R. & Springer, T. A. (1991). Characterization of ICAM-2 and evidence for a third counter-receptor for LFA-1. *Journal of Experimental Medicine*, **174**, 253–67.

De Waal Malefyt, R., Abrams, J., Bennett, B., Figdor, C. G. & De Vries, J. E. (1991). Interleukin 10 inhibits cytokine synthesis by human monocytes: an autoregulatory role of IL-10 produced by monocytes. *Journal of Experimental Medicine*, **174**, 1209–20.

Defilippi, P., Silengo, L., Tarone, G. (1992). Alpha 6 beta 1 integrin (laminin receptor) is down-regulated by tumor necrosis factor alpha and interleukin-1 beta in human endothelial cells. *Journal of Biological Chemistry*, **267**, 18303–7.

Delia, D., Lampugnani, M. G., Resnati, M., Dejana, E., Aiello, A., Fontanella, E., Soligo, D., Pierotti, M. A. & Greaves, M. F. (1993). CD34 expression is regulated reciprocally with adhesion molecules in vascular endothelial cells *in vitro*. *Blood*, **81**, 1001–8.

Doukas, J. & Pober, J. S. (1990). IFN-γ enhances endothelial activation induced by tumor necrosis factor but not IL-1. *Journal of Immunology*, **145**, 1727–33.

Duijvestijn, A. M., Schreiber, A. B. & Butcher, E. C. (1986). Interferon-γ regulates an antigen specific for endothelial cells involved in lymphocyte traffic. *Proceedings of the National Academy of Sciences USA*, **83**, 9114–18.

Dustin, M. L., Rothlein, R., Bhan, A. K., Dinarello, C. A. & Springer, T. A. (1986). Induction by IL-1 and interferon-γ: tissue distribution, biochemistry and function of a natural adherence molecule (ICAM-1). *Journal of Immunology*, **137**, 245–54.

Edwards, M. J., Heniford, B. T. & Miller, F. N. (1992). Mast cell degranulation inhibits IL-2-induced microvascular protein leakage. *Journal of Surgical Research*, **52**, 429–35.

Elices, M. J., Osborn, L., Takada, Y., Crouse, C., Luhowskyj, S., Hemler, M. E. & Lobb, R. (1990). VCAM-1 on activated endothelium interacts with the leukocyte integrin VLA-4 at a site distinct from the VLA-4/fibronectin binding site. *Cell*, **60**, 577–84.

Elliott, M. J., Gamble, J. R., Park, L. S., Vadas, M. A. & Lopez, A. F. (1991). Inhibition of human monocyte adhesion by interleukin-4. *Blood*, **77**, 2739–45.

Emeis, J. J. & Kooistra, T. (1986). Interleukin 1 and lipopolysaccharide induce an inhibitor of tissue-type plasminogen activator *in vivo* and in cultured endothelial cells. *Journal of Experimental Medicine*, **163**, 1260–6.

Epperson, D. E., Arnold, D., Spies, T., Cresswell, P., Pober, J. S. & Johnson, D. R. (1992). Cytokines increase transporter in antigen processing-1 expression more rapidly than HLA class I expression in endothelial cells. *Journal of Immunology*, **149**, 3297–301.

Galéa. P., Thibault, G., Lacord, M., Bardos, P., Lebranchu, Y. (1993). IL-4, but not tumor necrosis factor-α, increases endothelial cell adhesiveness for lymphocytes by activating a cAMP-dependent pathway. *Journal of Immunology*, **151**, 588–96.

Gamble, J. R., Khew-Goodall, Y., Vadas, M. A. (1993). Transforming growth factor-beta inhibits E-selectin expression on human endothelial cells. *Journal of Immunology*, **150**, 4494–503.

Gamble, J. R. & Vadas, M. A. (1988). Endothelial adhesiveness for blood neutrophils is inhibited by transforming growth factor-β. *Science*, **242**, 97–9.

Gauldie, J., Richards, C., Harnish, D., Lansorp, P. & Baumann, H., (1987). Interferon β_2/B-cell stimulatory factor type 2 shares identity with monocyte-derived hapatocyte-stimulating factor and regulates the major acute phase protein response in liver cells. *Proceedings of the National Academy of Sciences USA*, **84**, 7251–5.

Gazzinelli, R. T., Oswald, I. P., Hieny, S., James, S. L. & Sher, A. (1993). The microbicidal activity of interferon-γ-treated macrophages against *Trypanosoma cruzi* involves an L-arginine dependent, nitrogen oxide-mediated mechanism inhibitable by interleukin-10 and transforming growth factor-β. *European Journal of Immunology*, **22**, 2501–6.

Goldblum, S. E., Brann, T. W., Ding, X., Pugin, J. & Tobias, P. S. (1994). Lipopolysaccharide (LPS)-binding protein and soluble CD14 function as accessory molecules for LPS-induced changes in endothelial barrier function, *in vitro*. *Journal of Clinical Investigation*, **93**, 692–702.

Graber, N., Gopal, T. V., Wilson, D., Beall, L. D., Polte, T. & Newman, W. (1990). T-cells bind to cytokine activated endothelial cells via a novel sialoglycoprotein and endothelial leukocyte adhesion molecule-1. *Journal of Immunology*, **145**, 819–30.

Gross, S. S., Jaffe, E. A., Levi, R. & Kilbourn, R. G. (1991). Cytokine activated endothelial cells express an isotype of nitric oxide synthase which is tetrahydrobiopterin-dependent, calmodulin-independent and inhibited by arginine analogs with a rank-order of potency characteristic of activated macrophages. *Biochemical and Biophysical Research Communications*, **178**, 823–9.

Hanemaaijer, R., Koolwijk, P., Le Clercq, L., De Vree, W. J A. & Van Hinsbergh, V. W. M. (1993). Regulation of matrix metalloproteinase expression in human vein and microvascular endothelial cells: effects of tumour necrosis factor alpha, interleukin 1 and phorbol ester. *Biochemical Journal*, **296**, 803–9.

Hashimoto, Y., Hirohata, S., Kashiwado, T., Itoh, K. & Ishii, H. (1992). Cytokine regulation of hemostatic property and IL-6 production of human endothelial cells. *Inflammation*, **16**, 613–31.

Hemmi, S., Böhni, R., Stark, G., Di Marco, F. & Aguet, M. (1994). A novel member of the interferon receptor family complements functionality of the murine interferon γ receptor in human cells. *Cell*, **76**, 803–10.

Herbert, J. M., Savi, P., Laplace, M. C. & Lale, A. (1992). IL-4 inhibits LPS-, IL-1β- and TNFα-induced expression of tissue factor in endothelial cells and monocytes. *FEBS Letters*, 310, 31–3.

Herbert, J. M., Savi, P., Laplace, M. C., Lale, A., Dol, F., Dumas, A., Labit, C. & Minty, A. (1993). IL-4 and IL-13 exhibit comparable abilities to reduce pyrogen-induced expression of procoagulant activity in endothelial cells and monocytes. *FEBS Letters*, **328**, 268–70.

Hettmannsperger, U., Detmar, M., Owsianowski, M., Tenorio, S., Kammler, H. J. & Orfanos, C. E. (1992). Cytokine-stimulated human dermal microvascular endothelial cells produce interleukin 6 – inhibition by hydrocortisone, dexamethasone, and calcitriol. *Journal of Investigative Dermatology*, **99**, 531–6.

Howell, G., Pham, P., Taylor, D., Foxwell, B. & Feldman, M. (1991). Interleukin 4 induces interleukin 6 production by endothelial cells: synergy with interferon-γ. *European Journal of Immunology*, **21**, 97–101.

Ioffreda, M. D., Albelda, S. M., Elder, D. E., Radu, A., Leventhal, L. C., Zweiman, B. & Murphy, G. F. (1993). TNFα induces E-selectin expression and PECAM-1 (CD31) redistribution in extracutaneous tissues. *Endothelium*, **1**, 47–54.

Jackson, B. A., Goldstein, R. H., Roy, R., Cozzani, M., Taylor, L. & Polgar, P. (1993). Effects of transforming growth factor beta and interleukin-1 beta on expression of cyclooxygenase 1 and 2 and phospholipase A2 mRNA in lung fibroblasts and endothelial cells in culture. *Biochemical and Biophysical Research Communications*, **197**, 1465–74.

Jirik, F. R., Podor, T. J., Hirano, T., Kishimoto, T., Loskutoff, D. J., Carson, D. A. & Lotz, M. (1989). Bacterial lipopolysaccharide and inflammatory mediators augment IL-6 secretion by human endothelial cells. *Journal of Immunology*, **142**, 144–7.

Jones, D. A., Carlton, D. P., McIntyre, T. M., Zimmerman, G. A. & Prescott, S. M. (1993). Molecular cloning of human prostaglandin endoperoxide synthase type II and demonstration of expression in response to cytokines. *Journal of Biological Chemistry*, **268**, 9049–54.

Kapiotis, S., Besemer, J., Bevec, D., Valent, P., Bettelheim, P., Lechner, K. & Speiser, W. (1991). Interleukin-4 counteracts pyrogen-induced downregulation of thrombomodulin in cultured human vascular endothelial cells. *Blood*, **78**, 410–15.

Keelan, E. T. M., Licence, S. T., Peters, A. M., Binns, R. M. & Haskard, D. O. (1994). Characterization of E-selectin expression *in vivo* with use of a radiolabeled monoclonal antibody. *American Journal of Physiology*, **266**, H279–90.

Kilbourn, R. G. & Belloni, R. (1990). Endothelial cell production of nitrogen oxides in response to interferon γ in combination with tumor necrosis factor, interleukin 1 or endotoxin. *Journal of the National Cancer Institute*, **82**, 772–6.

Kishimoto, T. (1989). The biology of interleukin-6. *Blood*, **74**, 1–10.

Knowles, R. G. & Moncada, S. (1994). Nitric oxide synthases in mammals. *Biochemical Journal*, **298**, 249–58.

Koenig, A., Yakisan, E., Reuter, M., Huang, M., Sykora, K. W., Corbacioglu, S. & Welte, K. (1994). Differential regulation of stem cell factor mRNA expression in human endothelial cells by bacterial pathogens: and *in vitro* model of inflammation. *Blood*, **83**, 2836–43.

Kojima, S., Tadenuma, H., Inada, Y. & Saito, Y. (1989). Enhancement of plasminogen activator activity in cultured endothelial cells by granulocyte colony-stimulating factor. *Journal of Cellular Physiology*, **138**, 192–6.

Kong, X. J. & Fanburg, B. L., (1992). Regulation of Cu, Zn-superoxide dismutase in bovine pulmonary artery endothelial cells. *Journal of Cellular Physiology*, **153**, 491–7.

Korpelainin, E. I., Gamble, J. R., Smith, W. B., Goodall, G. J., Qiyu, S., Woodcock, J. M., Dottore, M., Vadas, M. A. & Lopez, A. (1993). The receptor for interleukin 3 is selectively induced in human endothelial cells by tumor necrosis factor alpha and potentiates interleukin 8 secretion and neutrophil transmigration. *Proceedings of the National Academy of Sciences USA*, **90**, 11137–41.

Kurihara, H., Yoshizumi, M., Sugiyama, T., Takaku, F., Yanagisawa, M., Masaki, T., Hamoki, M., Kato, H. & Yazaki, Y. (1989). Transforming growth factor-β stimulates the expression of endothelin mRNA by vascular endothelial cells. *Biochemical and Biophysical Research Communications*, **159**, 1435–40.

Kurt-Jones, E. A., Fiers, W., Pober, J. S., (1987). Membrane interleukin 1 induction on human endothelial cells and dermal fibroblasts. *Journal of Immunology*, **139**, 2317–24.

Lafrenie, R. M., Podor, T. J., Buchanan, M. R. & Orr, F. W. (1992). Up-regulated biosynthesis and expression of endothelial cell vitronectin receptor enhances cancer cell adhesion. *Cancer Research*, **52**, 2202–8.

Lapierre, L. A., Fiers, W. & Pober, J. S. (1988). Three distinct classes of regulatory cytokines control endothelial cell MHC antigen expression: interactions with immune (γ) interferon differentiate the effects of tumor necrosis factor and lymphotoxin from those of leukocyte (α) and fibroblast (β) interferons. *Journal of Experimental Medicine*, **167**, 794–804.

Larner, A. C., David, M., Feldman, G. M., Igarashi, K., Hackett, R. H., Webb, D. S. A., Sweitzer, S. M., Petricoin III, E. F. & Finbloom, D. S. (1993). Tyrosine phosphorylation of DNA binding proteins by multiple cytokines. *Science*, **261**, 1730–3.

Leeuwenberg, J. F. M., von Asmuth, E. J. U., Jeunhomme, T. M. A. A. & Buurman, W. A. (1990). IFN-γ regulates the expression of the adhesion molecule ELAM-1 and IL-6 production by human endothelial cells *in vitro*. *Journal of Immunology*, **145**, 2110–14.

Libby, P. & Hansson, G. K. (1991). Involvement of the immune system in human atherogenesis: current knowledge and unanswered questions. *Laboratory Investigation*, **64**, 5–15.

Libby, P., Ordovas, J. M., Auger, K. R., Robbins, A. H., Birinyi, L. K. & Dinarello, C. A. (1986). Endotoxin and tumor necrosis factor induce interleukin-1 gene expression in adult human vascular endothelial cells. *American Journal of Pathology*, **124**, 179–86.

Liew, F. Y., Li, F., Severn, A., Millott, S., Schmidt, J., Salter, M. & Moncada, S. (1991). A possible novel pathway of regulation by murine T helper type-2 (T_h-2) cells of a T_h-1 cell activity via the modulation of nitric oxide synthase activity on macrophages. *European Journal of Immunology*, **21**, 2489–94.

Locksley, R. M., Heinzel, F. P., Shepard, H. M., Agosti, J., Eessalu, T. E., Aggarwal, B. B. & Harlan, J. M. (1987). Tumor necrosis factor α and β differ in their capacities to generate interleukin 1 release from human endothelial cells. *Journal of Immunology*, **139**, 1891–5.

Loetscher, H., Pan, Y-U. E., Lahm, H-W., Gentz, R., Brockhaus, M., Tabuchi, H. & Lesslauer, W. (1990). Molecular cloning and expression of the human 55 Kd tumor necrosis factor receptor. *Cell*, **61**, 351–9.

Mackay, F., Loetscher, H., Stueber, D., Gehr, G. & Lesslauer, W. (1993). Tumor necrosis factor alpha (TNF-alpha)-induced cell adhesion to human endothelial cells is under dominant control of one TNF receptor type, TNF-R55. *Journal of Experimental Medicine,* **177**, 12877–86.

McMahan, C., Slack, J. L., Mosley, B., Cosman, D., Lupton, S. D., Brunton, L. L., Grubin, C. E., Wignell, J. M., Jenkins, N. A., Brannan, C. I., Copeland, N. G., Huebner, K., Croce, C. M., Cannizzarro, L. A., Benjamin, D., Dower, S. K., Spriggs, M. K., Sims, J. E. (1991). A novel IL-1 receptor cloned from B cells by mammalian expression is expressed in many cell types. *EMBO Journal*, **10**, 2821–32.

Maier, J. A., Hla, T. & Maciag, T. (1990). Cycloxygenase in an immediate-early gene induced by interleukin-1 in human endothelial cells. *Journal of Biological Chemistry*, **265**, 10805–8.

Maier, J. A. M., Statuto, M. & Ragnotti, G. (1994). Endogenous interleukin 1 alpha must be transported to the nucleus to exert its activity in human endothelial cells. *Molecular and Cellular Biology*, **14**, 1845–51.

Maier, J. A. M., Voulalas, P., Roeder, D. & Maciag, T. (1990). Extension of the life-span of human endothelial cells by an interleukin-1α antisense oligomer. *Science*, **249**, 1570–4.

Mantovani, A., Bussolino, F. & Dejana, E. (1992). Cytokine regulation of endothelial cell function. *FASEB Journal*, **6**, 2591–9.

Martin, N. B., Jamieson, A. & Tuffin, D. P. (1993). The effect of interleukin-4 on tumour necrosis factor-alpha induced expression of tissue factor and plasminogen activator inhibitor-1 in human umbilical vein endothelial cells. *Thrombosis and Haemostasis*, **70**, 1037–42.

Maruo, N., Morita, I., Ishizaki, Y., Murota, S. I. (1992*a*). Inhibitory effects of interleukin 6 on prostaglandin I_2 production in cultured bovine vascular endothelial cells. *Archives of Biochemistry and Biophysics*, **292**, 600–4.

Maruo, N., Morita, I., Shirao, M. & Murota, S. I. (1992*b*). IL-6 increases endothelial permeability *in vitro*. *Endocrinology*, **131**, 710–14.

Massagué, J. (1990). The transforming growth factor-β family. *Annual Review of Cell Biology*, **6**, 597–641.

May, M. J., Entwistle, E., Humphries, M. J. & Ager, A. (1993). VCAM-1 is a CS1 peptide-inhibitable adhesion molecule expressed by lymph node high endothelium. *Journal of Cell Science*, **106**, 109–19.

Merlin, G., Falcoff, E. & Aguet, M. (1985). ^{125}I-labelled human interferons alpha, beta and gamma: comparative receptor binding data. *Journal of General Virology*, **66**, 1149–51.

Minty, A., Chalon, R., Derocq, J-M., Dumont, X., Guillemot, J-C., Kaghad, M., Labit, C., Leplatois, P., Liauzun, P., Miloux, B., Minty, C., Casellas, P., Loison, G., Lupker, J., Shire, D., Ferrara, P. & Caput, D. (1993). Interleukin-13 is a new human lymphokine regulating inflammatory and immune responses. *Nature*, 362, 248–50.

Moutabarrik, A., Nakanishi, I., Namiki, M., Hara, T., Matsumoto, M., Ishibashi, M., Okuyama, A., Zaid, D. & Seya, T. (1993). Cytokine-mediated regulation of the surface expression of complement regulatory proteins, CD46(MCP), CD55(DAF), and CD59 on human vascular endothelial cells. *Lymphokine and Cytokine Research*, **12**, 167–72.

Muller, G., Behrens, J., Nussbaumer, V., Bohlen, P. & Birchmeier, W. (1987). Inhibitory action of transforming growth factor β on endothelial cells. *Proceedings of the National Academy of Sciences USA*, **84**, 5600–4.

Muller, J. M., Ziegler-Heitbrock, H. W. L. & Bauerle, P. A. (1993). Nuclear factor kappa B, a mediator of lipopolysaccharide effects. *Immunobiology*, **187**, 233–56.

Nachman, R. L., Hajjar, K. A., Silverstein, R. L. & Dinarello, C. A. (1986). Interleukin 1 induces endothelial cell synthesis of plasminogen activator inhibitor. *Journal of Experimental Medicine*, **163**, 1595–600.

Nawroth, P. P. & Stern, D. M. (1986). Modulation of endothelial cell hemostatic properties by tumor necrosis factor. *Journal of Experimental Medicine*, **163**, 740–5.

Needham, L., Pearson, J. D. & Hellewell, P. G. (1991). Adhesion of granulocytes, monocytes and related cell lines. In Gordon, J. L., ed. *Vascular Endothelium: Interactions with Circulating Cells*, pp. 61–89. Amsterdam: Elsevier.

Osborn L., Hession, C., Tizard, R., Vassallo, C., Luhowskyj, S., Chi-Rosso, G. & Lobb, R. (1989). Direct expression cloning of vascular cell adhesion molecule 1, a cytokine-induced endothelial protein that binds to lymphocytes. *Cell*, **59**, 1203–11.

Paleolog, E. M., Crossman, D. C., McVey, J. H. & Pearson, J. D. (1990). Differential regulation by cytokines of constitutive and stimulated secretion of von Willebrand factor from endothelial cells. *Blood*, **75**, 688–95.

Paleolog, E. M. & Pearson, J. D. (1990). Differential regulation by cytokines of constitutive and stimulated secretion of von Willebrand factor from human endothelial cells. In Zilla, P., Fasol, R. & Callow, A. eds. *Applied Cardiovascular Biology 1989*, pp. 189–193. Basel: Karger.

Pearson, J. D. (1993). The control of production and release of haemostatic factors in the endothelial cell. *Ballière's Clinical Haematology*, **6**, 629–51.

Pearson, J. D. (1994). Endothelial cell biology. In Bloom, A. L., Forbes, C. D., Thomas, D. P. & Tuddenham, E. G. D., eds. *Haemostasis and Thrombosis*, 3rd edn. pp. 219–232. Edinburgh: Churchill Livingstone.

Picker, L. J. (1994). Control of lymphocyte homing. *Current Opinion in Immunology*, **6**, 394–406.

Pober, J. S. (1988). Cytokine-mediated activation of vascular endothelium: physiology and pathology. *American Journal of Pathology*, **133**, 426–33.

Pober, J. S., Bevilacqua, M. P., Mendrick, D. L., Lapierre, L. A., Fiers, W. & Gimbrone, M. A. Jr. (1986*a*). Two distinct monokines, interleukin-1 and tumor necrosis factor, each independently induce biosynthesis and transient expression of the same antigen on the surface of cultured human vascular endothelial cells. *Journal of Immunology*, **136**, 1680–7.

Pober, J. S., Collins, T., Gimbrone, M. A. Jr., Cotran, R. S., Gitlin, J. D., Fiers, W., Clayberger, C., Krensky, A. M., Burakoff, J. J. & Reiss, C. S. (1983). Lymphocytes recognize human vascular endothelial and dermal fibroblast Ia antigens induced by recombinant immune interferon. *Nature*, **305**, 726–9.

Pober, J. S. & Cotran, R. S. (1990). Cytokines and endothelial cell biology. *Physiological Reviews*, **70**, 427–51.

Pober, J. S., Gimbrone, M. A. Jr., Lapierre, L. A., Mendrick, D. L., Fiers, W., Rothlein, R. & Springer, T. A. (1986*b*). Overlapping patterns of activation of human endothelial cells by interleukin 1, tumor necrosis factor, and immune interferon. *Journal of Immunology*, **137**, 1893–6.

Pober, J. S., Slowik, M. R., De Luca, L. G. & Ritchie, A. J. (1994). Elevated cyclic AMP inhibits endothelial cell synthesis and expression of TNF-induced endothelial leukocyte adhesion molecule-1, and vascular cell adhesion molecule-1, but not intercellular adhesion molecule-1. *Journal of Immunology*, **150**, 5114–23.

Pugin, J., Schurer-Maly, C. C., Leturcq, D., Moriarty, A., Ulevitch, R. J. & Tobias, P. S. (1993). Lipopolysaccharide activation of human endothelial and epithelial cells is mediated by lipopolysaccharide-binding protein and soluble CD14. *Proceedings of the National Academy of Sciences USA* **90**, 2744–8.

Radomski, M. W., Palmer, R. M. J. & Moncada, S. (1990). Glucocorticoids inhibit the expression of an inducible, but not the constitutive, nitric oxide synthase in vascular endothelial cells. *Proceedings of the National Academy of Sciences USA*, **87**, 10043–7.

Rajagopalan, V., Essex, D. W., Shapiro, S. S. & Konkle, B. A. (1992). Tumor necrosis factor-α modulation of glycoprotein Ibα expression in human endothelial and erythroleukemia cells. *Blood*, **80**, 153–61.

Read, M. A., Cordle, S. R., Veach, R. A., Carlisle, C. D. & Hawiger, J. (1993). Cell-free pool of CD14 mediates activation of transcription factor NF-kappa B by lipopolysaccharide in human endothelial cells. *Proceedings of the National Academy of Sciences USA*, **90**, 9887–91.

Read, M. A., Whitley, M. Z., Williams, A. J. & Collins, T. (1994). NF-kB and IkBα: an inducible regulatory system in endothelial activation. *Journal of Experimental Medicine*, **179**, 503–12.

Ripoche, J., Mitchell, J. A., Erdei, A., Madin, C., Moffatt, B., Mokoena, T., Gordon, S. & Sim, R. B. (1988). Interferonγ induces synthesis of complement alternative pathway proteins by human endothelial cells in culture. *Proceedings of the National Academy of Sciences USA*, **83**, 4167–72.

Rollins, B. J. & Pober, J. S. (1991). Interleukin-4 induces the synthesis and secretion of MCP-1/JE by human endothelial cells. *American Journal of Pathology*, **138**, 1315–19.

Rosenkranz-Weiss, P., Sessa, W. C., Milstien, S., Kaufman, S., Watson, C. A. & Pober, J. S. (1994). Regulation of nitric oxide synthesis by proinflammatory cytokines in human umbilical vein endothelial cells. Elevations in tetrahydrobiopterin levels enhance endothelial nitric oxide synthase specific activity. *Journal of Clinical Investigation*, **93**, 2236–43.

Ruegg, C., Postigo, A. A., Sikorski, E. E., Butcher, E. C., Pytela, R. & Erle, D. J. (1992). Role of integrin $\alpha 4\beta 7/\alpha 4\beta P$ in lymphocyte adherence to fibronectin and VCAM-1 in homotypic cell clustering. *Journal of Cell Biology*, **117**, 179–89.

Ryan, G. B. & Majno, G. (1977). Acute inflammation. *American Journal of Pathology*, **86**, 183–276.

Ryan, J., Brett, J., Tijburg, P., Bach, R. R., Kisiel, W., Stern, D. (1992). Tumor necrosis factor-induced endothelial tissue factor is associated with subendothelial matrix vesicles but is not expressed on the endothelial surface. *Blood*, **80**, 966–74.

Saksela, O., Moscatelli, D. & Rifkin, D. B. (1987). The opposing effects of basic fibroblast growth factor and transforming growth factor beta on the regulation of plasminogen activator activity in capillary endothelial cells. *Journal of Cell Biology*, **105**, 957–63.

Sato, N. & Miyajima, A. (1994). Multimeric cytokine receptors: common versus specific functions. *Current Opinion in Cell Biology*, **6**, 174–9.

Schall, T. J., Lewis, M., Koller, K. J., Lee, A., Rice, G. C., Wong, G. H. W., Gatanaga, T., Granger, G. A., Leutz, R., Raab, H., Kohr, W. J. & Goeddel, D. V. (1990). Molecular cloning and expression of a receptor for human tumor necrosis factor. *Cell*, **61**, 361–70.

Schleef, R. R., Bevilacqua, M. P., Sawdey, M., Gimbrone, M. A., Loskutoff, D. J. (1988). Interleukin 1 and tumor necrosis factor activation of vascular endothelium: effects on plasminogen activator inhibitor and tissue-type plasminogen activator. *Journal of Biological Chemistry*, **263**, 5797–803.

Schoedon, G., Schneemann, M., Blau, N., Edgell, C. J. S. & Schaffner, A. (1993). Modulation of human endothelial cell tetrahydrobiopterin synthesis by activating and deactivating cytokines: new perspectives on endothelium-derived relaxing factor. *Biochemical and Biophysical Research Communications*, **196**, 1343–8.

Schroder, J. M. & Christophers, E. (1989). Secretion of novel and homologous neutrophil-activating peptides by LPS-stimulated human endothelial cells. *Journal of Immunology*, **142**, 244–51.

Sepp, N. T., Gille, J., Li, L. J., Caughman, S. W., Lawley, T. J. & Swerlick, R. A. (1994). A factor in human plasma permits persistent expression of E-selectin by human endothelial cells. *Journal of Investigative Dermatology*, **102**, 445–50.

Shalaby, M. R., Sundan, A., Loetscher, H., Brockhus, M., Lesslauer, W. & Espevik, T. (1990). Binding and regulation of cellular functions by monoclonal antibodies against tumor necrosis factor receptors. *Journal of Experimental Medicine*, **172**, 1517–20.

Shingu, M., Nagai, Y., Isayama, T., Naono, T., Nobunaga, M. & Nagai, Y. (1993). The effects of cytokines on metalloproteinase inhibitors (TIMP) and collagenase production by human chondrocytes and TIMP production by synovial cells and endothelial cells. *Clinical and Experimental Immunology*, **94**, 145–9.

Sica, A., Matsushima, K., Van Damme, J., Wang, J. M., Polentarutti, N., Dejana, E., Colotta, F., Mantovani, A. (1990*a*). IL-1 transcriptionally activates the neutrophil chemotactic factor/IL-8 gene in endothelial cells. *Immunology*, **69**, 548–53.

Sica, A., Wang, J. M., Colotta, F., Dejana, E., Mantovani, A., Oppenheim, J. J., Larsen, C. G., Zachariae, C. O. C. & Matsushima, K. (1990*b*). Monocyte chemotactic and activating factor gene expression induced in endothelial cells by IL-1 and TNF. *Journal of Immunology*, **144**, 3034–8.

Sieff, C. A., Niemeyer, C. M., Mentzer, S. J. & Faller, D. V. (1988). Interleukin 1, tumor necrosis factor and the production of granulocyte-macrophage colony-stimulating factor by cultured mesenchymal cells. *Blood*, **72**, 1316–23.

Sikorski, E. E., Hallmann, R., Berg, E. L. & Butcher, E. C. (1993). The Peyer's patch high endothelial receptor for lymphocytes, the mucosal vascular addressin, is induced on a murine endothelial cell line by tumor necrosis factor-α and IL-1. *Journal of Immunology*, **151**, 5234–50.

Sims, J. E., March, C. J., Cosman, D., Widmer, M. B., MacDonald, H. R., McMahan, C. J., Grubin, C. E., Wignall, J. M., Jackson, J. L., Call, S. M., Friend, D., Alpert, A. R., Gillis, S., Urdal, D. L. & Dower, S. K. (1988). cDNA expression cloning of the IL-1 receptor a member of the immunoglobulin superfamily. *Science*, **241**, 585–9.

Sironi, M., Breviario, F., Proserpio, P., Biondi, A., Vecchi, A., Van Damme, J., Dejana, E. & Mantovani, A. (1989). IL-1 stimulates IL-6 production in endothelial cells. *Journal of Immunology*, **142**, 549–53.

Sironi, M., Munoz, C., Pollicino, T., Siboni, A., Sciacca, F. L., Bernasconi, S., Vecchi, A., Colotta, F. & Mantovani, A. (1993). Divergent effects of interleukin-10 on cytokine production by mononuclear phagocytes and endothelial cells. *European Journal of Immunology*, **23**, 2692–5.

Smith, C. A., Davis, T., Anderson, D., Solam, L., Beckman, M. P., Jerzy, R., Dower, S. K., Cosman, D. & Goodwin, R. G. (1990). A receptor for tumor necrosis factor defines an unusual family of cellular and viral proteins. *Science*, **248**, 1019–23.

Soh, J., Donnelly, R. J., Kotenko, S., Mariano, T. M., Cook, J. R., Wang, N., Emanuel, S., Schwartz, B., Miki, T. & Pestka, S. (1994). Identification and sequence of an accessory factor required for activation of the human interferon γ receptor. *Cell*, **76**, 803–10.

Springer, T. A. (1994). Traffic signals for lymphocyte recirculation and leukocyte emigration: the multistep paradigm. *Cell*, **76**, 301–14.

Stern, D. M., Bank, I., Nawroth, P. P., Cassimeris, J., Kisiel, W., Fenton, J. W. III, Dinarello, C., Chess, L. & Jaffe, E. A. (1985). Self-regulation of procoagulant events on the endothelial cell surface. *Journal of Experimental Medicine*, **162**, 1223–35.

Strieter, R. M., Kunkel, S. L., Showell, H. J., Remick, D. G., Phan, S. H., Ward, P. A. & Marks, R. M. (1989*a*). Endothelial cell gene expression of a neutrophil chemotactic factor by TNF-alpha, LPS and IL-1 α. *Science*, **243**, 1467–9.

Strieter, R. M., Wiggins, R., Phan, S. H., Wharram, B. L., Showell, H. J., Remick, D. G., Chensue, S. W. & Kunkel, S. L. (1989*b*). Monocyte chemotactic protein gene expression by cytokine-treated human fibroblasts and endothelial cells. *Biochemical and Biophysical Research Communications*, **162**, 694–9.

Suga, S. I., Itoh, H., Komatsu, Y., Ogawa, Y., Hama, N., Yoshimasa, T. & Nakao, K. (1993). Cytokine-induced C-type natriuretic peptide (CNP) secretion from vascular endothelial cells – evidence for CNP as a novel autocrine/paracrine regulator from endothelial cells. *Endocrinology*, **133**, 3038–41.

Suzuki, H., Shibono, K., Okane, M., Kono, I., Matsui, Y., Yamane, K. & Kashiwagi, H. (1989). Interferon-γ modulates messenger RNA levels of c-sis (PDGF-B chain), PDGF-A chain and IL-1α genes in human vascular endothelial cells. *American Journal of Pathology*, **134**, 35–43.

Suzuki, K., Tatsumi, H., Satoh, S., Senda, T., Nakata, T., Fujii, J. & Taniguchi, N. (1993). Manganese-superoxide dismutase in endothelial cells: localization and mechanism of induction. *American Journal of Physiology*, **265**, H1173–8.

Takehara, K., LeRoy, E. C. & Grotendorst, G. R. (1987). TGF-β inhibition of endothelial cell proliferation: alteration of EGF binding and EGF-induced growth-regulatory (competence) gene expression. *Cell*, **49**, 415–22.

Thornhill, M. H. & Haskard, D. O. (1990). IL-4 regulates endothelial cell activation by IL-1, tumor necrosis factor or IFN-γ. *Journal of Immunology*, **145**, 865–72.

Thornhill, M. H., Kyan-Aung, U. & Haskard, D. O. (1990). IL-4 increases human endothelial cell adhesiveness for T cells but not for neutrophils. *Journal of Immunology*, **144**, 3060–5.

Thornhill, M. H., Wellicome, S. M., Mahiouz, D. L., Lanchbury, J. S. S., Kyan-Aung, U. & Haskard, D. O. (1991). Tumor necrosis factor combines with IL-4 or IFN-γ to selectively enhance endothelial cell adhesiveness for T cells. The contribution of vascular cell adhesion molecule-1-dependent and -independent binding mechanisms. *Journal of Immunology*, **146**, 592–8.

Toi, M., Harris, A. L. & Bicknell, R. (1991). Interleukin-4 is a potent mitogen for capillary endothelium. *Biochemical and Biophysical Research Communications*, **174**, 1287–93.

Van de Kar, N. C. A. J., Monnens, L. A. H., Karmali, M. A. & Van Hinsbergh, V. W. M. (1992). Tumor necrosis factor and interleukin-1 induce expression of the verocytotoxin receptor globotriaosylceramide on human endothelial cells: implications for the pathogenesis of the hemolytic uremic syndrome. *Blood*, **80**, 2755–64.

Vassalli, P. (1992). The pathophysiology of tumor necrosis factors. *Annual Review of Immunology*, **10**, 411–52.

Vicart, P., Testut, P., Schwartz, B., Llorens Cortes, C., Perdomo, J. J., Paulin, D. (1993). Cell adhesion markers are expressed by a stable human endothelial cell line transformed by the SV40 large T antigen under vimentin promoter control. *Journal of Cellular Physiology*, **157**, 41–51.

Visner, G. A., Chesrown, S. E., Monnier, J., Ryan, U. A. & Nick, H. S. (1992). Regulation of manganese superoxide dismutase: IL-1 and TNF induction in pulmonary artery and microvascular endothelial cells. *Biochemical and Biophysical Research Communications*, **188**, 453–62.

Wagner, C. R., Vetto, R. M. & Burger, D. R. (1984). The mechanisms of antigen presentation by endothelial cells. *Immunobiology*, **168**, 453–69.

Warner, S. J. C., Auger, K. R. & Libby, P. (1987). Interleukin induces interleukin 1. II. Recombinant human interleukin 1 induces interleukin 1 production by adult human vascular endothelial cells. *Journal of Immunology*, **139**, 1911–17.

Wedgewood, J. F., Hatam, L. & Bonagura, V. R. (1988). Effect of interferon-γ and tumor necrosis factor on the expression of class I and class II major histocompatibility molecules by cultured human umbilical vein endothelial cells. *Cellular Immunology*, **111**, 1–9.

Wojta, J., Zoellner, H., Callicchio, M., Filonzi, E. L., Hamilton, J. A. & McGrath, K. (1994). Interferon-α2 counteracts interleukin-1α-stimulated expression of urokinase-type plasminogen activator in human foreskin microvascular endothelial cells *in vitro*. *Lymphokine and Cytokine Research*, **13**, 133–8.

Wojta, J., Zoellner, H., Gallicchio, M., Hamilton, J. A. & McGrath, K. (1992). Gamma-interferon counteracts interleukin-1 alpha stimulated expression of urokinase-type plasminogen activator in human endothelial cells *in vitro*. *Biochemical and Biophysical Research Communications*, **188**, 463–9.

Wolf, F. W., Marks, R. M., Sarma, V., Byers, M. G., Katz, R. W., Shows, T. B. & Dixit, V. M. (1992). Characterization of a novel tumor necrosis factor-alpha-induced endothelial primary response gene. *Journal of Biological Chemistry*, **267**, 1317–26.

Wrana, J. L., Attisano, L., Wieser, R., Ventura, F. & Massagué, J. (1994). Mechanism of activation of the TGFβ receptor. *Nature*, **370**, 341–7.

Wright, S. D., Ramos, R. A., Tobias, P. S., Ulevitch, R. J. & Mathison, J. C. (1990). CD14, a receptor for complexes of lipopolysaccharide (LPS) and LPS binding protein. *Science*, **249**, 1431–3.

Yoshizumi, M., Kourembanas, S., Temizer, D. H., Cambria, R. P., Quertermous, T. & Lee, M. E. (1992). Tumor necrosis factor increases transcription of the heparin-binding epidermal growth factor-like growth factor gene in vascular endothelial cells. *Journal of Biological Chemistry*, **267**, 9467–9.

Yoshizumi, M., Kurihara, H., Morita, T., Yamashita, T., Oh-Hashi Sugiyama, T., Takaku, F., Yanagisawa, M., Masaki, T. & Yazaki, Y. (1990). Interleukin 1 increases the production of endothelin-1 in cultured endothelial cells. *Biochemical and Biophysical Research Communications*, **166**, 324–9.

Yoshizumi, M., Perrella, M. A., Burnett, J. C. Jr. & Lee, M. E. (1993). Tumor necrosis factor downregulates an endothelial nitric oxide synthase mRNA by shortening its half life. *Circulation Research*, **73**, 205–9.

Yu, C-L., Haskard, D. O., Johnson, A. R. & Ziff, M. (1985). Human γ interferon increases binding of T lymphocytes to endothelial cells. *Cellular Immunology*, **62**, 554–60.

Zavoico, G. G., Ewenstein, B. M., Schafer, A. I. & Pober, J. S. (1989). IL-1 and related cytokines enhance thrombin-stimulated PGI_2 production in cultured endothelial cells without affecting thrombin-stimulated von Willebrand factor secretion or platelet-activating factor biosynthesis. *Journal of Immunology*, **142**, 3993–9.

Zoellner, H., Cebon, J., Layton, J. E., Stanton, H. & Hamilton, J. A. (1993). Contrasting effects of interleukin-4 on colony-stimulating factor and interleukin-6 synthesis by vascular endothelial cells. *Lymphokine and Cytokine Research*, **12**, 93–9.

Zsebo, K. M., Yuschenkoff, V. N., Schiffer, S., Chang, D., McCall, E., Dinarello, C. A., Brown, M. A., Altrock, B. & Bagby, G. C. Jr. (1988). Vascular endothelial cells and granulopoiesis: interleukin-1 stimulates release of G-CSF and GM-CSF. *Blood*, **71**, 99–103.

–3–
Interactions between granulocytes and endothelium

SUSSAN NOURSHARGH

Introduction

An inflammatory response is associated with alterations in vascular tone and blood flow, enhanced vascular permeability and the extravasation of leukocytes from the blood into the extravascular tissue. It may be beneficial to host defence or detrimental, resulting in an inflammatory disorder. Acute inflammation is of short duration and characterized by an infiltration of neutrophils, whilst a chronic inflammatory response involves the accumulation of lymphocytes, monocytes and, in certain allergic reactions, eosinophils. These processes of leukocyte accumulation *in vivo* are initiated by the local generation of inflammatory stimuli, and mediated by a series of adhesive interactions between circulating leukocytes and vascular endothelial cells lining post-capillary venules. In recent years, much progress has been made in our understanding of the molecular basis of these adhesive events. This chapter will discuss the mechanisms involved in leukocyte accumulation *in vivo*, focusing on mechanisms used by neutrophils and eosinophils.

Adhesion molecules

Table 3.1 lists the currently known adhesion molecules believed to be involved in the interaction of neutrophils and eosinophils with endothelial cells. These molecules belong to four structural groups which are discussed below.

Integrins expressed on leukocytes

Integrins are a large family of heterodimeric glycoproteins composed of non-covalently associated α and β subunits. These molecules play an important role in mediating cell–cell interactions and the interaction of cells with extracellular matrix proteins such as fibronectin, vitronectin and laminin (Albelda & Buck, 1990). The integrin family can be subdivided into

Table 3.1. *Characterized adhesion molecules involved in leukocyte/endothelial cell interaction*

Leukocyte	Endothelial cell
Integrins	*Ig superfamily*
CD11a/CD18 (LFA-1)	ICAM-1 (CD54)
CD11b/CD18 (MAC-1)	ICAM-2 (CD102)
CD11c/CD18 (p150, 95)	VCAM-1 (CD106)
CD11d/CD18	PECAM-1 (CD31)
VLA-4 ($\alpha_4\beta_1$; CD49d/CD29)	*Selectins*
($\alpha_4\beta_7$)	E-selectin (CD62E)
	P-selectin (CD62P)
Ig Superfamily	
ICAM-3 1CD50)	*Carbohydrates*
PECAM-1 (CD31)	sLe^x
	sLe^a and related structures
Selectins	
L-selectin (CD62L)	*Sialomucins*
	MAdCAM-1
Carbohydrates	GlyCAM-1
sLe^x	CD34
sLe^a	
and related structures	
Sialomucins	
PSGL-1	

classes based on the β subunits (8 characterized), which can be associated with one or more α subunits (15 characterized). With respect to leukocyte/ endothelial cell interactions, the most important members of the family are the β_2 integrins (CD11a/CD18, CD11b/CD18, CD11c/CD18, CD11d/ CD18) and the β_1 integrin VLA-4 ($\alpha_4\beta_1$, CD49d/CD29).

The CD11/CD18 glycoproteins are exclusively expressed on circulating leukocytes, often referred to as leukocyte integrins, and play an important role in the rapid adhesion of leukocytes to protein-coated surfaces and endothelial cells. The importance of these molecules in leukocyte adhesion has been demonstrated *in vitro* by the use of neutralizing monoclonal antibodies. Such studies have shown that the enhanced adhesion of neutrophils and eosinophils to cultured endothelial cells following stimulation of the leukocytes with chemoattractants or activation of the endothelial cells with cytokines, is CD18-dependent (Smith *et al.*, 1988; Lamas, Mulroney & Schleimer, 1988). In addition, the importance of the β_2 integrins was clearly illustrated following the characterization of a rare, autosomal recessive immunodeficiency disease called leukocyte adhesion deficiency (LAD) (Anderson & Springer, 1987). This syndrome, which has now been described in more than 50 patients, is associated with severe, life-threatening, bacterial infections. These clinical symptoms are believed to be due to the fact that the neutrophils from these patients fail to accumulate at sites of inflammation *in vivo* and are unresponsive with respect to all adhesion related responses *in vitro*. It is now known that these behavioural abnormalities are due to an inherited defect in the synthesis of CD18, the β chain of the β_2 integrins.

The well-characterized endothelial cell ligands for the CD11/CD18 glycoproteins belong to the immunoglobulin superfamily (see below). Intercellular adhesion molecule-1 (ICAM-1) is an important ligand for CD11a/CD18 and CD11b/CD18, and has been shown to mediate neutrophil and eosinophil adhesion *in vitro* (Smith *et al.*, 1989; Kyan-Aung *et al.*, 1991; Bochner *et al.*, 1991). CD11a/CD18 also interacts with ICAM-2, although the importance of this pathway in granulocyte adhesion *in vitro* and accumulation *in vivo* is less clear. CD11c/CD18 interacts with a molecule on stimulated endothelial cells which has yet to be fully characterized (Stacker & Springer, 1991) and the endothelial cell ligand for CD11d/CD18 is unknown.

In contrast to the CD11/CD18 complex which is expressed on all leukocytes, the β_1 integrin VLA-4 is expressed on all haematopoietic cells except the neutrophil. The well-characterized ligands for VLA-4 are the CS1 domain of fibronectin and the endothelial cell adhesion molecule vascular cell adhesion molecule-1 (VCAM-1, see below) (Guan & Hynes, 1990; Elices *et al.*, 1990), although the existence of other ligands has been suggested (Pulido *et al.*, 1991; Vonderheide & Springer, 1992). The VLA-4/VCAM-1 interaction, a second example of an interaction between the immunoglobulin and integrin superfamilies, mediates adhesion of lymphocytes and monocytes to stimulated endothelial cells (reviewed Chapter 4; also see Carlos *et al.*, 1990; Shimizu *et al.*, 1990). In addition, the interaction of VLA-4 with VCAM-1 mediates the adhesion of eosinophils to endothelial cells (Weller *et al.*, 1991; Walsh *et al.*, 1991), though the process of eosinophil transendothelial cell migration appears to involve the CD18/ICAM-1 pathway (Ebisawa *et al.*, 1992; Kuijpers *et al.*, 1993) as has been suggested for neutrophils (Smith *et al.*, 1989). The integrin $\alpha_4\beta_7$ is also expressed on all leukocytes except neutrophils and appears to weakly interact with the VLA-4 ligands VCAM-1 and fibronectin although its principal ligand is believed to be MAdCAM (mucosal vascular addressin cell adhesion molecule)-1. The role of $\alpha_4\beta_7$ in granulocyte migration is currently under investigation.

Following cellular stimulation, by chemoattractants or extracellular matrix proteins, there is a rapid increase in the surface expression of leukocyte β_2 integrins. This increase in expression, which on neutrophils can be up to 10-fold with respect to CD11b/CD18, is a result of mobilization of intracellular pools (Todd *et al.*, 1984; Miller *et al.*, 1987). In addition to this regulatory event, activation of cells is associated with a change in the avidity of integrins for their ligands (Hynes, 1992). This phenomenon, which has been termed affinity modulation, involves an agonist-induced conversion of integrins from an inactive state to an active form capable of interacting with ligands. Activation of the β_2 integrins is a rapid and reversible response (peaking within 5–10 minutes and returning to basal level by about 30 minutes), which may be controlled by a series of protein phosphorylation events (Hynes, 1992), although the exact mechanism is poorly understood. Other studies have suggested that the cytoplasmic tail of the β_2 chain has a role in the control of functional activity (Hibbs *et al.*, 1991). In neutrophils, affinity of CD11b/CD18 is apparently regulated by the *de novo* generation of a lipid factor called integrin modulating factor-1 (IMF-1) (Hermanowski-Vosatka *et al.*, 1992). Although there is much evidence for stimulated changes in avidity of VLA-4 expression on T-lymphocytes (Shimizu *et al.*, 1990), the occurrence of this event has yet to be fully investigated with respect to the eosinophil. Interestingly, a recent study has shown that the α chain cytoplasmic domain plays a critical role in regulating the constitutive avidity and agonist-stimulated activity of VLA-4 (Kassner & Hemler, 1993).

As well as responding to external cellular stimulation, increasing evidence indicates that integrins mediate information transfer into cells, acting as signalling receptors in a variety of cell types (Hynes, 1992). For example, in neutrophils, leukocyte integrins can generate signals stimulating cell spreading (Berton *et al.*, 1992), activation of the respiratory burst (Nathan *et al.*, 1989; Berton *et al.*, 1992) and production of LTB_4 (Graham *et al.*, 1993). With respect to the eosinophil, cross-linking of CD11a, CD11b, CD18 and VLA-4 by immobilized monoclonal antibody (mAb) caused activation of eosinophil respiratory burst and spreading (Laudanna *et al.*, 1993). In addition, adhesion to fibronectin, via VLA-4, triggers the generation of cytokines IL-3 and GM-CSF resulting in prolonged eosinophil survival in culture (Anwar *et al.*, 1993). Further, activation of VLA-4 by mAb 8A2, a recently characterized 'activating' CD29 mAb (Kovach *et al.*, 1991), stimulates adherence of eosinophils to fibronectin-coated plates whilst inhibiting eosinophil migration across fibronectin and endothelial cell-covered filters (Kuijpers *et al.*, 1993). These findings have been attributed to the 'freezing' of the VLA-4 molecule in its high avidity state resulting in prolonged adhesion and hence inhibition of migration (Kuijpers *et al.*, 1993).

Members of the immunoglobulin superfamily

A number of molecules with key roles in leukocyte/endothelial cell interactions belong to the immunoglobulin (Ig) superfamily. These molecules are

ICAM-1, ICAM-2, VCAM-1, platelet-endothelial cell adhesion molecule-1 (PECAM-1) and MAdCAM-1 which are all expressed on endothelial cells either constitutively and/or induced following cellular activation. Members of the Ig family have structural features first defined for immunoglobulins, characterized by repeated domains arranged within two sheets of anti-parallel β-strands stabilized by disulfide bonds (Williams & Barclay, 1988).

ICAM-1 (CD54) is a heavily glycosylated protein with a molecular weight of about 90kD. ICAM-1, containing five tandem extracellular domains, designated D1-D5 beginning at the N terminus, is constitutively expressed on vascular endothelial cells and other cell types such as fibroblasts, macrophages and lymphocytes (Dustin *et al.*, 1986). On endothelial cells, the expression of ICAM-1 can be enhanced in a slow (maximum level obtained at 18–24 hours) and protein synthesis dependent manner by cytokines such as IL-1, TNF and IFN-γ and by bacterial lipopolysaccharides (LPS). ICAM-2, a truncated form of ICAM-1, containing two Ig-domains, is also expressed on endothelial cells under basal conditions, however this expression is not altered on stimulated endothelial cells (Staunton, Dustin & Springer, 1989). CD11a/CD18 and CD11b/CD18 are both ligands for ICAM-1 (Rothlein *et al.*, 1986; Marlin & Springer, 1987; Smith *et al.*, 1989) whilst ICAM-2 only appears to interact with CD11a/CD18 (de Fougerolles *et al.*, 1991). Recent studies have shown that CD11a/CD18 can also interact with ICAM-3, a recently cloned member of the Ig family expressed on leukocytes but not endothelial cells (Fawcett *et al.*, 1992; de Fougerolles & Springer, 1992).

VCAM-1, also a glycosylated molecule, with a molecular weight of about 110 kD, contains either six or seven Ig domains, the longer form being predominant both *in vitro* and *in vivo* (Osborn *et al.*, 1989; Hession *et al.*, 1991). A low level of VCAM-1 expression is detected on unstimulated endothelial cells which can be greatly increased following endothelial cell activation by certain cytokines such as IL-1 and TNF, and LPS (maximum expression detected at 8–24 hours, depending on the stimulus used). The expression of VCAM-1, as found with ICAM-1, is not restricted to endothelial cells and can be detected on numerous cell types, such as macrophages and dendritic cells, in inflamed tissues. Interestingly, the expression of VCAM-1, but not ICAM-1 or endothelial selectins, can be enhanced by IL-4 (Thornhill, Kyan-Aung & Haskard, 1990; Schleimer *et al.*, 1992). These results suggest that the release of IL-4 by lymphocytes at sites of inflammation initiates a specific VCAM-1-mediated recruitment of leukocytes. This is of particular importance since the principal ligand for VCAM-1, as noted above, is the β_1 integrin VLA-4 expressed on all leukocytes but the neutrophil (Elices *et al.*, 1990), suggesting a role in the progression of an inflammatory response as neutrophil accumulation is replaced by mononuclear cells and eosinophils. Such a shift in the accumulation of specific leukocyte population usually occurs as the inflammatory lesion enters either the repair/resolution stage or progresses to a chronic inflammatory response.

Two other members of the Ig superfamily implicated in leukocyte-endothelial cell interactions are MAdCAM-1 (see Chapter 4) and PECAM-1 which is expressed on all cells in the vasculature, i.e. leukocytes, platelets and endothelial cells (reviewed in Delisser, Newman & Albeida, 1994). On endothelial cells, the expression of PECAM-1 is concentrated at cell–cell junctions where it plays a role in neutrophil transendothelial migration.

Selectins and their carbohydrate sialomucin ligands

Selectins are a family of molecules with an NH_2 terminal lectin-like domain, an epidermal growth factor repeat, a number of modules similar to those found in certain complement binding proteins, a membrane spanning region and a short cytoplasmic COOH-terminal domain (Lasky, 1992). To date, three members of the selectin family have been described, namely L-, P- and E-selectin.

L-selectin, originally described as a lymphocyte homing receptor, is now known to be present on the cell surface of all leukocytes and can mediate their adhesion to cytokine-activated endothelial cells via an inducible molecule on vascular endothelial cells (Spertini *et al.*, 1991*b*). The cell surface expression of L-selectin is very sensitive to cellular stimulation, exhibiting a rapid increase in affinity followed by shedding from the cell surface (Spertini *et al.*, 1991*a*; Kishimoto *et al.*, 1989). Neutrophils and eosinophils that have emigrated into sites of inflammation express a lower level of L-selectin than blood leukocytes (Kishimoto *et al.*, 1989; Mengelers *et al.*, 1993).

P-selectin is a 140 kD molecule found within secretory granules of platelets (α-granules) and endothelial cells (Weibel–Palade bodies). Following cellular activation, P-selectin is rapidly translocated to the cell surface where it mediates adhesive interactions with leukocytes (Lasky, 1992). With respect to endothelial cells, stimuli that induce the rapid expression of P-selectin include thrombin, leukotriene C_4 (LTC_4), histamine and H_2O_2 (McEver *et al.*, 1989; Patel *et al.*, 1991). Interestingly, in a recent study TNF was shown to induce the expression of P-selectin on mouse endothelial cells with a similar kinetics to that of TNF-induced E-selectin expression (Weller, Isenmann & Vestweber, 1992). These findings suggest that P-selectin may be expressed via two distinct mechanisms, a rapid secretion of stored molecules from granules and a cytokine-mediated slow expression of newly synthesized molecules.

E-selectin is a 95–115 kD molecule which appears to be mainly restricted to activated endothelial cells. Cultured endothelial cells stimulated by TNF, IL-1 or LPS express E-selectin in a slow (maximum level by 4–6 hours) and protein synthesis dependent manner (Bevilacqua *et al.*, 1987). This molecule, which was originally shown to mediate the adhesion of neutrophils to cytokine- or LPS-activated endothelial cells (Bevilacqua *et al.*, 1987), is now known to be involved in the adhesion of monocytes, a subpopulation of memory T lymphocytes, basophils and eosinophils (Picker *et al.*, 1991*a*; Carlos *et al.*, 1991; Shimizu *et al.*, 1991; Bochner *et al.*, 1991; Weller *et al.*, 1991; Luscinskas *et al.*, 1991). There is compelling evidence that selectins can interact with carbohydrate ligands (Lasky, 1992). The carbohydrate structures that have received much attention are oligosaccharides related to sialyl Lewis^x (sLe^x) and sialyl Lewis^a (sLe^a), found on the cell surface of both leukocytes and endothelial cells. All three selectins appear to interact with sLe^x and sLe^a though with different binding profiles (Foxall *et al.*, 1992; Berg *et al.*, 1992; Handa *et al.*, 1991). Interestingly, L-selectin appears to have a role in presenting sLe^x as a ligand to P- and E-selectin (Picker *et al.*, 1991*b*). L-selectin also interacts with a ligand on cytokine-activated endothelial cells but the nature of this molecule is as yet unknown (Spertini *et al.*, 1991*b*). Other carbohydrate structures implicated as ligands for selectins include phosphorylated mono- and polysaccharides and sulfated polysaccharides; (Lasky, 1992 and see Chapter 4). To date, three L-selectin mucin ligands (MAdCAM-1, GlyCAM-1 and CD34) and P-selectin glycoprotein ligand (PSGL-1), which also recognizes E-selectin, have been cloned.

As with integrins, there is some evidence indicating that binding of selectins to their ligands activates target cells. E-selectin up-regulates leukocyte integrins and in soluble form is reportedly chemotactic for neutrophils (Lo *et al.*, 1991). In contrast, P-selectin alone, when incorporated into model membranes or when expressed by transfected cells, does not induce neutrophil priming (Lorant *et al.*, 1993). Further, using an *in vitro* flow system, P-selectin can mediate neutrophil rolling but does not induce their firm adhesion, which is dependent on leukocyte integrins (Lawrence & Springer, 1991). However, the co-expression of P-selectin with platelet activating factor (PAF) on thrombin- or LTC_4-activated endothelial cells causes neutrophil priming, shape change and CD11/CD18 activation (Lorant *et al.*, 1993). In this respect, the elevations in neutrophil cytoplasmic free Ca^{2+} induced by thrombin- or IL-1-activated endothelial cells, via the expression of P- and E-selectin, respectively, are mediated by endothelial associated PAF (Kuijpers *et al.*, 1991; Lorant *et al.*, 1993). Such results have suggested that endothelial selectins, as well as mediating adhesion, may facilitate leukocyte/endothelial cell interactions via membrane bound molecules that induce cell activation (Zimmerman, Prescott & McIntyre, 1992).

The selectin family of adhesion molecules has been implicated in the very early stages of leukocyte/endothelial cell recognition and adhesion, i.e. the phenomenon of leukocyte rolling. Lipid bilayers containing P-selectin support neutrophil rolling under flow conditions *in vitro* (Lawrence &

Springer, 1991). Further, a number of elegant *in vivo* studies support this concept with respect to all three selectin molecules (discussed below). The importance of the selectin ligand, sLe^x, expression on leukocytes, in leukocyte accumulation *in vivo* was dramatically demonstrated recently following the identification of two cases of a second distinct leukocyte adhesion deficiency. This syndrome, termed LAD II as opposed to LAD I (CD18-deficient), involves similar clinical symptoms and defects in neutrophil adhesion *in vitro* to those seen with CD18-deficient leukocytes (Etzioni *et al.*, 1992). For example, LAD II neutrophils are unable to adhere to endothelial cells when stimulated with LTB_4 and exhibit a reduced level of motility. Despite the similarities between LAD I and LAD II neutrophils, neutrophils from LAD II patients have a normal expression of CD18 but do not express sLe^x on their cell surface. Since LAD II patients have deficiencies in a number of fucosylated carbohydrates, generated via independent synthesis pathways, it is believed that the clinical symptoms reflect a general defect in fucose metabolism (Etzioni *et al.*, 1992).

Mechanisms of granulocyte accumulation *in vivo*

Leukocyte accumulation *in vivo* is initiated following the generation of inflammatory stimuli, which may be generated in tissue fluid (e.g. complement derived proteins such as C5a), released from host cells (e.g. cytokines, PAF and LTB_4), or derived from invading microbes (e.g. formylated chemotactic peptides and LPS) (for review see Nourshargh, 1993). Mediators of leukocyte accumulation can be broadly classified into three categories, (1) stimuli that act directly on leukocytes, such as C5a and LTB_4, (2) stimuli that act on endothelial cells rendering them adhesive for leukocytes, such as IL-1 and TNF, and (3) stimuli that act indirectly by inducing the release of further mediators, e.g. LPS and IL-1 can cause the release of the potent neutrophil chemoattractant, IL-8, from cells such as tissue macrophages, fibroblasts and endothelial cells. Clearly, there is overlap between these groups as a particular mediator may fall into more than one category. The mechanism by which inflammatory mediators induce localized leukocyte accumulation *in vivo* is still unclear and despite much research a fundamental question that remains controversial concerns the site of action of chemoattractants. Although there is much *in vitro* evidence indicating the presence of high affinity chemoattractant receptors on both the neutrophil and eosinophil (for review see Nourshargh, 1993) there are also a number of *in vitro* studies indicating the existence of chemoattractant receptors on endothelial cells (Hoover *et al.*, 1984). One possible mechanism that has received much attention recently is that chemoattractants may be presented to leukocytes within the vascular lumen via receptors on endothelial cells (Rot, 1992). Such a mechanism, for which there is both *in vitro* and *in vivo* evidence (Rotrosen, Malech & Gallin, 1987; Colditz & Movat, 1984; Rot, 1992; Tanaka *et al.*, 1993), supports the possibility of an active role for vascular endothelial cells in chemoattractant-induced leukocyte accumulation *in vivo*. However, although the site of action of chemoattractant mediators in inducing neutrophil and eosinophil accumulation *in vivo* remains unclear, it has been demonstrated that a receptor-mediated event on the neutrophil is crucial in neutrophil accumulation in response to chemoattractants *in vivo* (Nourshargh & Williams, 1990).

The accumulation of leukocytes at sites of inflammation is mediated by the adhesive interaction of leukocytes to venular endothelial cells. This process appears to involve multiple sequential steps. The initial interaction is that of a weak reversible adhesion between leukocytes and endothelial cells resulting in the rolling of leukocytes along the venular wall. These rolling cells can then become activated by chemotactic stimuli expressed/bound on the cell surface of endothelial cells (Rot, 1992) or in solution generated at the site of inflammation. This activation step, induced by inflammatory stimuli, leads to a functional activation of the leukocytes as well as a change in their cell surface expression of adhesion molecules enabling rolling leukocytes to establish a firm adhesive bond with the vessel wall. Interestingly, the firm attachment of leukocytes to venular endothelial cells itself appears to trigger a secondary activation event within the leukocytes, and perhaps the endothelial cell, which may mediate the flattening of the leukocyte over the endothelium, enabling it to find and penetrate interendothelial cell junctions. This is followed by the interaction of the leukocytes with the perivascular basement membrane, which may involve leukocyte receptors for extracellular matrix proteins and granular proteolytic enzymes.

An elegant technique for investigating the *in vivo* events within a microvascular bed is by the use of intravital microscopy. This procedure allows the direct viewing of the microcirculation within translucent tissues such as the mesentery in anaesthetized animals. Using this technique, a number of studies have addressed the involvement of adhesion molecules in the different stages of leukocyte accumulation *in vivo* (Table 3.2). Functional blockers of L-selectin have been shown to inhibit leukocyte rolling in mesenteric venules in rabbits (von Andrian *et al.*, 1991, 1992) and rats (Ley *et al.*, 1991). Further, L-selectin transfected cell lines roll within mesenteric venules (von Andrian *et al.*, 1993*b*; Ley, Tedder & Kansas, 1993). The L-selectin-mediated neutrophil rolling appears to be only partly dependent on the molecule's lectin domain (von Andrian *et al.*, 1993*b*; Ley, Tedder & Kansas, 1993). In addition, a monoclonal antibody recognizing canine P-selectin has recently been shown to inhibit leukocyte rolling within canine mesenteric venules (Dore *et al.*, 1993). P-selectin has also been implicated in neutrophil rolling under flow conditions in an *in vitro* model (Lawrence &

Table 3.2. *Involvement of adhesion molecules in leukocyte behaviour as investigated by intravital microscopy* in vivo

	References
Rolling	
Spontaneous rolling inhibited by anti-L-selectin mAb, DREG 200, in rabbit mesenteric venules	von Andrian *et al.* (1991)
Spontaneous rolling inhibited by anti-L-selectin polyclonal Ab and a recombinant soluble L-selectin chimaera in rat mesenteric venules	Ley *et al.* (1991)
IL-1-induced rolling of human neutrophils in rabbit mesenteric venules inhibited by anti-L-selectin mAb, DREG 56, and by enzymatic removal of L-selectin	von Andrian *et al.* (1992)
LAD II neutrophils (sLe^x-deficient), rolled poorly in mesenteric venules of IL-1-treated rabbits	von Andrian *et al.* (1993*a*)
Spontaneous rolling inhibited by anti-P-selectin mAb, MD6, in canine mesenteric venules	Dore *et al.* (1993)
L-selectin transfected cells rolled within rabbit and rat mesenteric venules	Ley *et al.* (1993), von Andrian *et al.* (1993*b*)
IL-1-induced rolling of human neutrophils within rabbit mesenteric venules reduced by anti-sLe^x mAbs, CSLEX-1 and HECA-452	von Andrian *et al.* (1993*b*)
Firm adhesion and extravasation	
LTB_4- or zymosan activated serum-induced neutrophil adherence and extravasation in rabbit tenuissimus muscle venules inhibited by anti-CD18 mAb 60.3	Arfors *et al.* (1987)
Zymosan activated serum-induced neutrophil adherence in rabbit mesenteric venules inhibited by mAbs recognizing CD18 (R15.7), CD11a (R7.1), CD11b (LM2) and ICAM-1 (R6.5)	Argenbright *et al.* (1991)
Spontaneous adhesion of neutrophils to rabbit and cat mesenteric venules inhibited by anti-CD18 mAb IB4	von Andrian *et al.* (1991) Perry & Granger (1991)
LTB_4-induced adhesion and extravasation of human neutrophils within rabbit mesenteric venules blocked when rolling was inhibited	von Andrian *et al.* (1992)
LAD I neutrophils (CD18-deficient) failed to adhere to rabbit mesenteric venules in response to LTB_4	von Andrian *et al.* (1993*a*)

Springer, 1991). Since there is also evidence for the involvement of E-selectin in leukocyte rolling (Olofsson *et al.*, 1994), it is now generally believed that the rolling phenomenon is mediated by members of the selectin family. Recently, L-selectin and VLA-4 have been implicated in eosinophil rolling *in vivo* (Sriramarao *et al.*, 1994). An important point to note is that the rolling responses investigated in the studies described above were either 'spontaneous', detected in surgically prepared tissues, or induced by pretreating the animals with IL-1. There is as yet no direct evidence for the involvement of selectins in chemoattractant-induced neutrophil rolling. However, since chemoattractants such as C5a and IL-8 can induce rapid neutrophil accumulation *in vivo* a mechanism must exist to account for the rapid chemoattractant-induced leukocyte rolling. Possible mechanisms are upregulation of P-selectin and/or a rapid increase in the avidity of L-selectin for its endothelial cell ligand (Spertini *et al.*, 1991*a*, Foreman *et al.*, 1994). However, there is as yet no *in vivo* evidence for these proposals.

In contrast to the effects of anti-selectin reagents, monoclonal antibodies (mAbs) recognizing CD18 have no inhibitory effect on leukocyte rolling but prevent the subsequent firm adhesion of leukocytes to venular endothelial cells (Arfors *et al.*, 1987; von Andrian *et al.*, 1991; Argenbright, Letts & Rothlein, 1991; Perry & Granger, 1991). An anti-ICAM-1 mAb was also very effective at inhibiting chemoattractant-induced adhesion of leukocytes to venular walls within the rabbit mesenteric microvasculature (Argenbright, Letts & Rothlein, 1991). Interestingly, the CD18-mediated firm adhesion of neutrophils is inhibited when the rolling response is blocked (von Andrian *et al.*, 1992). These results clearly demonstrate that a selectin-mediated rolling is an essential prerequisite in the cascade of adhesive events leading to an integrin-mediated leukocyte emigration. This proposal is further illustrated in a recent study investigating the behaviour of neutrophils from patients suffering from leukocyte adhesion deficiency syndromes within the rabbit mesenteric microvasculature (von Andrian *et al.*, 1993*a*). LAD I neutrophils (CD18-deficient), exhibited normal rolling in animals pretreated with IL-1 but were incapable of establishing firm adhesion or emigrating across the vessel wall in response to LTB_4. In the same model, LAD II neutrophils (sLe^x-deficient) rolled poorly and were unable to adhere firmly to venules under normal shear force. However, under static conditions, LAD II neutrophils responded to LTB_4 by adhering to and emigrating across the vessel wall.

Anti-inflammatory effects of anti-adhesion reagents

The availability of adhesion molecule blockers, especially cross-reacting mAbs, suitable for use in animal models, has led to studies investigating the role of adhesion molecules in inflammatory processes *in vitro*. The majority of the early studies, due to the availability of appropriate antibodies, addressed the involvement of the CD11/CD18 complex in the process of neutrophil accumulation and neutrophil-dependent oedema formation and tissue damage in numerous *in vivo* models (for review see Nourshargh, 1992). Monoclonal antibody 60.3, the first anti-CD18 mAb to be investigated *in vivo* in rabbit models, inhibits neutrophil accumulation and neutrophil-dependent oedema induced by preformed inflammatory stimuli (Rampart & Williams, 1988; Arfors *et al.*, 1988; Nourshargh *et al.*, 1989) or in response to allergic inflammatory reactions in skin (Nourshargh *et al.*, 1989); it also blocks neutrophil accumulation into subcutaneously implanted polyvinyl sponges (Price, Beatty & Corpuz, 1987) and inflamed lungs (Doerschuk *et al.*, 1990). Anti-CD18 mAbs also have protective effects in models of ischaemia-reperfusion (for review see Nourshargh, 1992), meningitis (Tuomanen *et al.*, 1989), endotoxic shock (Thomas *et al.*, 1992), burns (Bucky *et al.*, 1991) and haemorrhagic shock (Vedder *et al.*, 1988; Mileski *et al.*, 1990). The key endothelial cell ligand for CD11/CD18, ICAM-1, has also been implicated in inflammatory processes *in vivo*. The first of such studies demonstrated that an anti-ICAM-1 antibody, R6.5, inhibited neutrophil accumulation into PMA-induced inflamed rabbit lungs (Barton *et al.*, 1989). In primates, mAb R6.5 suppressed T-cell-mediated injury in renal allograft rejection (Cosimi *et al.*, 1990) and attenuated antigen-induced airway eosinophilia and hyper-responsiveness in a model of asthma (Wegner *et al.*, 1990). As found with anti-CD18 reagents, mAbs recognizing ICAM-1 are protective in models of ischaemia-reperfusion injury (Seekamp *et al.*, 1993; Yamazaki *et al.*, 1993).

More recently, an anti-L-selectin mAb, MEL 14, was found to inhibit neutrophil accumulation into inflamed peritoneum in mice (Jutila *et al.*, 1989; Watson, *et al*,, 1991). Similar results have also been obtained using a soluble immunoglobulin chimaera containing the L-selectin extracellular domain, suggesting that soluble forms of adhesion molecules may be effective inhibitors of leukocyte accumulation *in vivo* (Watson *et al.*, 1991). In primates, an E-selectin antibody inhibits neutrophil accumulation into airways and late-phase airway obstruction following antigen challenge in a model of extrinsic asthma (Gundel *et al.*, 1991). Further, E-selectin has been implicated in the process of neutrophil accumulation and injury in IgG immune complex-mediated lung inflammation in rats (Mulligan *et al.*, 1991). In contrast, an anti-P-selectin mAb was without an effect on inflammatory responses induced by immune complexes, but significantly suppressed neutrophil accumulation and injury induced by intravenous cobra venom factor (CVF) (Mulligan *et al.*, 1992). In the latter model, which involves an acute lung injury due to systemic complement activation and is CD11/CD18 and ICAM-1 dependent (Mulligan *et al.*, 1993*b*), expression of

P-selectin was detected on the pulmonary vasculature within 5–10 minutes of the CVF infusion (Mulligan *et al.*, 1992). The CVF-induced lung injury was also reduced following the infusion of sLe^x, a ligand for P-selectin (Mulligan *et al.*, 1993*a*). Anti-P-selectin mAbs are also protective in models of reperfusion injury (Weyrich *et al.*, 1992; Winn *et al.*, 1993) and inhibit leukocyte/platelet interaction and fibrin deposition *in vivo* (Palabrica *et al.*, 1992).

In contrast to the relatively large number of studies investigating neutrophil accumulation *in vivo*, very few have examined the adhesive events mediating eosinophil accumulation. Wegner and colleagues were the first group to address this, and report that in a primate model of asthma, an anti-ICAM-1 mAb, but not an anti-E-selectin mAb, attenuated antigen-induced airway eosinophilia and hyperresponsiveness (Wegner *et al.*, 1990; Gundel *et al.*, 1991). Recently, it has been shown that a mAb recognizing VLA-4 effectively inhibits eosinophil accumulation in allergic and nonallergic inflammatory reactions in guinea-pig skin (Weg *et al.*, 1993). Responses investigated were a passive cutaneous anaphylaxis reaction and responses elicited by PAF, LTB_4, C5a des Arg, arachidonic acid or zymosan particles. These results suggested, for the first time, a role for VLA-4 in eosinophil accumulation *in vivo*. In more recent studies we have found that the same antibody partially inhibits eosinophil accumulation into guinea-pig airways induced by intravenous Sephadex particles (Das *et al.*, 1995). In this model, the lung eosinophilia was totally blocked when the animals were treated with a combination of mAbs to VLA-4 and CD18, indicating a necessity for both molecules in eosinophil extravasation *in vivo* as has been indicated in *in vitro* studies (Ebisawa *et al.*, 1991; Kuijpers *et al.*, 1993). Anti-VLA-4 mAbs also inhibit the accumulation of lymphocytes into dermal sites of delayed and contact hypersensitivity reactions in rats and mice (Chisholm, Williams, & Lobb, 1993; Issekutz, 1991). Interestingly, although neutrophils do not express VLA-4 on their cell surface, an anti-VLA-4 mAb has been shown to partially suppress neutrophil accumulation in immune complex-mediated lung injury in rats (Mulligan *et al.*, 1993*c*). This is believed to be due to an inhibitory effect on resident macrophages resulting in a reduction in the release of cytokines such as IL-1 and TNF which participate in the development of this inflammatory reaction (Mulligan & Ward, 1992). Similarly, anti-VLA-4 mAbs inhibit neutrophil accumulation in a murine model of contact hypersensitivity, suggesting that neutrophil accumulation in this model is at least partly dependent on VLA-4 expressing cells (Chisholm *et al.*, 1993).

Summary

The adhesive interaction of granulocytes with venular endothelial cells is an essential step in the process of granulocyte accumulation at sites of inflammation *in vivo*. The tremendous advances made in the field of adhesion molecules have led to a better understanding of the molecular events involved. Anti-adhesive reagents have demonstrated the importance of certain adhesion pathways in granulocyte accumulation *in vivo* and have indicated the effectiveness of anti-adhesion agents as potential anti-inflammatory drugs. It is generally believed that characterization of the regulatory mechanisms mediating the coordinated expression and/or activation of leukocyte and endothelial cell adhesion molecules will lead to the identification of novel targets for the development of more specific anti-inflammatory reagents.

Acknowledgements

The author is supported by The Wellcome.

References

Albelda, S. M. & Buck, C. A. (1990). Integrins and other cell adhesion molecules. *FASEB Journal*, **4**, 2868–80.

Anderson, D. C. & Springer, T. A. (1987). Leukocyte adhesion deficiency: an inherited defect in the MAC-1, LFA-1 and p150,95 glycoproteins. *Annual Review in Medicine*, **38**, 175–94.

Anwar, A. R. F., Moqbel, R., Walsh, G. M., Kay, A. B. & Wardlaw, A. J. (1993). Adhesion to fibronectin prolongs eosinophil survival. *Journal of Experimental Medicine*, **177**, 839–43.

Arfors, K.-E., Lundberg, C., Lindbom, L., Lundberg, K., Beatty, P. G. & Harlan, J. M. (1987). A monoclonal antibody to the membrane glycoprotein complex CD18 inhibits polymorphonuclear leukocyte accumulation and plasma leakage *in vivo*. *Blood*, **69**, 338–40.

Argenbright, L. W., Letts, L. G. & Rothlein, R. (1991). Monoclonal antibodies to the leukocyte membrane CD18 glycoprotein complex and to intercellular adhesion molecule-1 inhibit leukocyte-endothelial adhesion in rabbits. *Journal of Leukocyte Biology*, **49**, 253–7.

Barton, R. W., Rothlein, R., Ksiazer, J. & Kennedy, C. (1989). The effect of anti-intercellular adhesion molecule-1 on phorbol-ester-induced rabbit lung inflammation. *Journal of Immunology*, **143**, 1278–82.

Berg, E. L., Magnan, J., Warnock, R. A., Robinson, M. K. & Butcher, E. C. (1992). Comparison of L-selectin and E-selectin ligand specificities: the L-selectin can bind the E-selectin ligands sialyl-Le[a]. *Biochemical Biophysical Research Communications*, **184**, 1048–55.

Berton, G., Laudanna, C., Sorio C. & Rossi, F. (1992). Generation of signals activating neutrophil functions by leukocyte integrins: LFA-1 and gp150/95, but not CR3, are able to stimulate the respiratory burst of human neutrophils. *Journal of Cell Biology*, **116**, 1007–17.

Bevilacqua, M. P., Pober, J. S., Mendrick, D. L., Cotran, R. S. & Gimbrone, M. A. (1987). Identification of an inducible endothelial-leukocyte adhesion molecule. *Proceedings of the National Academy of Sciences USA*, **84**, 9238–42.

Bochner, B. S., Luscinskas, F. W., Gimbrone, M. A., Newman, W., Sterbinsky, S. A., Derse-Anthony, C. P., Klunk, D. & Schleimer, R. P. (1991). Adhesion of human basophils, eosinophils, and neutrophils to interleukin 1-activated human vascular endothelial cells:

contributions of endothelial cell adhesion molecules. *Journal of Experimental Medicine*, **173**, 1553–6.

Bucky, L. P., Vedder, N. B., Hong, H-Z., May, J. W. & Ehrlich, H. P. (1991). A monoclonal antibody which blocks neutrophil adhesion prevents second degree burns from becoming third degree. *American Burn Association*, 133.

Carlos, T., Kovach, N., Schwartz, B., Rosa, M., Newman, B., Wayner, E., Benjamin, C., Osborn, L., Lobb, R. & Harlan, J. (1991). Human monocytes bind to two cytokine-induced adhesive ligands on cultured human endothelial cells: endothelial–leukocyte adhesion molecule-1 and vascular cell adhesion molecule-1. *Blood*, **77**, 2266–71.

Carlos, T. M., Schwartz, B. R., Kovach, N. L., Yee, E., Rosso, M., Osborn, L., Chi-Rosso, G., Lobb, R. & Harlan, J. M. (1990). Vascular cell adhesion molecule-1 mediates lymphocyte adherence to cytokine-activated cultured human endothelial cells. *Blood*, **76**, 965–70.

Chisholm, P. L., Williams, C. A. & Lobb, R. R. (1993). Monoclonal antibodies to the integrin α-4 subunit inhibit the murine contact hypersensitivity response. *European Journal of Immunology*, **23**, 682–8.

Colditz, I. G. & Movat, H. Z. (1984). Desensitization of acute inflammatory lesions to chemotaxins and endotoxin. *Journal of Immunology*, **133**, 2163–8.

Cosimi, A. B., Conti, D., Delmonico, F. L., Preffer, F. I., Wee, S-L., Rothlein, R., Faanes, R. & Colvin, R. B. (1990). *In vivo* effects of monoclonal antibody to ICAM-1 (CD54) in nonhuman primates with renal allografts. *Journal of Immunology*, **144**, 4604–12.

de Fougerolles, A. R., Stacker, S. A., Schwarting, R. & Springer, T. A. (1991). Characterization of ICAM-2 and evidence for a third-counter-receptor for LFA-1. *Journal of Experimental Medicine*, **174**, 253–67.

de Fougerolles, A. R. & Springer, T. A. (1992). Intercellular adhesion molecule 3, a third adhesion counter-receptor for lymphocyte function-associated molecule 1 on resting lymphocytes. *Journal of Experimental Medicine*, **175**, 185–90.

Das, A. M., Williams, T. J., Lobb, R. R. & Nourshargh, S. (1995). Lung eosinophilia is dependent on IL-5, and the adhesion molecules CD18 and VLA-4 in a guinea-pig model. Immunology, 84, 41–6.

Delisser, H. M., Newman, P. J. & Albelda, S. A. (1994). Molecular and functional aspects of PECAM-1/CD31. *Immunology Today*, **15**, 490–5.

Doerschuk, C. M., Winn, R. K., Coxson, H. O. & Harlan, J. M. (1990). CD18-dependent and -independent mechanisms of neutrophil emigration in the pulmonary and systemic microcirculation of rabbits. *Journal of Immunology*, **144**, 2327–33.

Dore, M., Korthuis, R. J., Granger, D. N., Entman, M. L. & Smith, C. W. (1993). P-selectin mediates spontaneous leukocyte rolling *in vivo*. *Blood*, **82**, 1308–16.

Dustin, M. L., Rothlein, R., Bahn, A. K., Dinarello, C. A. & Springer, T. A. (1986). Induction by IL-1 and interferon-gamma: tissue distribution, biochemistry and function of a natural adherence molecule (ICAM-1). *Journal of Immunology*, **137**, 245–54.

Ebisawa, M., Bochner, B. S., Georas, S. N. & Schleimer, R. P. (1992). Eosinophil transendothelial migration induced by cytokines. 1. Role of endothelial and eosinophil adhesion molecules in IL-1β-induced transendothelial migration. *Journal of Immunology*, **149**, 4021–8.

Elices, M. J., Osborn, L., Takada, Y., Crouse, C., Luhowskyj, S., Hemler, M. E. & Lobb, R. R. (1990). VCAM-1 on activated endothelium interacts with the leukocyte integrin VLA-4 at a site distinct from the VLA-4/fibronectin binding site. *Cell*, **60**, 577–84.

Etzioni, A., Frydman, M., Pollack, S., Avidor, I., Phillips, M. L., Paulson, J. C. & Gershoni-Baruch, R. (1992). Brief report: recurrent severe infections caused by a novel leukocyte adhesion deficiency. *New England Journal of Medicine*, **327**, 1789–92.

Fawcett, J., Holness, C. L. L., Needham, L. A., Turley, H., Gatter, K. C., Mason, D. Y. &

Simmons, D. L. (1992). Molecular cloning of ICAM-3, a third ligand for LFA-1, constitutively expressed on resting leukocytes. *Nature*, **360**, 481–4.

Foreman, K. E., Vaporciyan, A. A., Bonish, B. K., Jones, M. L., Johnson, K. J., Glovsky, M. M., Eddy, S. M. & Ward, P. A. (1994). C5a-induced expression of P-selectin in endothelial cells. *Journal of Clinical Investigation*, **94**, 1147–55.

Foxall, C., Watson, S. R., Dowbenko, D., Fennie, C., Lasky, L. A., Kiso, M., Hasegawa, A., Asa, D. & Brandley, B. K. (1992). The three members of the selectin receptor family recognize a common carbohydrate epitope, the sialyl Lewis oligosaccharide. *Journal of Cell Biology*, **117**, 895–902.

Graham, I. L., Lefkowith, J. B., Anderson, D. C. & Brown, E. J. (1993). Immune complex-stimulated neutrophil LTB_4 production is dependent on β_2 integrins. *Journal of Cell Biology*, **120**, 1509–17.

Guan, J.-L. & Hynes, R. O. (1990). Lymphoid cells recognise an alternatively spliced segment of fibronectin via the integrin receptor $\alpha_4\beta_1$. *Cell*, **60**, 53–61.

Gundel, R. H., Wegner, C. D., Torcellini, C. A., Clarke, C. C., Haynes, N., Rothlein, R., Smith, C. W. & Letts, L. G. (1991). Endothelial leukocyte adhesion molecule-1 mediates antigen-induced acute airway inflammation and late phase airway obstruction in monkeys. *Journal of Clinical Investigations*, **88**, 1407–11.

Handa, K., Neudelman, E. D., Stroud, M. R., Shiozawa, T. & Hakomori, S. (1991). Selectin GMP-140 (CD62; PADGEM) binds to sialosyl-Le^a and sialosyl-Le^x, and sulfated glycans modulate this binding. *Biochemical and Biophysical Research Communications*, **181**, 1223–30.

Hermanowski-Vosatka, A., Van Strijp, J. A. G., Swiggard, W. J. & Wright, S. D. (1992). Integrin modulating factor-1: a lipid that alters the function of leukocyte integrins. *Cell*, **68**, 341–52.

Hession, C., Tizard, R., Vassallo, C., Schiffer, S. B., Goff, D., Moy, P., Chi-Rosso, G., Luhowskyj, S., Lobb, R. & Osborn, L. (1991). Cloning of an alternate form of vascular cell adhesion molecule-1 (VCAM-1). *Journal of Biological Chemistry*, **266**, 6682–5.

Hibbs, M. L., Xu, H., Stacker, S. A. & Springer, T. A. (1991). Regulation of adhesion to ICAM-1 by the cytoplasmic domain of LFA-1 integrin beta subunit. *Science*, **251**, 1611–13.

Hoover, R. L., Karnofsky, M. J., Austen, K. F., Corey, E. J. & Lewis, R. A. (1984). Leukotriene B_4 action on endothelium mediates augmented neutrophil/endothelial adhesion. *Proceedings of the National Academy of Sciences USA*, **81**, 2191–3.

Hynes, R. O. (1992). Integrins: versatility, modulation, and signalling in cell adhesion. *Cell*, **69**, 11–25.

Issekutz, T. B. (1991). Inhibition of *in vivo* lymphocyte migration to inflammation and homing to lymphoid tissues by the TA-2 monoclonal antibody. A likely role for VLA-4 *in vivo*. *Journal of Immunology*, **147**, 4178–84.

Jutila, M. A., Rott, L., Berg, E. L. & Butcher, E. C. (1989). Function and regulation of the neutrophil MEL-14 antigen *in vivo*: comparison with LFA-1 and MAC-1. *Journal of Immunology*, **143**, 3318–24.

Kassner, P. D. & Hemler, M. E. (1993). Interchangeable α chain cytoplasmic domains play a positive role in control of cell adhesion mediated by VLA-4, a β_1 integrin. *Journal of Experimental Medicine*, **178**, 649–60.

Kishimoto, T. K., Jutila, M. A., Berg, E. L. & Butcher, E. C. (1989). Neutrophil MAC-1 and MEL-14 adhesion proteins inversely regulated by chemotactic factors. *Science*, **245**, 1238–41.

Kovach, N. L., Carlos, T. M., Yee, E. & Harlan, J. M. (1991). A monoclonal antibody to β_1 integrin (CD29) stimulates VLA-dependent adherence of leukocytes to human umbilical vein endothelial cells and matrix components. *Journal of Cell Biology*, **116**, 499–509.

Kuijpers, T. W., Hakkert, B. C., Hoogerwerf, M., Leeuwenberg, J. F. M. & Roos, D. (1991). Role of endothelial leukocyte adhesion molecule-1 and platelet-activating factor in neutrophil adherence to IL-1-prestimulated endothelial cell. Endothelial leukocyte adhesion molecule-1-mediated CD18 activation. *Journal of Immunology*, **147**, 1369–76.

Kuijpers, T. W., Mul, E. P. J., Blom, M., Kovach, N. L., Gaeta, F. C. A., Tollefson, V., Elices, M. J. & Harlan, J. M. (1993). Freezing adhesion molecules in a state of high-avidity binding blocks eosinophil migration. *Journal of Experimental Medicine*, **178**, 279–84.

Kyan-Aung, U., Haskard, D. O., Poston, R. N., Thornhill, M. H. & Lee, T. H. (1991). Endothelial leukocyte adhesion molecule-1 and intercellular adhesion molecule-1 mediate the adhesion of eosinophils to endothelial cells *in vitro* and are expressed by endothelium in allergic cutaneous inflammation *in vivo*. *Journal of Immunology*, **146**, 521–8.

Lamas, A. M., Mulroney, C. M. & Schleimer, R. P. (1988). Studies on the adhesive interaction between purified human eosinophils and cultured vascular endothelial cells. *Journal of Immunology*, **140**, 1500–5.

Lasky, L. A. (1992). Selectins: Interpreters of cell-specific carbohydrate information during inflammation. *Science*, **258**, 964–9.

Laudanna, C., Melotti, P., Bonizzato, C., Piacentini, G., Boner, A., Serra, M. C. & Berton, G. (1993). Ligation of member of the β_1 or the β_2 subfamilies of integrins by antibodies triggers eosinophil respiratory burst and spreading. *Immunology*, **80**, 273–80.

Lawrence, M. B. & Springer, T. A. (1991). Leukocytes roll on a selectin at physiologic flow rates: distinction from and prerequisite for adhesion through integrins. *Cell*, **65**, 859–73.

Ley, K., Gaehtgens, P., Fennie, C., Singer, M. S., Lasky, L. A. & Rosen, S. D. (1991). Lectin-like cell adhesion molecule-1 mediates leukocyte rolling in mesenteric venules *in vivo*. *Blood*, **77**, 2553–5.

Ley, K., Tedder, T. F. & Kansas, G. S. (1993). L-selectin mediated leukocyte rolling in untreated mesenteric venules *in vivo* independent of E- or P-selectin. *Blood*, **82**, 1632–8.

Lo, S. K., Lee, S., Ramos, R. A., Lobb, R., Rosa, M., Chi-Rosso, G. & Wright, S. D. (1991). Endothelial-leukocyte adhesion molecule 1 stimulates the adhesive activity of leukocyte integrin CR3 (CD11b/CD18, MAC-1, $\alpha_m\beta_2$) on human neutrophils. *Journal of Experimental Medicine*, **173**, 1493–500.

Lorant, D. E., Topham, M. K., Whatley, R. E., McEver, R. P., McIntyre, T. M., Prescott, S. M. & Zimmerman, G. A. (1993). Inflammatory roles of P-selectin. *Journal of Clinical Investigations*, **92**, 559–70.

Luscinskas, F. W., Cybulsky, M. I., Kiely, J-M., Peckins, C. S., Davis, V. M. & Gimbrone, M. A. (1991). Cytokine-activated human endothelial monolayers support enhanced neutrophil transmigration via a mechanism involving both endothelial-leukocyte adhesion molecule-1 and intercellular adhesion molecule-1. *Journal of Immunology*, **146**, 1617–25.

Marlin, S. D. & Springer, T. A. (1987). Purified intercellular adhesion molecule-1 (ICAM-1) is a ligand for lymphocyte function-associated antigen 1 (LFA-1). *Cell*, **51**, 813–19.

McEver, R. P., Beckstead, J. H., Moore, K. L., Marshall-Carlson, L. & Bainton, D. F. (1989). GMP-140, a platelet α-granule membrane protein, is also synthesized by vascular endothelial cells and is localized in Weibel-Palade bodies. *Journal of Clinical Investigations*, **84**, 92–9.

Mengelers, H. J. J., Maikoe, T., Hooibrink, B., Kuijpers, T. W., Kreukniet, J., Lammers, J-W. J. & Koenderman, L. (1993). Down regulation of L-selectin expression on eosinophils recovered from bronchoalveolar lavage fluid after allergen provocation. *Clinical Experimental Allergy*, **23**, 196–204.

Mileski, W. J., Winn, R. K., Vedder, N. B., Pohlman, T. H., Harlan, J. M. & Rice, C. L. (1990). Inhibition of CD18-dependent neutrophil adherence reduces organ injury after hemorrhagic shock in primates. *Surgery*, **108**, 206–12.

Miller, L. J., Bainton, D. F., Borregard, N. & Springer, T. A. (1987). Stimulated mobilization of monocyte Mac-1 and P150,95 adhesion proteins from an intracellular vesicular compartment to the cell surface. *Journal of Clinical Investigations*, **80**, 535–44.

Mulligan, M. S. & Ward, P. A. (1992). Immune complex-induced lung and dermal vascular injury. Differing requirements for tumor necrosis factor-α and IL-1. *Journal of Immunology*, **149**, 331–9.

Mulligan, M. S., Varani, J., Dame, M. K., Lane, C. L., Smith, C. W., Anderson, D. C. & Ward, P. A. (1991). Role of endothelial-leukocyte adhesion molecule 1 (ELAM-1) in neutrophil-mediated lung injury in rats. *Journal of Clinical Investigations*, **88**, 1396–406.

Mulligan, M. S., Polley, M. J., Bayer, R. J., Nunn, M. F., Paulson, J. C. & Ward, P. A. (1992). Neutrophil-dependent acute lung injury. Requirement for P-selectin (GMP-140). *Journal of Clinical Investigations*, **90**, 1600–7.

Mulligan, M. S., Paulson, J. C., De Frees, S., Zheng, Z-L., Lowe, L. B. & Ward, P. A. (1993*a*). Protective effects of oligosaccharides in P-selectin-dependent lung injury. *Nature*, **364**, 149–51.

Mulligan, M. S., Smith, C. W., Anderson, D. C., Todd, R. F., Miyasaka, M., Tamatani, T., Issekutz, T. B. & Ward, P. A. (1993*b*). Role of leukocyte adhesion molecules in complement-induced lung injury. *Journal of Immunology*, **150**, 2401–6.

Mulligan, M. S., Wilson, G. P., Todd, R. F., Smith, C. W., Anderson, D. C., Varani, J., Issekutz, T. B., Myasaka, M., Tamatani, T., Rusche, J. R., Vaporciyan, A. A. & Ward, P. A. (1993*c*). Role of β_1, β_2, integrins and ICAM-1 in lung injury after deposition of IgG and IgA immune complexes. *Journal of Immunology*, **150**, 2407–17.

Nathan, C., Srimal, S., Farber, C., Sanchez, E., Kabbash, L., Asch, A., Gailit, J. & Wright, S. D. (1989). Cytokine-induced respiratory burst of human neutrophils: dependence on extracellular matrix proteins and CD11/CD18 integrins. *Journal of Cell Biology*, **109**, 1341–9.

Nourshargh, S. (1992). Adhesion molecules: potential targets for novel anti-inflammatory agents. In Barnes, P. J., ed. *New Drugs for Asthma, Volume II*, pp. 220–230. London: IBC Technical Services Ltd.

Nourshargh, S. (1993). Mechanisms of neutrophil and eosinophil accumulation *in vivo*. *American Review of Respiratory Diseases*, **148**, 560–4.

Nourshargh, S. & Williams, T. J. (1990). Evidence that a receptor operated event on the neutrophil mediates neutrophil accumulation *in vivo*: pretreatment of ^{111}In-neutrophils with pertussis toxin *in vitro* inhibits their accumulation *in vivo*. *Journal of Immunology*, **145**, 2633–8.

Nourshargh, S., Rampart, M., Hellewell, P. G., Jose, P. J., Harlan, J. M., Edwards, A. J. & Williams, T. J. (1989). Accumulation of ^{111}In-neutrophils in rabbit skin in allergic and non-allergic inflammatory reactions *in vivo*: inhibition by neutrophil pretreatment *in vitro* with a monoclonal antibody recognising the CD18 antigen. *Journal of Immunology*, **142**, 3193–8.

Olofsson, A. M., Arfors, K-E., Ramezani, L., Wolitsky, B. A. & Butcher, E. C. (1994). E-selectin mediates leukocyte rolling in interleukin-1 treated rabbit mesentery venules. *Blood*, **84**, 2749–58.

Osborn, L., Hession, C., Tizard, R., Cassallo, C., Luhowskyj, S., Chi-Rosso, G. & Lobb, R. (1989). Direct expression cloning of vascular cell adhesion molecule 1, a cytokine-induced endothelial protein that binds to lymphocytes. *Cell*, 59, 1203–11.

Palabrica, T., Lobb, R., Furie, B. C., Aronovitz, M., Benjamin, C., Hsu, Y-M., Sajer, S. A. & Furie, B. (1992). Leukocyte accumulation promoting fibrin deposition is mediated *in vivo* by P-selectin on adherent platelets. *Nature*, **359**, 848–51.

Patel, K. D., Zimmerman, G. A., Prescott, S. M., McEver, R. P. & McIntyre, T. M. (1991). Oxygen radicals induce human endothelial cells to express GMP-140 and bind neutrophils. *Journal of Cell Biology*, **112**, 749–59.

Perry, M. A. & Granger, D. N. (1992). Role of CD11/CD18 in shear rate-dependent leukocyte-endothelial cell interactions in cat mesenteric venules. *Journal of Clinical Investigations*, **87**, 1798–1804.

Picker, L. J., Kishimoto, T. K., Smith, C. W., Warnock, R. A. & Butcher, E. C. (1991*a*). ELAM-1 is an adhesion molecule for skin-homing T cells. *Nature*, **349**, 796–838.

Picker, L. J., Warnock, R. A., Burns, A. R., Doerschuk, C. M., Berg, E. L. & Butcher, E. C. (1991*b*). The neutrophil selectin LECAM-1 presents carbohydrate ligands to the vascular selectins ELAM-1 and GMP-140. *Cell*, **66**, 921–33.

Price, T. H., Beatty, P. G. & Corpuz, S. R. (1987). *In vivo* inhibition of neutrophil function in the rabbit using monoclonal antibody to CD18. *Journal of Immunology*, **139**, 4174–7.

Pulido, R., Elices, M. J., Campanero, M. R., Osborn, L., Schiffer, S., Garcia-Pardo, A., Lobb, R., Hemler, M. E. & Sanchez-Madrid, F. (1991). Functional evidence for three distinct and independently inhibitable adhesion activities mediated by the human integrin VLA-4. *Journal of Biological Chemistry*, **266**, 10241–45.

Rampart, M. & Williams, T. J. (1988). Evidence that neutrophil accumulation induced by interleukin-1 requires both local protein biosynthesis and neutrophil CD18 antigen expression *in vivo*. *British Journal of Pharmacology*, **94**, 1143–8.

Rot, A. (1992). Endothelial cell binding of NAP-1/IL-8: role in neutrophil emigration. *Immunology Today*, **13**, 291–4.

Rothlein, R., Dustin, M. L., Marlin, S. D. & Springer, T. A. (1986). An intercellular adhesion molecule (ICAM-1) distinct from LFA-1. *Journal of Immunology*, **137**, 1–5.

Rotrosen, D., Malech, H. L. & Gallin, J. I. (1987). Formyl peptide leukocyte chemoattractant uptake and release by cultured human umbilical vein endothelial cells. *Journal of Immunology*, **139**, 3034–40.

Schleimer, R. P. Sterbinsky, S. A., Kaiser, J., Bickel, C. A., Klunk, D. A., Tomioka, K., Newman, W., Luscinskas, F. W., Gimbrone, M. A., McIntyre, B. W. & Bochner, B. S. (1992). IL-4 induces adherence of human eosinophils and basophils but not neutrophils to endothelium. Association with expression of VCAM-1. *Journal of Immunology*, **148**, 1086–92.

Seekamp, A., Mulligan, M. S., Till, G. O., Smith, C. W., Miyaska, M., Tamatani, T., Todd, R. F. & Ward, P. A. (1993). Role of β_2 integrins and ICAM-1 in lung injury following ischemia-reperfusion of rat hind limbs. *American Journal of Pathology*, **143**, 464–72.

Shimizu, Y., Van Seventer, G. A., Horgan, K. J. & Shaw, S. (1990). Roles of adhesion molecules in T-cell recognition: fundamental similarities between four integrins on resting human T cells (LFA-1, VLA-4, VLA-5, VLA-6) in expression, binding, and costimulation. *Immunology Review*, **114**, 109–43.

Shimizu, Y., Shaw, S., Graber, N., Gopal, T. V., Horgan, K. J., Van Seventer, G. A. & Newman, W. (1991). Activation-independent binding of human memory T cells to adhesion molecule ELAM-1. *Nature*, **349**, 799–802.

Smith, C. W., Rothlein, R., Hughes, B. J., Mariscalco, M. M., Rudloff, H. E., Schmalstieg, F. C. & Anderson, D. C. (1988). Recognition of an endothelial determinant for CD18-dependent human neutrophil adherence and transendothelial migration. *Journal of Clinical Investigations*, **82**, 1746–56.

Smith, C. W., Marlin, S. D., Rothlein, R., Toman, C. & Anderson, D. C. (1989). Co-operative interactions of LFA-1 and Mac-1 with intercellular adhesion molecule-1 in facilitating adherence and transendothelial migration of human neutrophils *in vitro*. *Journal of Clinical Investigations*, **83**, 2008–17.

Spertini, O., Kansas, G. S., Munro, J. M., Griffin, J. D. & Tedder, T. F. (1991*a*). Regulation of leukocyte migration by activation of the leukocyte adhesion molecule-1 (LAM-1) selectin. *Nature*, **349**, 691–4.

Spertini, O., Luscinskas, F. W., Kansas, G. S., Munro, J. M., Griffin, J. D., Gimbrone, M. A. & Tedder, T. F. (1991*b*). Leukocyte adhesion molecule-1 (LAM-1, L-selectin) interacts with an inducible endothelial cell ligand to support leukocyte adhesion. *Journal of Immunology*, **147**, 2565–73.

Spiramarao, P., von Andrian, U. H., Butcher, E. C., Bourdon, M. A. & Broide, D. H. (1994). L-selectin and very late antigen-4 integrin promote eosinophil rolling at physiological shear rates *in vivo*. *Journal of Immunology*, **153**, 4238–46.

Stacker, S. A. & Springer, T. A. (1991). Leukocyte integrin P150,95 (CD11c/CD18) functions as an adhesion molecule binding to a counter-receptor on stimulated endothelium. *Journal of Immunology*, **146**, 648–55.

Staunton, D. E., Dustin, M. L. & Springer, T. A. (1989). Functional cloning of ICAM-2, a cell adhesion ligand for LFA-1 homologous to ICAM-1. *Nature*, **339**, 61–7.

Tanaka, Y., Adams, D. H., Hubscher, S., Hirano, H., Siebenlist, U. & Shaw, S. (1993). T-cell adhesion induced by proteoglycan-immobolized cytokine MIP-1β. *Nature*, **361**, 79–82.

Thomas, J. R., Harlan, J. M., Rice, C. L. & Winn, R. K. (1992). Role of leukocyte CD11/CD18 complex in endotoxic and septic shock in rabbits. *Journal of Applied Physiology*, **73**, 1510–16.

Thornhill, M. H., Kyan-Aung, U. & Haskard, D. O. (1990). IL-4 increases human endothelial cell adhesiveness for T cells but not for neutrophils. *Journal of Immunology*, **144**, 3060–5.

Todd, R. F., Arnaout, M. A., Rosin, R. E., Crowley, C. A., Peters, W. A. & Babior, B. M. (1984). Subcellular location of the large subunit of Mol (Mol_a; formerly gp 110), a surface glycoprotein associated with neutrophil adhesion. *Journal of Clinical Investigations*, **74**, 1280–90.

Tuomanen, E. I., Saukkonen, K., Sande, S., Cioffe, C. & Wright, S. D. (1989). Reduction of inflammation, tissue damage and mortality in bacterial meningitis in rabbits treated with monoclonal antibodies against adhesion-promoting receptors of leucocytes. *Journal of Experimental Medicine*, **170**, 959–68.

Vedder, N. B., Winn, R. K., Rice, C. L., Chi, E. Y., Arfors, K. E. & Harber, J. M. (1988). A monoclonal antibody to the adherence-promoting leukocyte glycoprotein, CD18, reduces organ injury and improves survival from hemorrhagic shock and resuscitation in rabbits. *Journal of Clinical Investigations*, **81**, 939–44.

von Andrian, U. H., Chambers, J. D., McEvoy, L. M., Bargatze, R. F., Arfors, K-E. & Butcher, E. C. (1991). Two-step model of leukocyte-endothelial cell interaction in inflammation: distinct roles for LECAM-1 and the leukocyte β_2 integrins *in vivo*. *Proceedings of the National Academy of Sciences USA*, **88**, 7538–42.

von Andrian, U. H., Hansell, P., Chambers, J. D., Berger, E. M., Filho, I. T., Butcher, E. C. & Arfors, K-E. (1992). L-selectin function is required for β_2-integrin-mediated neutrophil adhesion at physiological shear rates *in vivo*. *American Journal of Physiology*, **263**, H1034–44.

von Andrian, U. H., Berger, E. M., Ramezani, L., Chambers, J. D., Ochs, H. D., Harlan, J. M., Paulson, J. C., Etzioni, A. & Arfors, K-E. (1993*a*). *In vivo* behavior of neutrophils from two patients with distinct inherited leukocyte adhesion deficiency syndromes. *Journal of Clinical Investigations*, **91**, 2893–7.

von Andrian, U. H., Chambers, J. D., Berg, E. L., Michie, S. A., Brown, D. A., Karolak, D., Ramezani, L., Berger, E. M., Arfors K-E. & Butcher, E. C. (1993*b*). L-selectin mediates neutrophil rolling in inflamed venules through sialyl Lewis^x-dependent and -independent recognition pathways. *Blood*, **82**, 182–91.

Vonderheide, R. H. & Springer, T. A. (1992). Lymphocyte adhesion through very late antigen 4: evidence for a novel binding site in the alternatively spliced domain of vascular cell adhesion molecule 1 and an additional $\alpha 4$ integrin counter-receptor on stimulated endothelium. *Journal of Experimental Medicine*, **175**, 1433–42.

Walsh, G. M., Mermod, J-J., Hartnell, A., Kay, A. B. & Wardlaw, A. J. (1991). Human eosinophil, but not neutrophil, adherence to IL-1 stimulated human umbilical vascular endothelial cells is $\alpha_4\beta_1$ (very late antigen-4) dependent. *Journal of Immunology*, **146**, 3419–23.

Watson, S. R., Fennie, C. & Lasky, L. A. (1991). Neutrophil influx in to an inflammatory site inhibited by a soluble homing receptor-IgG chimaera. *Nature*, **349**, 164–6.

Weg, V. B., Williams, T. J., Lobb, R. R. & Nourshargh, S. (1993). A monoclonal antibody recognising very late activation antigen-4 (VLA-4) inhibits eosinophil accumulation *in vivo*. *Journal of Experimental Medicine*, **177**, 561–6.

Wegner, C. D., Gundel, R. H., Reilly, P., Haynes, N., Letts, L. G. & Rothlein, R. (1990). Intercellular adhesion molecule-1 (ICAM-1) in the pathogenesis of asthma. *Science*, **247**, 456–9.

Weller, A., Isenmann, S. & Vestweber, D. (1992). Cloning of the mouse endothelial selectins. Expression of both E- and P-selectin is inducible by tumor necrosis factor α. *Journal of Biological Chemistry*, **267**, 15176–83.

Weller, P. F., Rand, T. H., Goelz, S. E., Chi-Rosso, G. & Lobb, R. R. (1991). Human eosinophil adherence to vascular endothelium mediated by binding to vascular cell adhesion molecule 1 and endothelial leukocyte adhesion molecule 1. *Proceedings of the National Academy of Sciences USA*, **88**, 7430–3.

Weyrich, A. S., Ma, X-L., Lefer, D. J., Albertine, K. H. & Lefer, A. M. (1992). *In vivo* neutralization of P-selectin protects feline heart and endothelium in myocardial ischemia and reperfusion injury. *Journal of Clinical Investigations*, **91**, 2620–9.

Williams, A. F. & Barclay, A. N. (1988). The immunoglobulin superfamily – domains for cell surface recognition. *Annual Review in Immunology*, **6**, 381–405.

Winn, R. K., Liggitt, D., Vedder, N. B., Paulson, J. C. & Harlan, J. M. (1993). Anti-P-selectin monoclonal antibody attenuates reperfusion injury to the rabbit ear. *Journal of Clinical Investigations*, **92**, 2042–7.

Yamazaki, T., Seko, Y., Tamatani, T., Miyasaka, M., Yagita, H., Okumura, K., Nagai, R. & Yazaki, Y. (1993). Expression of intercellular adhesion molecule-1 in rat heart with ischemia/reperfusion and limitation of infarct size by treatment with antibodies against cell adhesion molecules. *American Journal of Pathology*, **143**, 410–18.

Zimmerman, G. A., Prescott, S. M. & McIntyre, T. M. (1992). Endothelial cell interactions with granulocytes: tethering and signalling molecules. *Immunology Today*, **13**, 93–100.

–4–

The regulation of lymphocyte migration by vascular endothelium and its role in the immune response

ANN AGER

The immune response can be divided into several stages. The stimulation of naive lymphocytes by antigen is followed by the proliferation of lymphocytes and their differentiation into effector lymphocytes which eliminate antigen from infected tissues (cytotoxic cells, antibody or cytokine secreting cells), and memory cells, which enable the host to mount a secondary immune response. These distinct stages of the immune response are regulated by the ability of lymphocytes to migrate to different organs of the body. Lymphocytes enter most organs directly from the bloodstream and recent research has emphasized the crucial role that vascular endothelial cells (EC) play in sorting lymphocyte subpopulations for subsequent migration into tissues. Before discussing the molecular basis of interactions between lymphocytes and endothelial cells that regulate lymphocyte migration, I would like to consider the pivotal role that lymphocyte migration plays in the regulation of the immune response.

Lymphocyte migration and the regulation of the immune response

Immune responses are initiated when T lymphocytes contact antigenic peptides complexed with products of the major histocompatibility complex (MHC) on the surface of antigen presenting cells (APC). Engagement of the antigen receptor is not sufficient to elicit the full proliferative response of naive T lymphocytes and additional receptor-ligand interactions are required to co-stimulate T cells (Schwartz, 1992). The site of stimulation of naive lymphocytes is thought to be restricted to secondary lymphoid organs (lymph nodes and spleen) where specialized, dendritic APC express full costimulatory activity for T cells (Steinman, 1991). The frequency of antigen-specific lymphocytes in the body is extremely low, at one in 10^5 to one in 10^6, and the chances of encounter with APC must be maximized for lymphocytes with appropriate antigen receptors to be activated. This is achieved by the continuous, large-scale traffic of naive lymphocytes (T and B cells) from the blood into lymphoid organs (Gowans, 1959). Lymphocytes spend up to 16 hours migrating through these tissues and, if not selected by antigen on APC, regain access to the blood (either directly from the spleen or indirectly from lymph nodes via the efferent lymphatics) for subsequent redistribution to lymph nodes and spleen. Lymphoid organs are strategically placed throughout the body to sequester antigen gaining access via the extensive mucosal and epithelial surfaces of the body. The continuous traffic or recirculation of naive lymphocytes between lymphoid organs via the blood and lymphatics ensures widespread distribution of receptor specificities throughout the immune system.

Following encounter with antigen, lymphocytes are retained within lymphoid organs for several days, presumably on the surface of APC. During this period lymphocytes divide and differentiate into effector cells and memory cells. The progeny, which include blasts and non-cycling lymphocytes, exit the organ and regain access to the bloodstream. In comparison with naive lymphocytes, these cells show significantly altered migration pathways. An early finding was that lymphoblasts in S-phase of the cell cycle preferentially returned to the site of antigenic stimulation (Griscelli, Vassalli & McCluskey, 1969; Smith, Martin & Ford, 1980). This property has been termed organ-specific homing and, thus far, two regions within the immune system have been identified; peripheral (subcutaneous) lymph nodes and mucosal-associated lymphoid organs. Lymphoblasts migrate more efficiently than unactivated lymphocytes to non-lymphoid organs, particularly to sites of inflammation, also demonstrating organ specific homing such that peripheral lymph node blasts preferentially migrate to sites drained by peripheral lymph nodes, e.g. the skin, and mucosal lymph node blasts migrate to the gut wall (Rose, Parrott & Bruce, 1976; Smith *et al.*, 1980). Recently activated T lymphocytes that are no longer cycling, but can be identified by expression of the RO isoform of CD45 (see below), show similar migration pathways to lymphoblasts. The preferential migration of blasts and recently activated lymphocytes to non-lymphoid tissues and sites of inflammation optimizes antigen elimination from infected tissues. The precise role of organ-specific homing is unclear. It ensures that areas drained by involved lymph nodes will be surveyed for antigen. Organ-specific homing may reflect the generation of a different type of immune response in the gut than in the periphery and it is a measure of precursor cells that migrate there. For example, IgA plasmablasts in thoracic duct lymph have been shown to localize in the gut wall (Husband &

Gowans, 1978). Differences in the profile of cytokines secreted by activated T cells in these two sites have also been reported (Daynes *et al.*, 1990) which may reflect localization of Th1 versus Th2 lymphocytes.

The differentiation of lymphocytes into effector cells and memory cells is not completely understood since there are few markers available to distinguish between naive lymphocytes and those that have already encountered antigen. Memory cells, defined by their ability to transfer immunity, do recirculate from blood to lymph since they can be detected in thoracic duct lymph and in lymphoid organs distant from the site of immunization (Ford, 1975). Not all lymphocytes recirculate from blood lymph. $CD5^+$ B cells, which represent a distinct lineage of B cells that secretes natural and autoimmune antibodies, preferentially localize in the peritoneal cavity. Effector cells such as antibody secreting plasma cells do not recirculate, but localize in the medullary regions of lymphoid organs and in the bone marrow (Tew *et al.*, 1992). Other effector cells do not recirculate and this may be a common property of lymphocytes that have differentiated, but do not proliferate in response to antigen. The best example is the $\gamma\delta$ receptor bearing T lymphocyte that migrates directly from the blood and localizes in epithelial linings where these cells are thought to mediate first-line defence to invading organisms (Allison & Havran, 1991).

The migration of lymphocytes into tissues

Histological studies of lymphoid organs and sites of inflammation show the exquisite regulation of lymphocyte infiltration. The appearance of lymphocytes within an organ could result from random entry of all leukocytes and subsequent retention of lymphocytes, or from selective migration directly from the bloodstream. Research over the last few years has demonstrated the ability of vascular endothelial cells (EC) to sort lymphocytes from other populations of leukocyte for migration into tissues. Sorting is mediated by specific recognition between lymphocytes and the luminal surface of vascular EC, via complementary sets of adhesion molecules. EC express class I and class II MHC, particularly at sites of inflammation. It is possible that antigen-specific lymphocytes could be sorted by adhesion to EC via peptide/MHC complexes. However, studies of lymphocyte migration into lymph nodes (Drayson, 1986) and sites of inflammation (Hall, Hopkins & Orlors, 1977; Husband & Gowans, 1978) have shown that most of the infiltrating cells are not specific for antigen, suggesting that this pathway does not normally operate, rather that lymphocytes are recruited non-specifically and selected by antigen after gaining access to the tissues. The absolute level and activity of individual adhesion molecules vary on lymphocytes and EC depending on their states of activation. It is proposed that the differential migration of naive and antigen-activated lymphocytes described above is regulated by alterations in adhesion molecules on these two cell types. Substantial progress has been made in identifying some adhesion molecules involved in lymphocyte migration (see pp. 72–76).

Adhesive interactions arrest lymphocytes from flowing blood on to the luminal surface of EC, allowing optimal delivery of signals that mediate the directed migration of lymphocytes out of the vessel. However, extravasation does not always follow binding to the luminal surface of the blood vessel and is, therefore, an important step in the regulation of lymphocyte traffic (Bjerknes, Chang & Ottoway, 1986). Extravasation involves regulated adhesion to, and detachment of, lymphocytes from EC, subendothelial pericytes and the basal lamina, which together make up the vessel wall. Lymphocytes then migrate through the tissues to encounter APC and infected cells. T and B lymphocytes follow separate migration pathways within lymphoid organs such that they segregate into distinct T- and B-regions. Interactions with stromal cells in these regions are crucial for the regulation of lymphocyte activation and differentiation in response to antigen. In comparison with adhesive interactions between lymphocytes and the luminal surface of EC, the latter processes which regulate entry and migration through tissues are poorly understood.

Experimental approaches to the study of lymphocyte migration

A substantial challenge to workers in the field has been to understand the molecular basis of lymphocyte-EC recognition that regulates the differential migration of lymphocyte populations. Separate approaches have been taken to study this problem *in vivo* and *in vitro* which, until recently, have not overlapped significantly because these assays measure different processes. *In vivo* studies measure the number of lymphocytes that enter tissues and therefore depend on adhesive interactions in addition to those with vascular EC, whereas *in vitro* assays measure adhesive interactions between lymphocytes and EC only. Both assays measure a dynamic process and, thus, the results depend on the timing of observations made. I will consider results from *in vivo* studies in this and the following section and results from *in vitro* studies in the final sections of the chapter.

Studies of the lymphocyte

Adoptive transfer of labelled cells into rodents (mice and rats) and large animals (sheep and pigs) has been widely used to describe the kinetics of lymphocyte migration to distinct organs of the body. These studies used unseparated populations of lymphocytes from blood, lymphatics or collected directly from lymphoid organs (which comprise mainly unactivated cells) and showed that lymphocytes are cleared from the bloodstream within 30 minutes and preferentially localize in lymphoid organs over the following 2 to 24 hours (Smith & Ford, 1983). Although some cells could be detected in non-lymphoid organs, a direct comparison of size, and therefore the fraction of the cardiac output that flows through these organs, demonstrate that migration into lymphoid organs is at least 50-fold higher. The distribution of lymphocytes is not random since peripheral lymph nodes are enriched in T lymphocytes and gut-associated lymphoid organs, such as Peyer's patches, are enriched in B lymphocytes. The distribution of $CD4^+$ and $CD8^+$ T cell subsets also differs between these two regions of the immune system (Kraal, Weissman & Butcher, 1983). Whether the differential migration of lymphocyte subsets is regulated at the level of EC recognition (Stevens, Weissman & Butcher, 1982) or is due to enrichment following entry from the bloodstream (Westermann *et al.*, 1992, 1993) remains to be determined.

The recent demonstration that expression of specific isoforms of CD45 (leukocyte common antigen) by T lymphocytes indicates whether lymphocytes have recently been activated (CD45RO) or not (CD45RA) has allowed the migration pathways of these cells to be directly compared. Originally, the RO and RA isoforms of CD45 were used to identify memory and naive lymphocytes, respectively; CD45RO cells can re-express the RA isoform and, thus, CD45RO is probably a more accurate marker of recent activation instead of a memory phenotype (for discussion of topic, see Mackay, 1993). All lymphocytes entering and leaving a single lymph node have been studied by sampling the blood as well as the afferent and efferent lymphatics of popliteal lymph nodes in sheep (Mackay, Marsten & Dudler, 1990). These studies showed that CD45RO T lymphocytes preferentially migrate from blood vessels in the skin, gaining access to the draining lymph node indirectly via the afferent lymphatics. In comparison, CD45RA T lymphocytes migrate directly into lymph nodes via specialized high endothelial venules (HEV), and do not migrate from vessels in non-lymphoid organs. These results emphasize the efficiency with which CD45RA T cells are extracted by blood vessels in lymph nodes. The selective migration of CD45RO T cells into non-lymphoid organs is also shown by the accumulation of CD45RO cells in human skin and sites of inflammation (Pitzalis *et al.*, 1988). The differential migration of CD45RA and CD45RO T lymphocytes ensures that unactivated cells are delivered to lymphoid organs for efficient activation by 'professional' APC. Recently activated cells, in which the machinery for antigen elimination is upregulated (e.g. cytotoxicity or cytokine secretion), are delivered to sites of inflammation in which antigen is localized. It seems inefficient to prevent the migration of CD45RO T cells to lymphoid organs, since antigen will also be localized there. A difference between CD45RA and CD45RO T lymphocytes could be that RA cells preferentially migrate through lymphoid organs, whereas RO cells migrate through non-lymphoid organs as well. Recent studies in support of this hypothesis have shown that organ specific homing of T lymphocytes to either peripheral lymph nodes or gut-associated lymphoid organs, originally demonstrated in the sheep (Cahill *et al.*, 1977), is restricted to the CD45RO population (Mackay *et al.*, 1992).

The studies of lymphoblast migration are remarkably similar to those using CD45RO T cells. Since T lymphoblasts are, presumably, the immediate precursors to CD45RO T lymphocytes the similarity in result is, perhaps, not surprising. A prediction would be that, following activation, lymphocytes acquire adhesion molecules that mediate binding to EC in non-lymphoid organs. It has already been shown that several adhesion molecules are expressed at higher levels on CD45RO T lymphocytes than on CD45RA T cells in humans and sheep (Sanders, Makgoba & Shaw, 1988; Mackay *et al.*, 1990. In addition, the adhesion molecule L-selectin, which mediates migration to lymph nodes, is down-regulated on CD45RO T lymphocytes thus diverting these cells away from lymphoid organs. Activated lymphocytes may not lose the capacity to bind to HEV in lymph nodes, but the frequency of interaction with EC in non-lymphoid organs and sites of inflammation will be higher, owing to larger blood flow through these organs. Various models of inflammation have been used to demonstrate increased lymphocyte migration, including contact hypersensitivity, delayed type hypersensitivity, organ allografts and autoimmune diseases. Since the inflammatory process is dynamic, the types of lymphocytes infiltrating will depend on the time studied after onset of the inflammatory process as well as the type of inflammation. Further studies are required to determine whether lymphocyte subsets preferentially migrate into distinct types of inflammation (e.g. $CD4^+$, $CD8^+$ or B cells, T cells secreting cytokines of either Th1 of Th2 phenotype).

Studies of vascular endothelium

Vascular endothelium plays an active role in the recruitment of lymphocytes since the expression of adhesion molecules varies on EC according to its microenvironment. A type of activated endothelium lines the lymph node post-capillary venules that support the large-scale migration of naive lymphocytes from the blood (Gowans & Knight, 1964). In histological specimens these vessels display a cuboidal endothelial morphology, rather than the flattened morphology typical of non-specialized vessels, and hence have been termed high endothelial venules (HEV). HEV are also characterized by the presence of lymphocytes, but not other types of leukocyte, either attached to the luminal surface, or embedded in the vessel wall. Although their morphology is a distinguishing feature and readily used for identification, it is not a prerequisite for the large-scale migration of lymphocytes since lymph nodes in sheep and athymic animals do not have morphologically distinct HEV, yet lymphocyte traffic is substantial in these animals (Morris & Courtice, 1977; Fossum, Smith & Ford, 1983). The dynamic morphology of these vessels may regulate blood flow through the node, and/or the surface area of the endothelial lining, so interactions with lymphocytes are maximized. A common feature of HEV, irrespective of endothelial morphology, is the expression of adhesion molecules that are not normally expressed by other types of endothelium. Some of these molecules are thought to mediate organ-specific homing of lymphoid cells and have been termed vascular addressins. The highly adhesive capacity of HEV was first demonstrated using the frozen section assay, which measures the binding of lymphocytes to lymph node sections at low temperatures (4–8°C) (Stamper & Woodruff, 1976). Additional properties distinguishing HEV from other blood vessels include expression of non-specific esterase, and secretory vesicles by lining EC, and also an unusually thickened sub-endothelial basal lamina (Anderson, Anderson & Wyllie, 1976). Whether these properties play any role in regulating lymphocyte migration is unclear. Other properties of HEV that could regulate lymphocyte migration, such as the integrity of inter-EC junctions that would allow lymphocytes to extravasate, and the polarized secretion or retention of chemoattractants that could direct lymphocyte migration out of the vessel, have not been studied.

Studies of lymphocyte interactions with the luminal surface of HEV using intravital microscopy have shown that extravasation is a complex event which does not simply depend on a single, adhesive interaction. Lymphocytes continually contact the blood vessel surface and the majority detach within one second. If contact persists for more than 1–3 seconds, it is successful, in that the lymphocyte is arrested from blood flow for at least 30 seconds (Bjerknes *et al.*, 1986) and, presumably, proceeds to migrate out of the vessel. Separate studies have shown that lymphocyte migration across HEV is accompanied by dramatic changes in morphology as lymphocytes lose surface microvilli and adopt a smooth-surfaced morphology (van Ewijk, Brons & Rozing, 1975). Although the stimulus and intracellular signalling pathways that regulate lymphocyte migration are undetermined, G-protein linked receptors are thought to be involved. The migration of lymphocytes into lymph nodes *in vivo* is inhibited by pertussis toxin pre-treatment (Steen *et al.*, 1990); intravital microscopic analysis shows that pertussis toxin inhibits the formation of stable, adhesive contacts that precedes extravasation, but does not affect the number of short-lived contacts made initially (Bargatze & Butcher, 1993).

HEV are normally only found in lymph nodes. Blood vessels with a similar morphology have been reported at sites of chronic immune-mediated inflammation where they support increased traffic of lymphocytes from the blood, such as rheumatoid synovium and other autoimmune disorders (Freemont, 1988), also in experimentally induced granulomas (Smith, McIntosh & Morris, 1970; Freemont & Ford, 1985). Within lymph nodes, HEV, as defined by morphology and vascular addressin expression, are restricted to the paracortex in which T lymphocytes become sequestered, although post-capillary venules that are not specialized for lymphocyte traffic are found in other areas of the node. The precise origin of HEV is not clear. The morphology and adhesive capacity of HEV are dependent on the antigen load in that organ. The number of lymphocytes migrating into a single node increases up to four-fold following antigen administration. A combination of factors is responsible, including increased blood flow, an increase in the number of HEV and increased binding of lymphocytes to individual HEV (Anderson, Anderson & Wyllie, 1975; Drayson, Smith & Ford, 1981). Studies in which the afferent lymphatics have been ligated, preventing the influx of antigen and APC, have shown that the endothelial cells lining HEV flatten and lose their ability to bind lymphocytes *in vitro* and to support migration *in vivo*, within 1–3 days following deafferentization (Hendriks, Duivestijn & Kraal, 1987; Mebius *et al.*, 1991). A reasonable hypothesis would be that activated lymphocytes in the paracortical area of the node induce HEV phenotype and function in local post-capillary venules, via a direct effect on the endothelial lining. However, lymphocyte recirculation occurs constitutively in the absence of antigen in fetal (Pearson, Simpson-Morgan & Morris, 1976; Cahill *et al.*, 1979) and germ-free animals (Manolios, Geczy & Schreiber, 1988), which suggests that HEV can function in an antigen-free environment, perhaps at a reduced level of activity. The location of HEV appears crucial for the initiation of immune responses since dendritic APC localize to the T cell area. Unactivated lymphocytes migrating in via HEV are delivered directly to antigen already processed for presentation by cells with full co-stimulatory activity for T lymphocytes. These studies suggest that the extent of lymphocyte migration into individual lymphoid organs can be regulated via a direct effect of antigen on the capacity of blood vessels to support lymphocyte extravasation. Presumably this mechanism serves to maximize the immune response in a single node. Direct evidence in support of this hypothesis comes from studies using isolated, perfused rat spleens, in which the size of the antibody response to injected sheep red blood cells was directly related to the concentration of lymphocytes in the perfusate (Ford & Gowans, 1967).

Following activation, lymphocytes (either blasts or CD45RO T lymphocytes) migrate via non-specialized EC to sites of non-immune inflammation or to non-lymphoid organs where they will be stimulated on encountering antigen. Release of inflammatory cytokines from activated T cells will induce expression of adhesion molecules on local blood vessels, some of which may be the same as those expressed by lymph node HEV. Whether these vessels go on to express full HEV phenotype and function may depend on the continual production of inflammatory cytokines, as well as other factors such as those that regulate HEV within lymphoid organs. Further studies of HEV are required to determine their precise origin and function. The formation of HEV in pathological situations could prolong, rather than resolve, inflammation since CD45RA T lymphocytes may be delivered to non-lymphoid organs via these induced vessels. Activation of naive lymphocytes will then occur in an environment that may not be adapted to tolerate the potentially harmful products of immune activation, such as cytokines, cytotoxic cells, etc. Instead of resolving the immune response by clearing antigen from these sites, the immune response may persist due to the influx of a lymphocyte population that is normally excluded from non-lymphoid organs. This is particularly important in the context of autoimmunity when the focus of the immune response is towards self, as opposed to exogenous, antigen. Self-antigen may not be readily cleared from the body and is, thus, a source of constant antigenic stimulation. The ability to inhibit lymphocyte traffic to such sites may limit the pathology associated with autoimmune disorders.

Identification and function of adhesion molecules involved in lymphocyte-EC interactions

In the following two sections I will address the roles of individual adhesion molecules implicated in lymphocyte migration. I will not give detailed information on the structure of adhesion molecules but refer the reader to original references and reviews covering the selectins, the integrins and members of the immunoglobulin superfamily (Piggott & Power, 1993; see also Chapter 3) and the mucins (Shimizu & Shaw, 1993).

Significant advances in identifying adhesion molecules on different types of EC have been made using *in vitro* models. The generation of monoclonal antibodies, following immunization with purified populations of EC, has been crucial for their functional analysis *in vitro* and *in vivo*. The expression and function of adhesion molecules on HEV involved in organ-specific homing have been studied using the frozen section assay and lymphoma cell lines which adhere preferentially to HEV in either peripheral or mucosal lymph nodes. This assay is restricted to low temperatures; therefore, it will not measure adhesive interactions between lymphocytes and HEV which depend on activation (see pp. 76–80). Following immunization with lymph node stroma, the monoclonal antibodies MECA 79 and 367 were generated and shown to identify vascular addressins on HEV. MECA 79 antigen is expressed preferentially in peripheral lymph nodes of mice and humans and has been called a peripheral addressin (Streeter, Rouse & Butcher, 1988*b*). It defines a functional carbohydrate epitope which modifies several biochemically distinct molecules synthesized by HEV, and mediates binding to L-selectin on lymphocytes (Berg *et al.*, 1991). Previous studies using the monoclonal antibody MEL-14 had shown that L-selectin on mouse lymphocytes mediated binding to peripheral lymph node HEV and migration to peripheral lymph nodes *in vivo*; the molecule was therefore called a peripheral lymph node homing receptor. Although antibodies to L-selectin do not block adhesion to mucosal lymph nodes HEV *in vitro*, lymphocyte migration to mucosal lymph nodes *in vivo* is partially inhibited (Hamann *et al.*, 1991); thus L-selectin is not strictly a peripheral homing receptor. Three ligands for L-selectin have been identified. They have been termed mucins because their protein backbones are decorated with dense arrays of O-linked sugars. One is a 50 kD sulphated glycoprotein called GlyCAM-1 (Lasky *et al.*, 1992) and the second is a glycosylated, sulphated form of CD34 (Baumhueter *et al.*, 1993); both are synthesized by HEV in peripheral lymph nodes. The third is MAdCAM-1 (Berg *et al.*, 1993) which is selectively expressed in mucosal lymph nodes (see below). It is not known if MAdCAM-1 is sulphated, but it is predicted to express O-linked sugars. The extent of O-linked glycosylation of L-selectin ligands (up to 70% for GlyCAM-1) suggests that the functional epitope(s) may be presented in an aggregated or polyvalent form for high avidity interaction. L-selectin recognition is dependent on sulphation (Imai, Lasky & Rosen, 1993) and/or sialylation of carbohydrate residues in its ligands (True *et al.*, 1990).

Monoclonal antibody MECA367 identifies the 55 kD glycoprotein MAdCAM-1 (Briskin, McEvoy & Butcher, 1993), which is expressed by HEV in mucosal LN and by non-specialized venules in the lamina propria of the gut wall in mice. As well as binding to L-selectin, MAdCAM-1 binds to $\alpha_4\beta_7$ integrin on mouse lymphoid cells (Berlin *et al.*, 1993), which has been determined in separate studies to be a mucosal lymph node homing receptor (Holzmann & Weissman, 1989); MAdCAM-1 has therefore been termed a mucosal addressin (Streeter *et al.*, 1988*a*). In addition to a mucin-like domain, MAdCAM-1 contains several other potential adhesion domains, including sequences homologous to VCAM-1 and ICAM-1. Although the functional domain has not yet been identified, by analogy with the other α_4 subunit containing integrin VLA-4, it is likely to reside in the VCAM-1 homologous region. *In vivo* studies have demonstrated a clear role for α_4 subunit containing integrins (Issekutz, 1991) and $\alpha_4\beta_7$ directly (Hamann *et al.*, 1994) in lymphocyte migration to gut-associated lymphoid organs in rodents. Whether MAdCAM-1 regulates lymphocyte migration to other mucosal sites, such as the lungs or the reproductive tract, remains to be determined. MAdCAM-1 can be induced on EC at sites of inflammation in non-mucosal tissues (O'Neill *et al.*, 1991), which suggests that its role extends beyond that in mucosal homing. The function of MAdCAM-1 in species other than the mouse is undetermined since reagents are currently not available for these studies.

Variants of CD44 on the lymphocyte surface were originally identified as homing receptors for lymph nodes and inflamed synovium in humans (Jalkanen *et al.*, 1987). Recent studies have challenged a role of CD44 in lymphocyte migration to lymph nodes *in vivo* (Camp *et al.*, 1993) and in lymphocyte binding to cultured HEV (Yang & Binns, 1993) in rodents. Other adhesion molecules have been identified on HEV such as ICAM-1 and ICAM-2, which both bind to LFA-1 on the lymphocyte surface. These molecules are expressed by HEV in peripheral and mucosal lymph nodes, as well as by non-specialized vessels, and are therefore thought to play a secondary role in organ-specific homing. In comparison with L-selectin, LFA-1 plays a less important role in lymphocyte binding to HEV *in vitro* and in lymphocyte migration to lymph nodes *in vivo* (Hamann *et al.*, 1988). LFA-1 dependent interactions may contribute to the stabilization of adhesion or to the subsequent transendothelial migration of lymphocytes that follows binding to the surface of EC (see pp. 76–81). In comparison with lymphocyte migration to lymph nodes, the molecular basis of lymphocyte migration to the spleen is poorly understood. Lymphocytes migrate from capillaries in the marginal sinus which are not related to HEV and use different adhesion pathways which depend on recognition of glycosylated molecules on the lymphocyte surface (Berg *et al.*, 1992; Weston & Parish, 1992).

The regulation of lymphocyte migration to non-lymphoid organs has been studied using a different *in vitro* model which employs primary cultures of vascular EC. In contrast to the frozen section assay, lymphocyte interactions can be measured at physiological temperature using this assay; activation-dependent adhesion will therefore be detected. Although isolation and propagation of EC from post-capillary venules (i.e. the site at which leukocytes normally extravasate) are technically demanding, significant advances have been made using EC cultured from major blood vessels, in particular, human umbilical vein (HUV). The availability of cultured EC from rodents is limited and studies in mice and rats lag behind those in humans. Although the relationship between umbilical vein EC and post-capillary EC is unclear, the use of cultured HUVEC has identified several adhesion molecules involved in lymphocyte–EC interactions. An early observation was that the cytokines IL-1, IL-4, TNF, IFN-γ and other inflammatory stimuli such as endotoxin, which are likely to be produced at sites of non-immune and/or immune inflammation, alter the adhesive capacity of cultured HUVEC for distinct populations of leukocytes either by upregulation or by *de novo* expression of distinct sets of adhesion molecules (for review see Chapter 3; and Bevilacqua, 1993). For example, LPS, IL-1 and TNF induce *de novo* expression of E-selectin (formerly ELAM-1) which mediates binding of neutrophils and a subpopulation of T lymphocytes. IFN-γ, as well as LPS, IL-1 and TNF up-regulate expression of ICAM-1, which mediates LFA-1-dependent binding of neutrophils, lymphocytes and monocytes. IL-4 as well as LPS, IL-1, TNF and IFN-γ induce VCAM-1 expression, which mediates VLA-4 dependent binding of lymphocytes and monocytes. Finally, TNF, IL-1 and LPS induce expression of a ligand for L-selectin that mediates binding of lymphocytes, neutrophils and monocytes, although adhesion was only detectable under conditions in which the integrins were inhibited, e.g. at the low temperatures used in the frozen section assay (Spertini *et al.*, 1992; Brady *et al.*, 1992). A heparin-like ligand for L-selectin, which is distinct from those expressed by HEV, has been shown in several types of non-lymphoid EC including HUVEC (Norgard-Sumnicht, Varki & Varki, 1993). These *in vitro* observations have been supported by the detection of altered expression of E-selectin, ICAM-1, VCAM-1 and MECA 79 antigen by EC in different types of inflammation in humans and other species (for review see Pober & Cotran, 1991). In addition, lymphocyte migration to hypersensitivity lesions in rodents is inhibited by antibodies to L-selectin, α_4 integrin and LFA-1 (Dawson *et al.*, 1992; Chisholm, Williams & Lobb, 1993; Scheynius, Camp & Pure, 1993). Analyses of clinical material have shown that the profile of adhesion molecules expressed by EC does not necessarily reflect the composition of the leukocytic infiltrate seen (Koch *et al.*, 1991) which suggests that additional factors regulate lymphocyte migration out of the vessel and into the inflammatory site.

Further studies are required to correlate lymphocyte migration *in vivo* with adhesion molecule expression by HEV and cultured vascular EC. Some adhesion molecules identified *in vitro* have yet to be tested *in vivo*. Of those tested in both assays, some give conflicting results. This may be due, in part, to the heterogeneity of the lymphocyte population used, e.g. peripheral blood lymphocytes versus lymphocytes collected from lymphoid organs. The roles of homing receptors and addressins need to be re-assessed since these molecular interactions may be utilized by cells other than lymphocytes and in tissues not included in their proposed site of action. In a separate approach, neutrophil interactions with inflamed blood vessels have been modelled *in vitro* using cultured HUVEC and purified adhesion molecules. Results from these studies have generated a model of neutrophil interactions with vascular EC that involves multiple, sequential adhesive events. Although not yet substantiated for lymphocyte migration either to lymph nodes or to sites of inflammation, there are striking similarities in the types of adhesion molecule already implicated in these processes, such that a similar model is likely to apply (for discussion see Butcher, 1991). In the next section I will re-assess the roles of individual adhesion molecules (including homing receptors and addressins) implicated in lymphocyte–EC interactions in the context of the multistep adhesion cascade proposed to regulate neutrophil migration.

Multistep adhesion cascade and the regulation of leukocyte migration

An important consideration has been that adhesive interactions between leukocytes and EC take place in the presence of shear stresses at the vessel wall interface induced by flowing blood. This has been addressed by measuring binding events between neutrophils and either HUVEC or immobilized adhesion molecules under flow, as opposed to static, conditions. These studies have suggested that different stages of extravasation are governed by a distinct type of adhesion molecule, and that it is the combination of adhesion molecules used that regulates the specificity of leukocyte migration rather than any one adhesion molecule alone (see Chapter 3 and Zimmerman, Prescott & McIntyre, 1992).

Rolling

The initial binding of leukocytes to the luminal surface of the vessel wall is mediated by the selectins. The restricted expression of selectins by either leukocytes or EC emphasizes the role these molecules play in leukocyte migration. Selectins recognize carbohydrate epitopes which can be displayed by more than one type of molecule on the opposing cell surface, e.g. glycoproteins, glycolipids. It is proposed that selectins mediate low affinity, high avidity, tethering interactions which support reversible interactions between leukocytes and EC in the presence of flowing blood. This adhesive interaction classically manifests itself as rolling of neutrophils in inflamed blood vessels. Once these two cell types are in close proximity, additional stimuli operate to stabilize the interaction and promote directed leukocyte migration (see next step). The most important selectin in lymphocyte migration is leukocyte (L)-selectin (formerly LECAM-1, MEL14 antigen, $gp90^{mel\text{-}14}$). Although it was originally identified as a peripheral lymph node homing receptor in the mouse, L-selectin is widely expressed by the majority of circulating neutrophils and monocytes, yet homing to lymph nodes is specific for lymphocytes. L-selectin has also been implicated in the migration of neutrophils to inflamed peritoneum (Watson, Fennie & Lasky, 1991), presumably via induced expression of ligands on EC.

How does L-selectin regulate the differential migration of lymphocytes and neutrophils? The activity of L-selectin is independently regulated on lymphocytes and neutrophils. Selectin-dependent adhesion is generally thought to be activation independent, however, the affinity of L-selectin can be upregulated by leukocyte-specific stimuli (Spertini *et al.*, 1991). As found for other adhesion molecules, the cytoplasmic tail and its interaction with the actin cytoskeleton play important roles in regulating L-selectin function (Kansas *et al.*, 1993). L-selectin on lymphocytes and neutrophils recognizes distinct ligands on EC. Neutrophil L-selectin is differentially glycosylated, enabling it to bind to the two other members of the selectin family, E-selectin (formerly ELAM-1) and P-selectin (CD62, formerly GMP-140) (Picker *et al.*, 1991), which are expressed by inflamed EC and play an important role in neutrophil migration. The less important role of L-selectin in lymphocyte migration to Peyer's patches could reflect the fact that more activated lymphocytes, on which L-selectin expression is down-regulated and other adhesion molecules are up-regulated, migrate to this site since it is under continual antigenic challenge via the gastrointestinal tract. Although lymphocytes do not roll on the luminal surface of HEV to the same extent as neutrophils roll in inflamed blood vessels, lymphocytes and HEV do undergo reversible interactions or collisions which have the hallmark of selectin dependent adhesion as demonstrated *in vitro* (Lawrence & Springer, 1991).

Of the other selectins, E-selectin has been implicated in lymphocyte migration. A subpopulation of lymphocytes which localize in inflamed skin express a molecule called cutaneous lymphocyte associated antigen (CLA; identified by mAb HECA 452). $CD4^+$ T lymphocytes which express CLA bind to E-selectin via CLA (Picker *et al.*, 1991) in an activation-independent manner (Shimizu *et al.*, 1991). Whether the CLA/E-selectin interaction represents a further category of organ-specific homing, i.e. skin homing, remains to be determined. P-selectin has not been implicated in lymphocyte–EC interactions thus far, although a genetically engineered soluble form of P-selectin binds to a subpopulation of activated $CD4^+$ T lymphocytes and regulates cytokine production by these cells (Damle *et al.*, 1992).

Triggering

This is a rapid event which occurs within 1–3 seconds of initial contact with EC, and it mediates activation-dependent changes in a second type of adhesion molecule on the leukocyte surface, the integrins (see next step). This stage is associated with spreading and crawling of neutrophils over the endothelial surface, presumably in search of an exit site. A variety of stimuli have been shown to activate neutrophils in this way and some of these are classical chemoattractants, e.g. C5a and fMLP. Integrin activating stimuli are not drawn from a single family of molecules, but range from lipids, such as platelet activating factor (PAF), to cytokines and bacterial products such as fMLP. A unifying property of these stimuli may be the intracellular signalling events that they transduce. Chemoattractants for neutrophils induce cytoskeletal-dependent shape changes associated with cell locomotion which are inhibited by pertussin toxin. Thus far, all the known receptors for chemoattractants are G-protein linked, pertussis toxin inhibitable, seven membrane-spanning receptors. A second property is that integrin-activating stimuli demonstrate selectivity towards different populations of leukocytes, and have therefore been proposed to play a crucial role in the specificity of leukocyte migration. For example, different members of the chemokine family of low molecular weight chemoattractants show selective activity towards neutrophils (e.g. IL-8) versus lymphocytes and monocytes (e.g. RANTES, MIP-1α, MIP-1β) (Schall, 1991). Some stimuli induce down-regulation of L-selectin on neutrophils, which is proposed to facilitate integrin-mediated adhesion and/or subsequent transendothelial migration. To function at the luminal surface of the blood vessel, integrin-activating stimuli must be presented there in a cell-associated form. Chemokines contain binding sites for glycosaminoglycans and can, therefore, be immobilized on the luminal surface of EC by proteoglycans, such as heparin sulphate (Tanaka *et al.*, 1993*b*). Integrin-activating stimuli do not have to be synthesized by EC, although some chemokines are, but can be produced in the immediate microenvironment by bacteria or activated mononuclear cells as long as they have access to the surface of blood vessels for efficient activation of leukocyte integrins. A particularly effective stimulus for integrin activation on T lymphocytes is engagement of the antigen receptor (Shimizu *et al.*, 1990). As discussed above, there is little evidence to implicate processed antigen on the surface of EC in lymphocyte extravasation *in vivo*. However, the availability of transgenic mice expressing antigen receptors of defined specificities for peptide should allow this possibility to be tested. Thus far, two stimuli have been shown to activate integrins on lymphocytes. Antibodies to CD31 (PECAM-1) increase the affinity of VLA-4 on human T cell subsets (Tanaka *et al.*, 1992). The chemokine, MIP-1β, increases the affinity of VLA-4 for VCAM-1 on human CD8$^+$ T cells and is particularly effective when immobilized to a proteoglycan modified form of CD44 (Tanaka *et al.*, 1993*a*). In a separate study, EC cultured from rat lymph node HEV (see pp. 81–88) synthesize a soluble factor which induces pertussis toxin-inhibitable, locomotor morphology in unactivated lymphocytes, although its effect on integrins was not determined (Harris, 1991). The potential roles of these and other stimuli in the migration of lymphocytes to lymphoid organs and sites of inflammation remain to be determined.

Stable adhesion

This step completely arrests leukocytes from flowing blood, and allows optimal delivery of signals that stimulate migration out of the vessel wall. As discussed above, the adhesion of leukocytes to EC is mediated by integrins which have already been activated on the leukocyte surface. The ability of leukocyte integrins to exist in inactive and active states is important for interactions with vascular EC since it allows leukocytes to circulate in a non-adhesive state, but be recruited to the luminal surface of EC at sites where an appropriate integrin-activating stimulus is expressed. The switch between the two is a rapid event that does not depend on gene activation or protein synthesis; rapid reversal of an adhesive event would allow the leukocyte to move along a surface and on to the next surface during the process of extravasation. Integrin activation is an example of 'inside-out signalling' in that the conformation of an integrin at the cell surface is regulated by signals generated inside the cell by unrelated cell surface receptors (Springer, 1990). There are several possible mechanisms to explain activation of integrins including clustering in the cell membrane, conformational changes in the extracellular domain and association of cytoplasmic tails with cyto-skeletal components, all of which could induce higher affinity binding to ligand. As well as 'inside-out signalling', integrin activation may be induced by post-ligand binding events, or by alterations in divalent cation concentration at the cell surface. Research into mechanisms of integrin activation is substantial and beyond the scope of this chapter; I refer the reader to excellent reviews on the subject (Humphries, Mould & Tuckwell, 1993; Mobley, Reynolds & Shimizu, 1993).

Circulating lymphocytes constitutively express several members of the β_1 (VLA) integrin family including VLA-4, VLA-5 and VLA-6, as well as the β_2 integrin, LFA-1. The absolute levels of all these adhesion molecules are raised on CD45RO T lymphocytes in humans and sheep, and are proposed to regulate the migration pathways of these activated lymphocytes *in vivo*, although there is no direct evidence to support this hypothesis. The importance of β_2 integrins in neutrophil migration is supported by clinical data from patients with β_2 integrin deficiency (leukocyte adhesion deficiency – LAD), in which neutrophils fail to migrate to sites of inflammation. In comparison, LFA-1 is not absolutely required for lymphocyte migration since lymphocytes are found in lymph nodes and in inflammatory sites of LAD patients (Schwartz *et al.*, 1990). The β_1 integrin, VLA-4, has been implicated in lymphocyte migration to inflammatory sites via recognition of VCAM-1, which is induced on inflamed EC. The integrin(s) which would be predicted to regulate the migration of unactivated lymphocytes to lymph nodes via HEV (according to this model) has not yet been identified, although we have presented evidence in support of VLA-4 and VLA-5 from *in vitro* studies (see pp. 81–88). A VLA-4 related integrin, $\alpha_4\beta_7$, mediates homing of activated lymphocytes to mucosal lymph nodes; however, this integrin has not been implicated in homing to peripheral lymph nodes. Intraepithelial lymphocytes in the gut wall express a related integrin, which comprises the β_7 subunit associated with a novel α chain, α_{IEL} (Kilshaw & Murant, 1991). It is not clear whether this integrin regulates migration from the blood or subsequent localization of these lymphocytes in the epithelial lining. Leukocyte integrins have been referred to as activation-dependent adhesion molecules; however, some integrins function in the frozen section assay (Hamann *et al.*, 1988). It may therefore be more accurate to think of integrins in different states of activity, rather than in inactive and active conformations.

According to this model, these three steps are sufficient to mediate the adhesion of different types of leukocyte to EC that regulates their differential migration into tissues. I would now like to consider the events following adhesion that result in extravasation as the fourth step of the model.

Extravasation

This is a complex event which is poorly understood. The adhesion and de-adhesion of leukocytes to EC, subendothelial pericytes and the extracellular basal lamina may all be manifestations of one process of integrin-mediated adhesion under the control of a chemoattractant. Since the β_1 integrins recognize extracellular matrix components as well as cell surface ligands, one can envisage a role for these adhesion molecules in the migration of lymphocytes across the vessel wall and into the tissues. Thus, once initiated, extravasation is an automatic consequence of stable adhesion. However, there is evidence that migration across the vessel wall is regulated independently of adhesion. The time taken to migrate to the basal lamina of HEV is significantly longer in athymic animals in comparison with their euthymic littermates (Fossum *et al.*, 1988), although these blood vessels express similar levels of some adhesion molecules (Picker & Butcher, 1992). Antibody inhibition studies have shown that lymphocyte binding to the surface of HUVEC is mediated via VLA-4/VCAM-1 whereas transendothelial migration is mediated by LFA-1/ICAM-1 recognition (Oppenheimer-Marks *et al.*, 1991). A crucial event in extravasation must be the intracellular signalling pathways that regulate leukocyte locomotion, although these are poorly understood. For example, there may be cross-talk between adhesion molecules on the lymphocyte surface, analogous to the co-stimulation of T lymphocytes by antigen receptor and accessory molecules, which amplifies the response by activating locomotor capacity in lymphocytes. The selective migration of lymphocytes may therefore be governed, in part, by the intracellular signalling pathways that regulate locomotion in lymphocytes.

Discussion of the model

Lymphocytes, and not other leukocytes, are bound to the luminal surface of HEV in histological sections of lymph nodes. Lymphocytes are therefore probably selected for extravasation by adhesive interactions with the luminal surface of HEV, as proposed in the multistep adhesion cascade for neutrophil migration. There may be subtle differences in the integrins and/or activating stimuli (chemoattractants) used by naive versus activated lymphocytes, or B versus T-cell subpopulations which would regulate their differential migration described on pp. 67–72. Additional adhesion molecules have already been identified and/or implicated in lymphocyte–EC interactions (Toyama-Sorimachi, Miyake & Miyasaka, 1993; Salmi, Kalino & Jalkanen, 1993) but their precise roles remain to be determined. It is possible that the requirement for selectins in initial binding, and integrins in adhesion strengthening, may not be absolute. For example, CD44, which has also been implicated in lymphocyte migration, can interact directly with the cytoskeleton. CD44 therefore may perform a similar function to integrins in lymphocyte extravasation. E-selectin has been shown to act as a 'tethered chemoattractant' for neutrophils, in that it directly activates β_2 integrins via an unidentified ligand on the neutrophil surface (Leo *et al.*, 1991). In contrast to other adhesion molecules, GlyCAM-1 does not have a transmembrane domain. GlyCAM-1 secreted by HEV may function as a chemoattractant, inducing locomotor activity in responding lymphocytes. Several adhesion molecules which span the plasma membrane of lymphocytes or EC are detectable in plasma. The potential roles of soluble forms of these adhesion molecules in regulating leukocyte migration remain to be determined (Gearing & Newman, 1993). Although further work is required to understand the molecular basis of lymphocyte extravasation, the multistep adhesion cascade which regulates the selective adhesion of neutrophils to EC will probably be directly applicable to the lymphocyte. A prediction from this model is that adhesion molecules do not have to be selectively expressed by lymphocytes or by EC in particular organs, since it is the combination of adhesion molecules and chemoattractants that regulates the specificity of leukocyte migration. This model allows redundance in the use of adhesion molecules since more than one molecule may perform the same function.

An *in vitro* model of lymphocyte migration from the blood into lymph nodes

The success of using cultured vascular endothelial cells to model neutrophil–EC interactions prompted us to study lymphocyte–HEV interactions using a

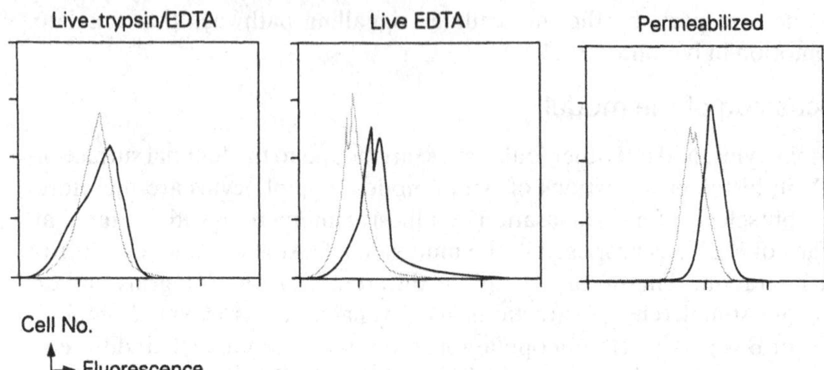

Fig. 4.1. Expression of GlyCAM-1 by cultured high endothelial cells. HEC were detached from tissue culture dishes by incubation in 0.025% EDTA in PBS for 10 min at 37 °C. Live cells were analysed for cell surface expression of GlyCAM-1; fixed and permeabilized cells for intracellular localization of GlyCAM-1. Cells were stained with a rabbit anti-peptide antisera to mouse GlyCAM-1 (Lasky *et al.*, 1992) and analysed by flow cytometry. GlyCAM-1 was detected on the surface of the majority of HEC as shown in the middle panel and the number of positive cells did not increase following permeabilization (right-hand panel). To check the specificity of GlyCAM-1 staining, HEC were incubated with 0.1% trypsin for 10 min prior to staining (left-hand panel). GlyCAM-1 was no longer detectable at the cell surface since it is degraded by trypsin. Solid lines: anti-peptide antisera to GlyCAM-1. Broken lines: rabbit IgG. Profiles show log fluorescence (10^0 to 10^4 channels on *x*-axis and cell number (0 to 500) on *y*-axis.

similar model. High endothelial cells (HEC) have been isolated from rat lymph nodes and propagated in long-term culture to study the regulation of HEV phenotype and interactions with lymphocytes. Using the rapid, selective uptake of inorganic sulphate to identify HEC, enriched cultures were isolated by collagenase digestion of peripheral (cervical or popliteal) lymph nodes from adult rats. As found for other types of EC, HEC demonstrate substantial proliferative capacity and can be maintained for up to 30 cell doublings after isolation (Ager, 1990). This provides large numbers of cells derived originally from lymph node high endothelium for subsequent analysis *in vitro*. Although maintained in the absence of a lymphoid microenvironment, cultured HEC express the HEV specific molecule GlyCAM-1 (Fig. 4.1), which is one of several sulphated metabolites synthesized by HEV. Since GlyCAM-1 expression is normally restricted to peripheral lymph nodes, these results suggest that high endothelium in adult animals is irreversibly committed to the phenotype of the host lymph node. Recent studies of vascular addressin expression *in vivo* support this proposal and demonstrate that commitment occurs during the late neonatal period (Mebius *et al.*, 1993).

Under static assay conditions, between 20- and 50-fold more lymphocytes adhere to cultured HEC than to either aortic EC, or aortic fibroblasts. In addition, cultured HEC actively support the transendothelial migration of lymphocytes (Ager & Mistry, 1988). This is a rapid event detectable within five minutes of plating lymphocytes on to cultured HEC and is dependent on a viable endothelial layer. In comparison, lymphocytes do not migrate across aortic EC layers or into three-dimensional biological matrices, such as type I collagen gels. Pulse-chase analyses using allotype marked lymphocytes have shown clearly that lymphocytes which bind to the surface of HEC (type I cells) and those which migrate (type II cells) represent one population at different stages of interaction with the HEC layer instead of two independent populations. In addition, up to 80% of lymphocytes bound to the surface of HEC migrate across the endothelial layer (Hourihan, Allen & Ager, 1993). The use of cultured HEC therefore allows the events following adhesion (i.e. step four of the model) to be analysed. Static adhesion assays allow analysis of triggering and stable adhesion (steps two and three), but flow conditions will be required to analyse selectin dependent interactions. We have used lymphocytes collected either from the thoracic duct, or directly from lymph nodes for these studies; no major differences are seen between the interactions of these two lymphocyte populations with cultured HEC, except that the levels of lymphocyte binding and migration are slightly higher for lymph node cells. The majority of these cells are not in cell cycle and analysis of HEC-adherent lymphocytes shows that at least 80% are resting, the remainder being lymphoblasts which are enriched by two–three fold. HEC-adherent lymphocytes comprise a mixture of $CD4^+$ and $CD8^+$ T cells as well as B cells. In comparison with the lymphocyte population plated, B cells are slightly enriched and $CD4^+$ T cells are slightly depleted, which suggests that migration of these lymphocyte subsets may be regulated independently. Consistent with the pulse-chase analysis, lymphocyte subsets are equally distributed in the surface bound and migrated populations (Ager & Mistry, 1988). This observation supports the proposal that lymphocyte subpopulations are selected for migration by adhesion to the surface of EC.

Lymphocyte binding and migration can be up-regulated by cytokine pretreatment of the endothelial layer; however, individual cytokines differ in their effects. IFN-γ, TNF-α and IL-1β pretreatment of HEC increase the total number of lymphocytes (type I + type II cells) that adhere, IFN-γ having the greatest effect. However, only IFN-γ and TNF-α increase the number of lymphocytes that migrate across HEC layers, again IFN-γ having the greater effect (Fig. 4.2). IL-1β does not affect the ability of HEC to support migration (May & Ager, 1992). These results show that binding to

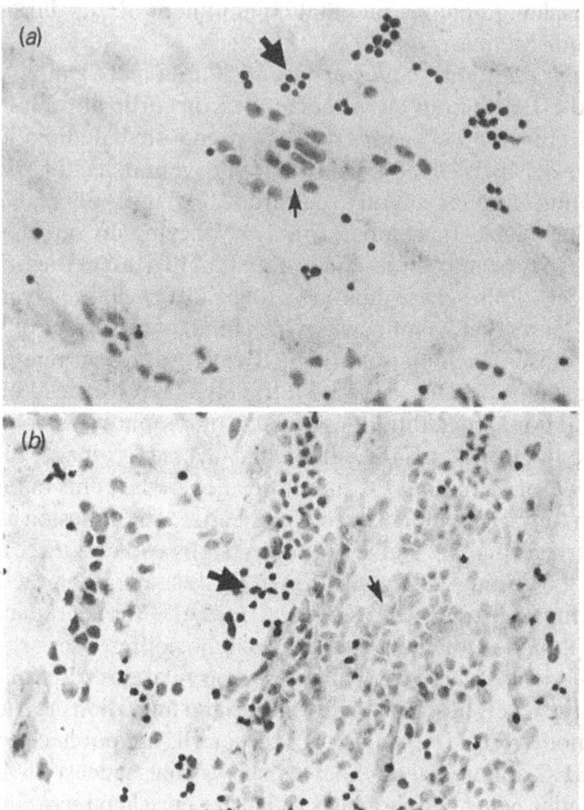

Fig. 4.2. Effect of interferon-γ on lymphocyte binding and trans-endothelial migration. Rat lymphocytes were incubated with either untreated (A) or IFN-γ treated (B) HEC for 60 min at 37 °C as previously described (May & Ager, 1992). HEC-adherent lymphocytes were identified as either type I, surface bound cells (large arrows) or type II, migrated cells (small arrows). IFN-γ up-regulates the total number of lymphocytes that adhere to cultured HEC (types I and II), but preferentially increases the number that migrate across the endothelial layer.

the surface of HEC and migration across the HEC layer are regulated independently. Although cultured HEC support a basal level of lymphocyte migration, this can be increased by cytokines, which may mimic a stimulus for HEV activity *in vivo*. We have not performed similar studies on non-specialized EC in the rat, however, results using HUVEC have documented increased transendothelial migration of lymphocytes following pre-treatment with both IFN-γ and IL-1 (Oppenheimer-Marks, Davis & Lipsky,

1990). The relative effects of these two cytokines were not determined in these studies, and therefore it is difficult to compare the results directly with our own.

Up to 70% of lymphocytes adhering to untreated and IFN-γ treated HEC do so via VLA-4 mediated recognition of VCAM-1 (May *et al.*, 1993). Cultured HEC constitutively express VCAM-1, its expression is up-regulated by IFN-γ and antibodies to VCAM-1 inhibit adhesion to the same extent as antibodies to VLA-4. HEV in rat lymph nodes also express significant levels of VCAM-1. These results suggest that this adhesive pathway may regulate the constitutive migration of unactivated lymphocytes to lymphoid organs. Since unactivated lymphocytes bind to immobilized ligands (May *et al.*, 1993), VLA-4 may adopt a partially active conformation on these cells; thus this integrin may not require a secondary stimulus (i.e. step 2) to mediate adhesion to HEC. An early finding using this model was that CS1 peptide, which encodes an alternative VLA-4 binding site in fibronectin, preferentially inhibited lymphocyte binding to the surface of cultured HEC, suggesting that an endothelial ligand may be a cell surface form of fibronectin. Subsequent studies have shown that CS1 peptide inhibits the binding of lymphocytes to immobilized VCAM-1 protein (May *et al.*, 1993). Detailed analysis reveals that CS1 peptide competitively inhibits binding of solubilized VLA-4 to VCAM-1 (Makarem *et al.*, 1994). These results suggest that CS1 peptide mimics an adhesion site in VCAM-1 which may be located in immunoglobulin domains one or four, which have both been shown to support VLA-4-dependent binding (Osborn, Vassallo & Benjamin, 1992).

Thus far, the VLA-4/VCAM-1 adhesion pathway has been implicated in the migration of lymphocytes to inflammatory sites. In a specific recall response in humans, the kinetics of induced VCAM-1, but not ICAM-1, correlated with T cells infiltrating the intestinal wall of coeliac patients following antigen challenge (Ensari *et al.*, 1993). Antibodies to VLA-4 inhibit development of EAE in rats (Yednock *et al.*, 1992), and contact hypersensitivity in mice (Ferguson & Kupper, 1993) following adoptive transfer of antigen specific T cells, although these studies did not demonstrate inhibition of lymphocyte migration directly. If VLA-4/VCAM-1 mediates lymphocyte migration to lymph nodes as well as to sites of inflammation, attempts to block this pathway in order to limit inflammation may have unwanted, immunosuppressive side-effects.

Other integrins on lymphocytes have been implicated in interactions with HEC. Antibodies to VLA-5 inhibit the adhesion of human PBL to a slightly greater extent than anti-VLA-4 antibodies or CS1 peptide. Analysis of type I and type II lymphocytes showed that, in comparison with antibodies to VLA-4, migration was preferentially blocked by antibodies to VLA-5, which suggests that fibronectin in the HEC layer may regulate the transendothelial migration of lymphocytes (Szekanecz, Humphries & Ager, 1992). Studies of LFA-1-dependent interactions have given equivocal results. Although cultured HEC constitutively express high levels of ICAM-1, antibodies to ICAM-1 or LFA-1 do not inhibit the adhesion of unactivated rat lymphocytes, even following IFN-γ activation of HEC (May & Ager, 1992; May *et al.*, 1993). In contrast, the adhesion of human PBL to rat HEC is partially inhibited by antibodies to β_2 integrins, although the effects were less than those with anti-β_1 integrin antibodies (Szekanecz *et al.*, 1992). Studies of human PBL interactions with HUVEC have shown that lymphocyte migration across the EC layer is restricted to previously activated lymphocytes and that it is blocked by antibodies to LFA-1. In fact, IL-2 activated rat lymphocytes do show LFA-1-dependent adhesion to cultured HEC (Pankonin, Reipert & Ager, 1992). It is possible that the differences we have seen between human PBL and rat lymphocytes reflect the numbers of recently activated lymphocytes in these two populations of cells. Although we have not determined the effects of antibodies to LFA-1 on the transendothelial migration of rat lymphocytes directly, the lack of effect on total lymphocyte adhesion to HEC suggests that unactivated lymphocytes employ either alternative or additional integrin(s) to migrate into lymph nodes.

Transendothelial migration of lymphocytes is not an automatic consequence of binding to the surface of HEC (Hourihan *et al.*, 1993). The number of lymphocytes that migrate is directly related to the concentration of lymphocytes plated on to the HEC layer. Lymphocytes which have already bound to the upper surface of HEC detach, rather than migrate across the endothelial layer, when non-adherent lymphocytes are removed by washing. If a chemoattractant is involved in this process, these results suggest that its activity may be regulated by lymphocyte–EC interactions in addition to those mediated by integrins. To study the mechanism of transendothelial migration, type I and type II lymphocytes have been collected and their properties compared. Type II lymphocytes show a three–four fold increase in ability to migrate across cultured HEC and this correlates with a transient increase in the affinity of VLA-4 for CS1 peptide. The integrin-activating stimulus remains to be determined, but our results suggest that it is tightly associated with the HEC surface and that it will be up-regulated by cytokines such as IFN-γ and TNF, but not IL-1. We suggest that it functions as a crucial migration signal that ensures the successful extravasation of lymphocytes following adhesion to the luminal surface of HEV. Of the integrin-activating stimuli identified for lymphocytes, engagement of CD31 on the lymphocyte surface is an unlikely candidate, since expression of CD31 is not a prerequisite for transendothelial migration (Bird *et al.*, 1993). We have been unable to up-regulate VLA-4 affinity by soluble extracts from cultured HEC; the tight association with the HEC surface suggests that it could be an immobilized chemokine. Further studies

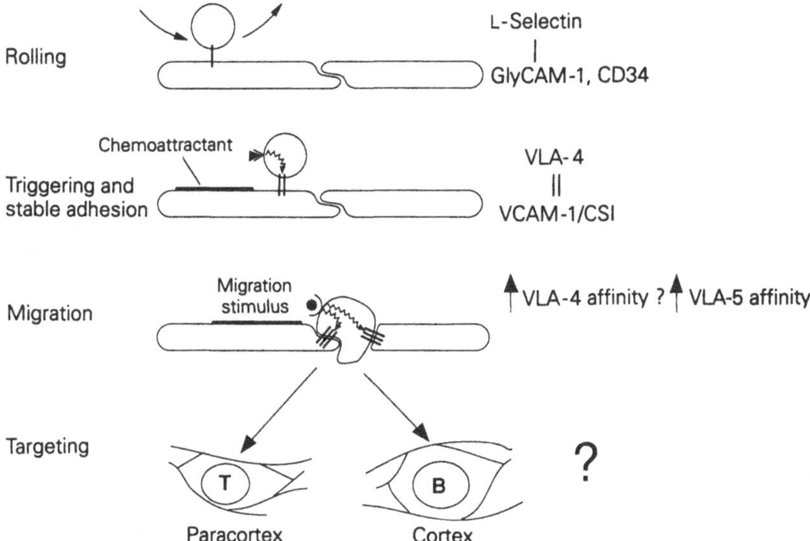

Fig. 4.3. Proposed model of lymphocyte interactions with lymph node high endothelium. The multistep adhesion cascade which regulates neutrophil interactions with inflamed EC is directly applicable to lymphocyte–HEV interactions. Studies using cultured HEC show that adhesion of unactivated lymphocytes to the luminal surface is mediated by VLA-4 recognition of a CS1 peptide-like adhesion site in VCAM-1. Transendothelial migration of lymphocytes is mediated via an increase in the affinity of VLA-4, and possibly VLA-5, following contact with the endothelial layer. The proposed migration stimulus may be analogous to the chemoattractant which triggers stable adhesion according to this model. The molecular basis of the differential migration of T and B lymphocytes, once they have entered lymphoid organs, is unknown.

are required to identify this stimulus, and to determine whether it is different from that utilized by lymphocytes to migrate to sites of inflammation. The altered adhesive capacity of lymphocytes following interactions with HEC may regulate the transendothelial migration of lymphocytes, in that β_1 integrins other than VLA-4 are also activated to bind ligands in the extracellular matrix underlying HEC, resulting in net movement across the endothelial layer.

Results using cultured HEC suggest that the multistep adhesion cascade proposed to regulate neutrophil migration is directly applicable to lymphocyte–HEV interactions (Fig. 4.3). VLA-4 is, at least, partially active on rat lymphocytes and may support some binding of lymphocytes to HEV in flowing blood, although binding will be increased by a chemoattractant. We propose that an integrin-activating stimulus operates on lymphocytes following contact with the surface of HEC and increases the affinity of VLA-4 and, possibly VLA-5, to mediate migration across the endothelial layer. The proposed migration stimulus may be analogous to a chemoattractant in this model. Further studies are required to determine the role of L-selectin/GlyCAM-1 interaction but we assume that it operates prior to integrins in this *in vitro* model.

As discussed earlier, the function of HEC is to deliver lymphocytes to APC in the lymph node. The altered adhesive capacity of lymphocytes following migration across HEC may mediate subsequent contact with APC. It is known that lymphocytes cluster with APC and that this event is crucial for the subsequent selection of antigen-specific lymphocytes. The molecular basis of this adhesive interaction is undetermined (Steinman, 1991).

General discussion

The critical role of vascular endothelium in the immune response has been discussed. This is dependent on the ability of EC to deliver unactivated lymphocytes to lymphoid organs for antigen recognition and activated lymphocytes to non-lymphoid organs and sites of inflammation for antigen elimination. When antigen is not completely cleared from the body, such as in autoimmune diseases, the ability to manipulate lymphocyte migration to involved sites may limit pathology. The identification of stimuli that induce vascular changes associated with HEV in these sites may also prove a useful way of controlling inflammation. Much attention has been paid to the adhesive interactions between lymphocytes and EC which mediate initial binding to the blood vessel surface, but further work is required to determine the molecular basis of lymphocyte migration across the vessel wall into lymphoid organs and sites of inflammation. The identification of adhesion molecules and chemoattractants that regulate lymphocyte migration will be important for the rational design of anti-inflammatory drugs that do not affect lymphocyte recirculation and, therefore, have immunosuppressive effects. The widespread use of some adhesion molecules by cells other than lymphocytes will limit their potential as selective inhibitors of lymphocyte migration. The apparently overlapping function of some adhesion molecules warrants further studies to identify which, if any, are redundant. The use of transgenes and targeted gene disruption in experimental animals should identify the precise roles of individual adhesion molecules in the migration of lymphocytes.

References

Ager, A. (1990). Isolation and culture of high endothelial venule endothelium from rat lymph nodes. In Warren, J. ed., *Endothelium: An Introduction to Current Research*. pp. 273–293, Wiley-Liss, Inc.

Ager, A. & Humphries, M. J. (1990). Use of synthetic peptides to probe lymphocyte-high endothelial cell interactions. Lymphocytes recognise a ligand on the endothelial surface which contains the CS1 adhesion motif. *International Immunology*, **2**, 921–8.

Ager, A. & Mistry, S. (1988). Interactions between lymphocytes and cultured high endothelial cells: an *in vitro* model of lymphocyte migration across high endothelial venule endothelium. *European Journal of Immunology*, **18**, 1265–74.

Allison, J. P. & Havran, W. L. (1991). The immunobiology of T cells with invariant $\gamma\delta$ antigen receptors. *Annual Review in Immunology*, **9**, 679–705.

Anderson, N. D., Anderson, A. O. & Wyllie, R. G. (1975). Microvascular changes in lymph nodes draining skin allografts. *American Journal of Pathology*, **81**, 131–53.

Anderson, N. D., Anderson, A. O. & Wyllie, R. G. (1976). Specialised structure and metabolic activities of high endothelial venules in rat lymphatic tissues. *Immunology*, **31**, 455–73.

Bargatze, R. F. & Butcher, E. C. (1993). Rapid G protein-regulated activation event involved in lymphocyte binding to high endothelial venules. *Journal of Experimental Medicine*, **178**, 367–72.

Baumhueter, S., Singer, M. S., Henzel, W., Hemmerich, S., Renz, M., Rosen, S. D. & Lasky, L. A. (1993). Binding of L-selectin to the vascular sialomucin CD34. *Science*, **262**, 436–8.

Berg, E. L., Robinson, M. K., Warnock, R. A. & Butcher, E. C. (1991). The human peripheral lymph node addressin is a ligand for LECAM-1, the peripheral lymph node homing receptor. *Journal of Cell Biology*, **114**, 343–9.

Berg, E. L., McEvoy, L. M., Berlin, C., Bargatze, R. F. & Butcher, E. C. (1993). L-Selectin mediated lymphocyte rolling on MAdCAM-1. *Nature*, **366**, 695–8.

Berg, van den T. K., Breve, J. J. P., Damoiseaux, J. G. M. C., Dopp, E. A., Kelm, S., Crocker, P. R., Dijkstra, C. D. & Kraal, G. (1992). Sialoadhesion in macrophages: its identification as a lymphocyte adhesion molecule. *Journal of Experimental Medicine*, **176**, 647–53.

Bevilacqua, M. P. (1993). Endothelial–leucocyte adhesion molecules. *Annual Review in Immunology*, **11**, 767–804.

Berlin, C., Berg, E. L., Briskin, M. J., Andrew, D. P., Kilshaw, P. J., Holzmann, B., Weissman, I. L., Hamann, A. & Butcher, E. C. (1993). $\alpha_4\beta_7$ Integrin mediates lymphocyte binding to the mucosal vascular addressin MAdCAM-1. *Cell*, **74**, 185–95.

Bird, I. N., Spragg, J. H., Ager, A. & Matthews, N. (1993). Studies of lymphocyte transendothelial migration: analysis of migrated cell phenotypes with regard to CD31 (PECAM-1), CD45RA and CD45RO. *Immunology*, **80**, 553–60.

Bjerknes, M., Chang, H. & Ottoway, C. A. (1986). Dynamics of lymphocyte–endothelial interactions *in vivo*. *Science*, **231**, 402–5.

Brady, H. R., Spertini, O., Jimenez, W., Brenner, B. M., Marsden, P. A. & Tedder, T. F. (1992). Neutrophils, monocytes and lymphocytes bind to cytokine-activated kidney glomerular endothelial cells through L-selectin *in vitro*. *Journal of Immunology*, **149**, 2437–44.

Briskin, M. J., McEvoy, L. M. & Butcher, E. C. (1993). MAdCAM-1 has homology to immunoglobulin and mucin-like adhesion receptors and to IgA1. *Nature*, **363**, 461–4.

Butcher, E. C. (1991). Leucocyte–endothelial cell recognition: three (or more) steps to specificity and diversity. *Cell*, 67, 1033–6.

Cahill, R. N. P., Poskitt, D. C., Frost, D. C. & Trnka, Z. (1977). Two distinct pools of recirculating T lymphocytes: migratory characteristics of nodal and intestinal lymphocytes. *Journal of Experimental Medicine*, **145**, 420–8.

Cahill, R. N. P., Poskitt, D. C., Hay, J. B., Heren, I. & Trnka, Z. (1979). The migration of lymphocytes in the fetal lamb. *European Journal of Immunology*, **9**, 251–3.

Camp, R. L., Scheynius, A., Johansson, C. & Pure, E. (1993). CD44 is necessary for optimal contact allergic responses but is not required for normal leucocyte extravasation. *Journal of Experimental Medicine*, **178**, 497–507.

Chisholm, P. L., Williams, C. A. & Lobb, R. R. (1993). Monoclonal antibodies to the integrin α_4 subunit inhibit the murine contact hypersensitivity response. *European Journal of Immunology*, **23**, 682–8.

Damle, N. K., Klussman, K., Dietsch, M. T., Motragheghpar, N. & Aruffo, A. (1992). GMP-140 (P-selectin/CD62) binds to chronically stimulated but not resting $CD4^+$ T lymphocytes and regulates their production of proinflammatory cytokines. *European Journal of Immunology*, **22**, 1789–93.

Daynes, R. A., Aranco, B. A., Dowell, T. A., Huang, K. & Dudley, D. (1990). Regulation of murine lymphokine production *in vivo*. III. The lymphoid tissue microenvironment exerts regulatory influences over T helper cell function. *Journal of Experimental Medicine*, **171**, 979–96.

Dawson, J., Sedgwick, A. D., Edwards, J. C. W. & Lees, P. (1992). The monoclonal antibody MEL-14 can block lymphocyte migration into a site of chronic inflammation. *European Journal of Immunology*, **22**, 1647–50.

Drayson, M. T. (1986). The entry of lymphocytes into stimulated lymph nodes: the site of selection of alloantigen-specific cells. *Transplantation*, **41**, 745–51.

Drayson, M. T., Smith, M. E. & Ford, W. L. (1981). The sequence of changes in blood flow and lymphocyte influx to stimulated rat lymph nodes. *Immunology*, **44**, 125–33.

Ensari, A., Ager, A., Marsh, M. N., Morgan, S. & Moriarty, K. J. (1993). Time-course of adhesion molecule expression in rectal mucosa of gluten-sensitive subjects after gluten challenge. *Clinical Experimental Immunology*, **92**, 303–7.

Ewijk, W. van, Brons, N. H. C. & Rozing, J. (1975). Scanning electron microscopy of homing and recirculating lymphocyte populations. *Cellular Immunology*, **19**, 245–61.

Ferguson, T. A. & Kupper, T. S. (1993). Antigen-independent processes in antigen-specific immunity. *Journal of Immunology*, **150**, 1172–82.

Ford, W. L. (1975). Lymphocyte migration and immune responses. *Progress in Allergy* Vol. 19, pp. 1–59 Basel: Karger.

Ford, W. L. & Gowans, J. L. (1967). The role of lymphocytes in antibody formation. II. The influence of lymphocyte migration on antibody formation in the isolated, perfused spleen. *Proceedings of the Royal Society B*, **168**, 244–62.

Fossum, S., Smith, M. E. & Ford, W. L. (1983). The recirculation of T and B lymphocytes in the athymic, nude rat. *Scandinavian Journal of Immunology*, **17**, 551–7.

Freemont, A. J (1988). Functional and biosynthetic changes in endothelial cells of vessels in chronically inflamed tissues: evidence for endothelial control of lymphocyte entry into diseased tissues. *Journal of Pathology* **155**, 225–30.

Freemont, A. J. & Ford, W. L (1985). Functional and morphological changes in post-capillary venules in relation to lymphocyte infiltration into BCG-induced granulomata in rat skin. *Journal of Pathology*, **147**, 1–12.

Gearing, A. J. H. & Newman, W. (1993). Circulating adhesion molecules in disease. *Immunology Today*, **14**, 506–12.

Gowans, J. L. (1959). The recirculation of lymphocytes from blood to lymph in the rat. *Journal of Physiology*, **146**, 54–69.

Gowans, J. L. & Knight, E. J. (1964). The route of recirculation of lymphocytes in the rat. *Proceedings of the Royal Society B*, **195**, 257–82.

Griscelli, C., Vassalli, P. & McCluskey, R. (1969). The distribution of large, dividing lymph node cells in syngeneic rats after intravenous injection. *Journal of Experimental Medicine*, **130**, 1427–51.

Hall, J. G., Hopkins, J. & Orlors, E. (1977). Studies on the lymphocytes of sheep. III. Destination of lymph borne immunoblasts in relation to their tissue of origin. *European Journal of Immunology*, **7**, 30–7.

Hamann, A., Andrew, D. P., Jablonski-Westrich, D., Holzmann, B. & Butcher, E. C. (1994). The role of α_4 integrins in lymphocyte homing to mucosal tissues *in vivo*. *Journal of Immunology*, **152**, 3282–93.

Hamann, A., Jablonski-Westrich, D., Duivestijn, A. M., Butcher, E. C., Baisch, H., Harder, R. & Thiele, H-G. (1988). Evidence of an accessory role of LFA-1 in lymphocyte-high endothelial cell interaction during homing. *Journal of Immunology*, **190**, 693–9.

Hamann, A., Jablonski-Westrich, D., Jonas, P. & Thiele, H-G. (1991). Homing receptors re-examined: mouse LECAM-1 is involved in lymphocyte migration to gut-associated lymphoid tissue. *European Journal of Immunology*, **21**, 2925–9.

Harris, H. (1991). The stimulation of lymphocyte mobility by cultured high endothelial cells and its inhibition by pertussis toxin. *International Immunology*, **3**, 535–42.

Hendriks, H. R., Duivestijn, A. M. & Kraal, G. (1987). Rapid decrease in lymphocyte adherence to high endothelial venules in lymph nodes deprived of afferent lymphatic venules. *European Journal of Immunology*, **17**, 1691–5.

Holzmann, B. & Weissman, I. L. (1989). Peyer's patch specific lymphocyte homing receptors consist of a VLA-4 like α chain associated with either of two integrin β chains, one of which is novel. *EMBO Journal*, **8**, 1735–41.

Hourihan, H., Allen, T. D. & Ager, A. (1993). Lymphocyte migration across high endothelium is associated with increases in $\alpha_4\beta_1$ integrin (VLA-4) affinity. *Journal of Cell Science*, **104**, 1049–59.

Humphries, M. J., Mould, A. P. & Tuckwell, D. S. (1993). Dynamic aspects of adhesion receptor function – integrins twist and shout. *BioEssays*, **15**, 391–7.

Husband, A. J. & Gowans, J. L. (1978). The origin and antigen dependent distribution of IgA-containing cells in the intestine. *Journal of Experimental Medicine*, **148**, 1146–60.

Imai, Y., Lasky, L. A. & Rosen, S. D. (1993). Sulphation requirement for GlyCAM-1, an endothelial ligand for L-selectin. *Nature*, **361**, 555–7.

Issekutz, T. B. (1991). Inhibition of *in vivo* lymphocyte migration to inflammation and homing to lymphoid tissues by the TA-2 monoclonal antibody. A likely role for VLA-4 *in vivo*. *Journal of Immunology*, **147**, 4178–84.

Jalkanen, S., Bargatze, R. F., de los Toyes, J. & Butcher, E. C. (1987). Lymphocyte recognition of high endothelium: antibodies to distinct epitopes of an 85–95 kD glycoprotein antigen differentially inhibit lymphocyte binding to lymph node, mucosal, or synovial endothelial cells. *Journal of Cell Biology*, **105**, 893–990.

Kansas, G. S., Ley, K., Munro, J. M. & Tedder, T. F. (1993). Regulation of leucocyte rolling and adhesion to high endothelial venules through the cytoplasmic domain of L-selectin. *Journal of Experimental Medicine*, **177**, 833–8.

Kilshaw, P. J. & Murant, S. J. (1991). Expression and regulation of β_7 (β_p) integrins on mouse lymphocytes: relevance to the mucosal immune system. *European Journal of Immunology*, **21**, 2591–7.

Koch, A. E., Burrows, J. C., Haines, K. G., Carlos, T. M., Harlan, J. M., Joseph, S. & Leibovich, S. (1991). Immunolocalisation of endothelial and leucocyte adhesion molecules in human rheumatoid and osteoarthritic synovial tissues. *Laboratory Investigations*, **64**, 313–20.

Kraal, G., Weissman, I. L. & Butcher, E. C. (1983). Differences in the *in vivo*, distribution and homing of T cell subsets to mucosal vs. non-mucosal lymphoid organs. *Journal of Immunology*, **130**, 1097–102.

Lasky, L. A., Singer, M. S., Dowbenko, D., Imai, Y., Henzel, W. J., Grimley, C., Fennie, C.,

Gillett, N., Watson, S. R. & Rosen, S. D. (1992). An endothelial ligand for L-selectin is a novel mucin-like molecule. *Cell*, **69**, 927–38.

Lawrence, M. B. & Springer, T. A. (1991). Leucocytes roll on a selectin at physiologic flow rates: distinction from and prerequisite for adhesion through integrins. *Cell*, **65**, 859–73.

Leo, S. K., Lee, S., Ramos, R. A., Lobb, R., Rosa, M., Chi-Rerso, G. & Wright, S. D. (1991). Endothelial-leucocyte adhesion molecule-1 stimulates the adhesive activity of leucocyte integrin CR3 on human neutrophils. *Journal of Experimental Medicine*, **173**, 1493–560.

Mackay, C. R. (1993). Immunological memory. *Advances in Immunology*, **53**, 217–65.

Mackay, C. R., Marsten, W. L. & Dudler, L. (1990). Naive and memory T cells show distinct pathways of lymphocyte recirculation. *Journal of Experimental Medicine*, **171**, 801–17.

Mackay, C. R., Marsten, W. L., Dudler, L., Spertini, O., Tedder, T. F. & Hein, W. R. (1992). Tissue-specific migration pathways of phenotypically distinct subpopulations of memory T cells. *European Journal of Immunology*, **22**, 887–95.

Markarem, R., Newham, P., Askari, J. A., Green, L. J., Clements, J., Edwards, M., Humphries, M. J. & Mould, A. P. (1994). Competitive binding of vascular cell adhesion molecule-1 and the HEPII/IIICS domain of fibronectin to the integrin $\alpha_4\beta_1$. *Journal of Biological Chemistry*, **269**, 4005–11.

Manolios, N., Geczy, C. L. & Schreiber, L. (1988). High endothelial venule morphology and function are inducible in germ-free mice: a possible role for interferon-γ. *Cellular Immunology*, **117**, 136–51.

May, M. J. & Ager, A. (1992). ICAM-1 independent lymphocyte transmigration across high endothelium: differential upregulation by IFN-γ, TNF-α and IL-1β. *European Journal of Immunology*, **22**, 219–26.

May, M. J., Entwistle, G., Humphries, M. J. & Ager, A. (1993). VCAM-1 is a CS1 peptide-inhibitable adhesion molecule expressed by lymph node high endothelium. *Journal of Cell Science*, **106**, 109–19.

Mebius, R. E., Streeter, P. R., Breve, J., Duivestijn, A. M. & Kraal, G. (1991). The influence of afferent lymphatic vessel interruption of vascular addressin expression. *Journal of Cell Biology*, **115**, 85–95.

Mebius, R. E., Breve, J., Kraal, G. & Streeter, P. R. (1993). Developmental regulation of vascular addressin expression: a possible role for site-associated environments. *International Immunology*, **5**, 443–9.

Mobley, J. L., Reynolds, P. J. & Shimizu, Y. (1993). Regulatory mechanisms underlying T cell integrin receptor function. *Seminars in Immunology*, **5**, 227–36.

Morris, B. & Courtice, F. C. (1977). Cells and immunoglobulins in lymph. *Lymphology*, **10**, 62–70.

Norgard-Sumnicht, K. E., Varki, N. M. & Varki, A. (1993). Calcium-dependent heparin-like ligands for L-selectin in non-lymphoid endothelial cells. *Science*, **261**, 480–3.

O'Neill, J. K., Butter, C., Baker, D. *et al.* (1991). Expression of vascular addressins and ICAM-1 by endothelial cells in the spinal cord during chronic relapsing experimental allergic encephalomyelitis in the Biozzi AB/H mouse. *Immunology*, **72**, 520–5.

Oppenheimer-Marks, N., Davis, L. S. & Lipsky, P. E. (1990). Human T lymphocyte adhesion to endothelial cells and transendothelial migration. Alteration of receptor use relates to the activation status of both the T cell and the endothelial cell. *Journal of Immunology*, **145**, 140–8.

Oppenheimer-Marks, N., Davis, L. S., Bogue, D. J., Ramberg, J. & Lipsky, P. E. (1991). Differential utilisation of ICAM-1 and VCAM-1 during the adhesion and transendothelial migration of human T lymphocytes. *Journal of Immunology*, **147**, 2913–21.

Osborn, L., Vassallo, C. & Benjamin, C. D. (1992). Activated endothelium binds lymphocytes through a novel binding site in the alternatively spliced domain of vascular cell adhesion molecule-1. *Journal of Experimental Medicine*, **176**, 99–107.

Pankonin, G., Reipert, B. & Ager, A. (1992). Interactions between IL-2 activated lymphocytes and vascular endothelium: binding to and migration across specialised and non-specialised endothelia. *Immunology*, **77**, 51–60.

Pearson, L. D., Simpson-Morgan, M. W. & Morris, B. (1976). Lymphopoiesis and lymphocyte recirculation in the sheep foetus. *Journal of Experimental Medicine*, **143**, 167–86.

Picker, L. J. & Butcher, E. C. (1992). Physiological and molecular mechanisms of lymphocyte homing. *Annual Review in Immunology*, **10**, 561–91.

Picker, L. J., Kishimoto, T. K., Smith, C. W., Warnock, R. A. & Butcher, E. C. (1991*a*). ELAM-1 is an adhesion molecule for skin homing T cells. *Nature*, **349**, 796–9.

Picker, L. J., Warnock, R. A., Burns, A. R., Doerschuk, C. M., Berg, E. L. & Butcher, E. C. (1991). The neutrophil selectin LECAM-1 presents carbohydrate ligands to the vascular selectins ELAM-1 and GMP-140. *Cell*, 66, 921–3.

Pigott, R. & Power, C. (1993). *The Adhesion Molecule Facts Book*. Academic Press Ltd.

Pitzalis, C., Kingsley, G., Haskard, D. & Panayi, G. (1988). The preferential accumulation of helper-induced T lymphocytes in inflammatory lesions: evidence for regulation by selective endothelial and homotypic adhesion. *European Journal of Immunology*, **18**, 1379–404.

Pober, J. S. & Cotran, R. S. (1991). Immunological interactions of lymphocytes with vascular endothelium. *Advances in Immunology*, **50**, 261–302.

Rose, M. L., Parrott, D. M. V. & Bruce, R. G. (1976). Migration of lymphoblasts to the small intestine. II. Divergent migration of mesenteric and peripheral immunoblasts to sites of inflammation in the mouse. *Cellular Immunology*, **17**, 36–46.

Salmi, M., Kalimo, K. & Jalkanen, S. (1993). Induction and function of vascular adhesion protein-1 at sites of inflammation. *Journal of Experimental Medicine*, **178**, 2255–60.

Sanders, M. E., Makgoba, M. W. & Shaw, S. (1988). Human naive and memory T cells: re-interpretation of helper–inducer and suppressor–inducer subsets. *Immunology Today*, **9**, 195–9.

Schall, T. J (1991). Biology of the RANTES/SIS cytokine family. *Cytokine*, **3**, 165–283.

Scheynius, A., Camp, R. L. & Pure, E. (1993). Reduced contact sensitivity reactions in mice treated with monoclonal antibodies to leucocyte function-associated molecule-1 and inter-cellular adhesion molecule-1. *Journal of Immunology*, **150**, 655–63.

Schwartz, B. R., Wayer, E. A., Carlos, T. M., Ochs, H. D. & Harlan, J. M. (1990). Identification of surface proteins mediating adherence of CD11/CD18-deficient lymphoblastoid cells to cultured human endothelium. *Journal of Clinical Investigation*, **85**, 2019–22.

Schwartz, R. H. (1992). Costimulation of T lymphocytes: the role of CD28, CTLA4 and B7/BB1 in interleukin 2 production and immunotherapy. *Cell*, **71**, 1065–68.

Shimizu, Y. & Shaw, S. (1993). Mucins in the mainstream. *Nature*, **366**, 630–1.

Shimizu, Y., Newman, W., Tanaka, Y. & Shaw, S. (1992). Lymphocyte interactions with endothelial cells. *Immunology Today*, **13**, 106–12.

Shimizu, Y., Shaw, S., Graber, N., Gopal, T. G., Horgan, K. J., van Seventer, G. A. & Newman, W. (1991). Activation-independent binding of human memory T cells to adhesion molecule ELAM-1. *Nature*, **349**, 799–802.

Shimizu, Y., van Seventer, G. A., Horgan, K. J. & Shaw, S. (1990). Regulated expression and function of three VLA (β1) integrin receptors on T cells. *Nature*, **345**, 250–3.

Smith, J. B., McIntosh, G. H. & Morris, B. (1970). The migration of cells through chronically inflamed tissues. *Journal of Pathology*, **100**, 21–9.

Smith, M. E. & Ford, W. L. (1983). The recirculating lymphocyte pool of the rat: a systematic description of the migratory behaviour of recirculating lymphocytes. *Immunology*, **49**, 83–93.

Smith, M. E., Martin, A. F. & Ford, W. L. (1980). Migration of lymphoblasts in the rat. *Monographs Allergy*, **16**, 203–32.

Spertini, O., Kansas, G. S., Munro, J. M., Griffin, J. D. & Tedder, T. F. (1991). Regulation of leucocyte migration by activation of leucocyte adhesion molecule-1 (LAM-1) selectin. *Nature*, **349**, 691–4.

Spertini, O., Luscinskas, F. W., Kansas, G. S. *et al.* (1992). Leucocyte adhesion molecule-1 (LAM-1, L-selectin) interacts with an inducible endothelial cell ligand to support leucocyte adhesion. *Journal of Immunology*, **147**, 2565–73.

Springer, T. A. (1994). Traffic signals for lymphocyte recirculation and leucocyte emigration: the multistep paradigm. *Cell*, **76**, 301–14.

Stamper, H. B. & Woodruff, J. J. (1976). Lymphocyte homing into lymph nodes: an *in vitro* demonstration of the selective affinity of recirculating lymphocytes for high endothelial venules. *Journal of Experimental Medicine*, **144**, 828–32.

Steen, P. D., Ashwood, E. R., Huang, K., Daynes, R. A., Ching, H-T. & Samlowski, W. E. (1990). Mechanisms of pertussis toxin inhibition of lymphocyte-HEV interactions. I. Analysis of lymphocyte homing receptor-mediated binding mechanisms. *Cellular Immunology*, **131**, 67–85.

Steinman, R. M. (1991). The dendritic cell system and its role in immunogenicity. *Annual Review of Immunology*, **9**, 271–96.

Stevens, S. K., Weissman, I. L. & Butcher, E. C. (1982). Differences in the migration of B and T lymphocytes: organ-selective localisation *in vivo* and the role of lymphocyte-endothelial cell recognition. *Journal of Immunology*, **128**, 844–51.

Streeter, P. R., Lakey-Berg, E., Rouse, B. T. N., Bargatze, R. F. & Butcher, E. C. (1988*a*). A tissue-specific endothelial cell molecule involved in lymphocyte homing. *Nature*, **331**, 41–6.

Streeter, P. R., Rouse, B. T. N. & Butcher, E. C. (1988*b*). Immunohistologic and functional characterisation of a vascular addressin involved in lymphocyte homing into peripheral lymph nodes. *Journal of Cell Biology*, **107**, 1853–62.

Szekanecz, Z., Humphries, M. J. & Ager, A. (1992). Lymphocyte adhesion to high endothelium is mediated by two β_1 integrin receptors for fibronectin, $\alpha_4\beta_1$ and $\alpha_5\beta_1$. *Journal of Cell Science*, **101**, 885–94.

Tanaka, Y., Albelda, S. M., Horgan, K. J., van Seventer, G. A., Shimizu, Y., Newman, W., Hallam, J., Newman, P. J., Buck, C. A. & Shaw, S. (1992). CD31 expressed on distinctive T cell subsets is a preferential amplifier of β_1 integrin mediated adhesion. *Journal of Experimental Medicine*, **176**, 245–53.

Tanaka, Y., Adams, D. H., Hubscher, S., Hirano, H., Siebentist, V. & Shaw, S. (1993a). T-cell adhesion induced by proteoglycan-immobilised cytokine MIP-1β. *Nature*, **361**, 79–82.

Tanaka, Y., Adams, D. H. & Shaw, S. (1993*b*). Proteoglycans on endothelial cells present adhesion-inducing cytokines to leucocytes. *Immunology Today*, **14**, 111–15.

Tew, J. G., Di Losa, R. M., Burton, G. F., Koses, M. H., Kupp, L. I., Masuda, A. & Szakal, A. K. (1992). Germinal centres and antibody production in bone-marrow. *Immunology Review*, **126**, 99–112.

Toyama-Sorimachi, N., Miyake, K. & Miyasaka, M. (1993). Activation of CD44 induces ICAM-1/LFA-1 independent, Ca^{2+}, Mg^{2+} -independent adhesion pathway in lymphocyte-endothelial cell interactions. *European Journal of Immunology*, **23**, 439–46.

True, D. D., Singer, M. S., Lasky, L. A. & Rosen, S. D. (1990). Requirement for sialic acid on the endothelial ligand of a lymphocyte homing receptor. *Journal of Cell Biology*, **111**, 2757–64.

Watson, S. R., Fennie, C. & Lasky, L. A. (1991). Neutrophil influx into an inflammatory site inhibited by a soluble homing receptor – IgG chimera. *Nature*, 349, 164–9.

Westermann, J., Blaschke, V., Zimmerman, G., Hirschfield, V. & Pabst, R. (1992). Random entry of circulating lymphocyte subsets into peripheral lymph nodes and Peyers patches: no evidence *in vivo* of a tissue-specific migration of B and T lymphocytes at the level of high endothelial venules. *European Journal of Immunology*, **22**, 2219–23.

Westermann, J., Persin, S., Matyas, J., van der Meide, P. & Pabst, R. (1993). IFN-γ influences the migration of thoracic duct B and T lymphocytes subsets *in vivo*. *Journal of Immunology*, **150**, 3843–52.

Weston, S. A. & Parish, C. R. (1992). Evidence that mannose recognition by splenic sinusoidal cells plays a role in the splenic entry of lymphocytes. *European Journal of Immunology*, **22**, 1975–82.

Yang, H. & Binns, R. M. (1993). CD44 is not directly involved in the binding of lymphocytes to cultured high endothelial cells from peripheral lymph nodes. *Immunology*, **79**, 418–24.

Yednock, T. A., Cannon, C., Fritz, L. C., Sanchez-Madrid, F., Steinman, L. & Karin, N. (1992). Prevention of experimental autoimmune encephalomyelitis by antibodies against $\alpha_4\beta_1$ integrin. *Nature*, **356**, 63–6.

Zimmerman, G. A., Prescott, S. M. & McIntyre, T. M. (1992). Endothelial cell interactions with granulocytes: tethering and signalling molecules. *Immunology Today*, **13**, 93–100.

–5–

Role of the vascular endothelium in immunologically mediated neurological disease

VIRGINIA CALDER and JOHN GREENWOOD

General introduction

The selective cellular barrier that separates the blood from the parenchyma of the nervous tissue has been increasingly implicated in the pathogenesis of diseases affecting central (CNS) and peripheral nervous systems (PNS). In recent years there has been particular interest in the potential role of these barriers in the development of diseases involving the immune system. The original doctrine of the nervous system being an immunologically privileged site has now been redefined to include the concept of a limited access of immune cells during their normal role of tissue surveillance. The role of the three vascular barrier sites, namely the blood–brain, blood–retinal and blood–nerve barriers (BBB, BRB and BNB, respectively) in the induction and propagation of disease processes can be divided into separate but related phenomena. First, the endothelial cells which form these barriers play a significant part in the recruitment of circulating immune cells. Secondly, they possess the potential to act as antigen presenting cells at the barriers and thirdly, leukocyte migration and the release of cytokines and other inflammatory agents leads to the disruption of the barrier, the formation of vasogenic oedema and secondary problems. Our current understanding of how these related phenomena are involved in various immunologically mediated diseases of the nervous system is outlined below. In this chapter we cover the most common of the immunologically mediated neurological diseases, and highlight the role of the vascular endothelial cell in this diverse range of clinical syndromes. Due to the magnitude of this field and the limited space available, comprehensive citation is not possible although recent and key papers are cited providing the reader with the opportunity to pursue the topic in greater detail.

Immunologically mediated human neurological diseases

Multiple sclerosis

Multiple sclerosis (MS) is a human demyelinating disease affecting the white matter of the CNS. There are various immunological abnormalities in MS which suggest an important role for T cells in its pathogenesis although the aetiology of this disease remains unknown. Although oligoclonal bands of immunoglobulins (Ig), detected by polyacrylamide gel electrophoresis in the cerebrospinal fluid (CSF), are a hallmark of MS, no disease-specific antigen has been isolated. It is therefore likely that the production of Ig by B cells is a bystander phenomenon, probably in response to the generation of myelin fragments. In contrast, T cells are thought to play a crucial role in the process of demyelination since many T cells (mainly $CD4^+$) can be found at the leading edge of the plaques and in the surrounding normal-appearing white matter. Immunohistological studies of plaque tissue have demonstrated the presence in early MS lesions of a focal accumulation of activated T cells around small venules. Enhanced levels of activated T cells expressing interleukin-2 receptors have also been observed in the CSF in MS (Bellamy *et al.*, 1985). Myelin degeneration in later MS lesions is associated with a marked perivenular inflammation consisting of T cells, B cells and macrophages. Recruitment of leukocytes from the circulation is therefore a pivotal event in the development of this and other immunologically mediated diseases.

An enhanced expression of histocompatibility leukocyte antigens (HLA) class II molecules has also been observed within the white matter on various CNS resident cells, including endothelial cells (Traugott, Scheinberg & Raine, 1985), perhaps induced by lymphokines such as interferon-γ (IFNγ) produced by the activated T cells within the plaques. Cerebral vascular endothelial cells isolated from human brain do not constitutively express HLA class II. However, it has been demonstrated that incubation with human IFNγ results in the expression of both HLA-DR and -DP antigens (McCarron *et al.*, 1991*b*) with approximately 40% of the endothelial cell population expressing the HLA-DR antigen. The possibility that class II-expressing endothelial cells can act as antigen presenting cells to stimulate further T cell activation within the CNS and hence perpetuate the disease has been the focus of many studies. In favour of this theory are the results from *in vitro* experiments using cultures of rat and mouse CNS-derived endothelium, as discussed later in this chapter.

Recent immunohistological studies have also highlighted the expression of adhesion molecules on perivascular endothelium in human CNS tissue. It has been found that some adhesion molecules are present on brain endothelium under normal conditions whilst others such as very late activation antigen-1 (VLA-1) are up-regulated under inflammatory conditions (Rossler *et al.*, 1992). It has also been demonstrated that cultures of human cerebral endothelial cells constitutively express low levels of intercellular adhesion molecule-1 (ICAM-1) with up-regulation following treatment with a combination of IFN-γ and tumour necrosis factor-α (TNF-α) (Wong & Dorovini-Zis, 1992). The presence of these adhesion molecules on the vessel walls as well as on parenchymal cells like astrocytes and microglia may guide inflammatory cells into and through the brain in the course of immune surveillance and inflammation.

Lymphokines have also been detected in MS lesions; both TNFα and TNFβ were identified in acute and chronic active MS lesions but were absent from chronic silent lesions (Selmaj *et al.*, 1991). It has also been found that CNS-derived endothelial cells can produce cytokines *in vitro*, further supporting a costimulatory role for these cells in immune-mediated demyelination. This work is described later in this chapter.

Posterior uveitis

Posterior uveitis is a significant cause of irreversible visual loss in man due to its deleterious effects on the retina and optic nerve, and accounts for 10% of blind registrations in adults of working age in the UK. Posterior uveitis may occur in isolation, or be associated with a systemic disease such as Behçet's disease or sarcoidosis. The clinical activity within the posterior segment of the eye can easily be monitored, and most forms of the disease have several features in common including vitreous inflammatory cells, retinal vasculitis and macular oedema. Immunohistological studies have demonstrated a predominance of $CD4^{+}$T cells infiltrating the retina and an increase in class II expression but very few B cells or neutrophils and no evidence of immune complex deposition (Lightman & Chan, 1990). Furthermore, cyclosporin A (CsA), an inhibitor of T cell activation, is often clinically effective in treating this chronic inflammatory disease (Towler, Whiting & Forrester, 1990). Recent studies have shown an increase in activated T cells in the blood, aqueous and vitreous samples from patients with all forms of posterior uveitis in comparison with normal volunteers (Deschênes, Char & Kaleta, 1988). Such findings suggest a pivotal role for activated T cells in the perpetuation of this condition yet there are many questions which remain unanswered as to the immunopathogenic mechanisms involved. What triggers T cell infiltration across the BRB? Are the T cells activated within the retina and, if so, which cells are presenting antigen to T cells and which antigen(s) are involved? Not surprisingly, endothelial cells have been implicated in these processes due to their ideal anatomical location at the BRB, their ability to express class II molecules and adhesion molecules and their production of cytokines.

Vitreous and/or retinochoroidal biopsies from patients with posterior uveitis have shown increased expression of HLA class II molecules on the retinal vascular endothelium (Fujikawa & Haugen, 1990). In another study of uveitic eyes, lymphocyte function-associated antigen-1 (LFA-1) was expressed on infiltrating lymphocytes and ICAM-1 was expressed on endothelial cells of retinal and choroidal blood vessels, and the retinal pigment epithelium in all six uveitic eyes, but in none of the normal control eyes. In the same study, ocular inflammatory cells stained strongly positive for TNFα in all eyes with uveitis, and four of six uveitic eyes showed mild staining for TNFβ and IFNγ (Whitcup *et al.*, 1992). These studies stress the importance of lymphocyte infiltration, and the important role that activated vascular endothelium plays in the pathogenesis of posterior uveitis.

Guillain–Barré syndrome

Acute inflammatory demyelinating polyradiculoneuropathy or Guillain–Barré syndrome (GBS) is an acute paralytic disease affecting the peripheral nervous system in man (recently reviewed by Rostami, 1993). GBS is characterized by acute progressive motor weakness of the extremities and of bulbar and facial musculature. Deep tendon reflexes are reduced or absent, and sensory symptoms are mild. Respiratory failure and autonomic dysfunction may be seen. The CSF shows increased protein and no or very few cells. The nerve conduction velocity is slowed, and the pathology shows segmental demyelination with mononuclear cell infiltration. Although the aetiology and pathogenesis of GBS is presently unclear, recent evidence supports the possibility that nerve injury in this disease is immunologically mediated. Various antibodies to peripheral nerve myelin and circulating immune complexes have been found in patients with GBS. Although the target antigen(s) for these antibodies are not well understood, neutral glycolipids cross-reactive with Forssman antigen and gangliosides are possible candidates.

The reactivity of T cells was recently examined in GBS, using P0 and P2 proteins of peripheral nerve myelin (Khalili-Shirazi *et al.*, 1992). The proliferative responses of blood mononuclear cells to myelin proteins and synthetic peptides derived from them were determined in patients with GBS, normal controls (NC) and patients with other neuropathies (ONP). Twelve out of 19 GBS patients responded to P0 or P2, 6 to P0 and its peptides only, 3 to P2 and its peptides only, and 3 to both P0 and P2 antigens. Responses to at least one of the antigens were also found in only 4/17 NC and 2/6 ONP. In conclusion immune responses in GBS appear to be heterogeneous but the early T cell responses to P0 protein, described here for the first time, may be important in the pathogenesis of some cases.

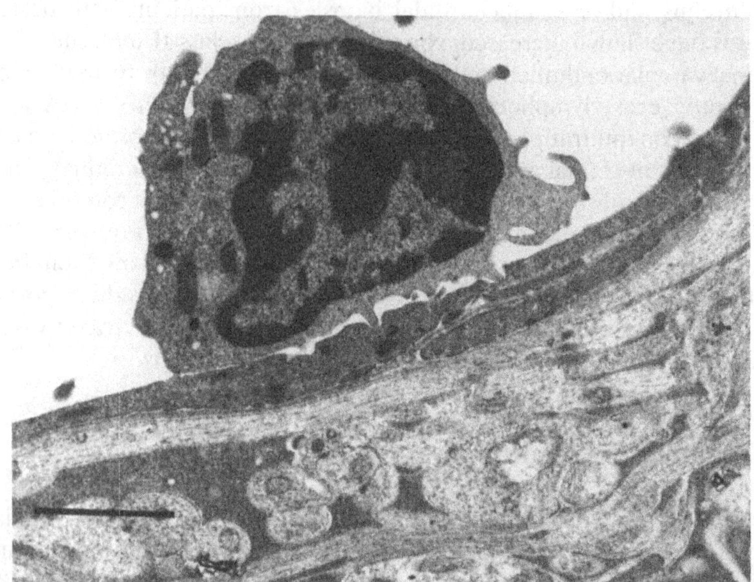

Fig. 5.1. Transmission electron micrograph of a leukocyte, possibly a T cell, adhering and probing the endothelial cell of a brain microvessel from a guinea-pig with toxoplasma. Bar = 2 μm. (Courtesy of Drs C. E. N. Pavesio & P. Gormley.)

Other immunologically mediated neurological diseases

There are also several infectious agents which are known to result in immunologically mediated neurological disease. Parasites such as toxoplasma are known to cause leukocyte infiltration into the nervous system (Fig. 5.1), and viruses infecting the CNS such as HIV, CMV and measles can also be associated with lymphocytic infiltration and subsequent damage to the nervous system. In an attempt to elucidate the mechanisms involved, experimental models such as Theiler's virus (for poliomyelitis) have been studied. Thus by *in situ* hybridization, Theiler's virus RNA was found in cells associated with vascular endothelium in the brains and spinal cords of infected mice (Zurbriggen & Fujinami, 1988). Theiler's virus RNA-positive endothelial cells were observed not only near the primary lesions but also away from demonstrable lesions in normal-appearing regions in the central nervous system. This suggests that endothelial cells could be involved in the disease but, as for many of these diseases, their role remains unclear. One possible role for endothelial cells has recently been suggested by the finding that ICAM-1 is an endothelial cell adhesion receptor for *Plasmodium falciparum* (Berendt *et al.*, 1989).

The aim of the rest of this chapter will be to focus on the results from experimental models which highlight the probable roles for endothelial cells in the human conditions.

Immunologically mediated experimental diseases

The experimental animal models of MS (experimental autoimmune encephalomyelitis; EAE), posterior uveitis (experimental autoimmune uveoretinitis; EAU) and GBS (experimental autoimmune neuritis; EAN) have provided valuable information on the basic mechanisms involved in immunologically mediated neurological disease. These diseases can be induced in certain species and strains following systemic immunization with appropriate site-specific antigens and in some species by adoptive transfer of antigen-specific activated $CD4^+$ T cells. Of fundamental importance to the pathogenesis of the human conditions is the infiltration of immunopathogenic T cells into the tissue, a process which is faithfully reproduced in these experimental diseases (Fig. 5.2). Irrespective of the initiating event, these diseases progress largely as the result of increasing numbers of inflammatory cells crossing the vascular barriers and entering the tissue. Associated with this enhanced cellular traffic there is a concomitant breakdown of barrier integrity and subsequent oedema formation. The blood–tissue barriers in controlling leukocyte migration therefore play an important role in orchestrating the development of these diseases. These basic phenomena have been extensively investigated in the experimental animal models of immune-mediated diseases of the nervous system and have led to a greater understanding of the human conditions.

In addition to the *in vivo* models of these diseases a considerable amount of data concerning the role of the vascular endothelium has been accumulated from *in vitro* studies. Recent developments of tissue culture methods for isolating nervous system vessels and the subsequent culture of endothelia has led to a rapid increase in our understanding of the molecular mechanisms of leukocyte adhesion and migration and on the role of major histocompatibility complex (MHC) expression in the disease process.

Properties of the vascular endothelia of the blood–tissue barriers

The vascular endothelia of the brain, retina and peripheral nerve are highly specialized and differ from the endothelia of other vascular beds. The fundamental property of nervous tissue endothelia is their ability to form a

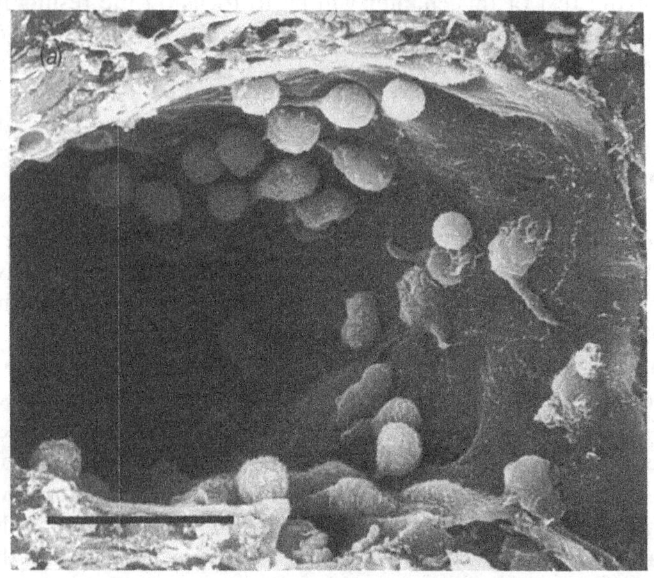

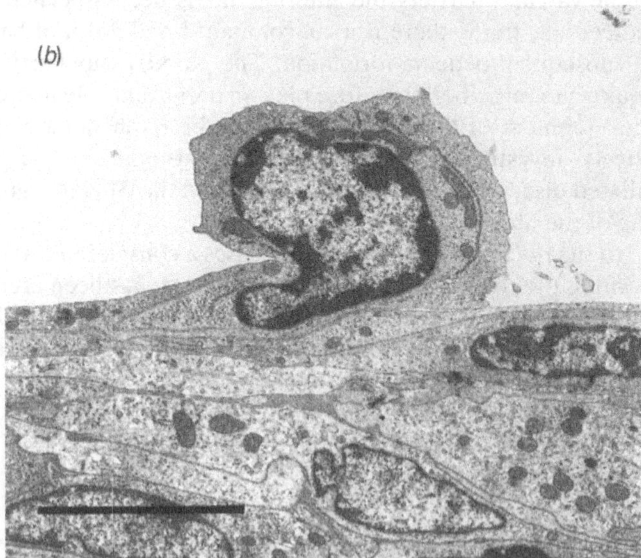

Fig. 5.2. (*a*) Scanning electron micrograph of leukocytes adhering to a vessel wall of retinal blood vessel from a rat with EAU. Bar = 20 μm. (*b*) Transmission electron micrograph of a leukocyte, probably a T cell, penetrating the blood vessel wall in the cerebellum of a guinea-pig with CREAE. Bar = 4 μm. (Courtesy of Dr P. Munro.)

highly selective barrier between the blood and the parenchyma. The ultrastructural correlate of this barrier is formed principally by the presence of tight junctions (TJ) which are composed of points of fusion of the membrane of adjacent endothelia; the zonula occludens. In addition to these specialized junctions the endothelial cells also express low levels of pinocytosis, no fenestrae and no transendothelial pores. As a result of these properties CNS microvessels have been shown *in vivo* to exhibit very high transvascular resistances of the order of 1500 Ω cm^2 (Butt & Jones, 1992). The induction of these special properties is thought to be brought about by their close relationship with astrocytes. Current opinion suggests that factors released from these perivascular cells prompt the endothelia to exhibit their specialized characteristics (Greenwood, 1991). However, definitive proof for this, namely the identification and isolation of the factor/s that are responsible, has yet to be achieved.

In addition to these morphological properties, nervous tissue endothelia are also characterized by their differential expression of both surface and intracellular molecules. Of paramount importance to the recruitment of leukocytes from the blood is the expression of cell adhesion molecules on the endothelial cell luminal membrane. Furthermore, the presence of MHC molecules on endothelial cells has led to speculation that these cells possess the potential for antigen presentation. Finally, the expression of receptors to inflammatory compounds such as histamine and the cytokines may also play a significant role in the response of the vascular barriers to inflammation.

Immunological role of the vascular endothelia of the blood–tissue barriers

Antigen presentation

A major question that has been addressed extensively is the antigen-presenting capabilities of endothelial cells of the nervous system. Because of their close proximity to circulating immune cells these cells have been the subject of attention in the search for a resident antigen presenting cell (APC) within the nervous sytem. To satisfy the criteria of an APC, the vascular endothelia must be able to express MHC class II molecules in association with antigenic epitopes and to generate the necessary co-stimulatory signals to lymphocytes.

As with all cells, endothelia from the nervous system express MHC class I and are thus able to interact with $CD8^+$ T cells in an MHC class I-restricted manner. Indeed, it has been shown that brain endothelial cells infected with virus can become the target for virus-specific, MHC-restricted cytotoxic T cell damage, a process which could potentially lead to a significant level of damage to the vascular bed. In Theiler's virus-induced demyelination, which is used as a model of MS, the virus gains access to the CNS by replicating in the cerebral endothelia. However, although damage to infected endothelial cells *in vitro* has been observed, the endothelia *in vivo* appear not to be damaged.

Under normal conditions nervous tissue endothelia do not express MHC class II molecules. These endothelia, however, have been shown to be capable of expressing class II molecules both *in vivo* and *in vitro* under the correct conditions. Whether these cells can still function as APCs and whether they possess all the requisite co-stimulatory signals to cause T cell proliferation and/or cytotoxicity *in vivo* is still a contentious issue. The weight of current evidence, however, suggests that nervous system endothelia are capable of expressing MHC class II molecules but lack the necessary costimulatory factors to induce significant T cell proliferation *in vivo*. (Compare this with the role of the vascular endothelium in allograft rejection, reviewed in Chapter 11).

Various studies have investigated the expression of MHC class II molecules on neural endothelia in inflamed tissue. Early studies with EAE indicated that MHC class II was induced on endothelia (Traugott *et al.*, 1985) even prior to inflammatory cell infiltration (Sobel *et al.*, 1984). The degree of resolution of these studies was such that it was not entirely clear whether class II expression was restricted to the endothelia or was limited to perivascular cells (Butter *et al.*, 1991) although luminal membrane expression of the Ia molecule has been reported ultrastructurally (Sobel, Natale & Schneeberger, 1987). These differences may well be species dependent since class II expression on endothelial cells is rarely observed in rat EAE (Vass *et al.*, 1986) whereas in chronic relapsing EAE (CREAE) in the guinea pig, expression of class II molecules has been demonstrated (Sobel *et al.*, 1987).

In *in vitro* studies, which offer greater experimental flexibility, the expression and induction of MHC molecules on nervous tissue endothelia and their ability to operate as APC has also been investigated. Both brain and retinal endothelial cells in culture express MHC class I constitutively but fail to express significant levels of class II (Male, Pryce & Hughes, 1987; Risau, Engelhardt & Wekerle, 1990; Liversidge, Sewell & Forrester, 1990). Following activation with cytokines such as IFN-γ and interleukin-1 (IL-1) the expression of class I molecules is enhanced and class II molecules are induced (Male & Pryce, 1988*a*;) with combinations of cytokines acting in both a synergistic (Male & Pryce, 1988*b*) and inhibitory manner (Tanaka & McCarron, 1990).

The potential for MHC class II molecule expression appears to be directly related to the susceptibility of a particular species or strain to experimental autoimmune diseases (Male & Pryce, 1988*c*; Jemison *et al.*, 1993). For example, the strains of rat (Lewis) and mouse (SJL/J) with the greatest capacity for MHC class II expression are also those in which EAE is most readily induced. What is not clear, however, is whether this is due to differences in the MHC regulatory genes, to other MHC-linked genes or to a differential ability to respond to cytokine stimulation.

It is now well accepted that endothelial cells of the nervous system are capable of presenting antigen to T cells *in vitro* since brain endothelia can become the target for antigen-specific, MHC class II restricted cell-mediated cytotoxic damage (Risau *et al.*, 1990; Sedgwick *et al.*, 1990; McCarron *et al.*, 1991*b*). Although these CNS endothelia appear to be capable of presenting antigen in a recognizable form to T cells, their ability to present the full complement of stimulatory signals to induce T cell proliferation remains unresolved. Initial reports indicated that CNS endothelia were able to induce T cell proliferation (McCarron *et al.*, 1985; Wilcox *et al.*, 1989; Myers, Dougherty & Ron, 1993) but conflicting results have also been reported (Pryce, Male & Sedgwick, 1989; Risau *et al.*, 1990). Whether these discrepancies are due to species differences or to the degree of endothelial cell purity is unclear, although it has been shown that smooth muscle cells and pericytes, which are potential contaminating cells, can express class II MHC and induce T cell proliferation (Hart *et al.*, 1987; Fabry *et al.*, 1990). In recent studies (unpublished) we have found that with certain T cell/endothelial cell ratios both cerebral and retinal endothelial cells are capable of inducing $CD4^+$ T cell proliferation in a class II restricted manner, albeit at a lower level than with professional APCs. Thus, although endothelial cells of the nervous system are capable of presenting antigen and inducing T cell proliferation they are not as proficient as classical APCs. This uncertainty, however, has led to the investigation of other cell types, such as microglia and smooth muscle/pericytes, as being the principal resident APCs in the nervous system.

Leukocyte adhesion to and migration across the vascular barriers

To fulfil their role in immune surveillance, leukocytes must be able to cross blood vessel walls and enter the tissue beyond. This function is believed to be performed with limited impediment at the majority of vascular beds. Within the nervous system, however, the influx and traffic of leukocytes is restricted by the presence of the specialized endothelia of the blood–tissue barriers. Until recently, these barriers were thought to completely obstruct the passage of leukocytes from the blood into the tissue under normal conditions. It is now believed that activated lymphocytes, and possibly other leukocytes such as monocytes, are able to traverse the normal blood–tissue barriers and enter the nervous system in limited numbers (Hickey, Hsu &

Kimura, 1991; Lassmann *et al.*, 1993). This low rate of influx into the nervous tissue is thought to be due primarily to a restricted expression of vascular adhesion molecules which limits the capture of leukocytes from the circulating blood. In certain disease conditions of the nervous system, however, leukocyte migration across the vasculature is strikingly up-regulated and is a major factor determining the development and outcome of immunologically mediated diseases of the nervous system.

For leukocytes to leave the circulation and enter the nervous system, their passage in the blood must be halted by the formation of complex adhesive interactions between the circulating immune cell and the endothelia. These interactions are mediated by a diverse group of molecules, collectively referred to as adhesion molecules, expressed on the surface of both the leukocyte and endothelia. The general processes governing leukocyte recruitment from the blood have been investigated extensively and have been reviewed comprehensively elsewhere (see Chapters 3 and 4). Our current understanding is that, at the vascular barriers of the nervous system, the same basic principles of leukocyte adhesion and migration are also thought to operate. Extravasation of leukocytes is believed to involve three basic stages.

1. The margination of circulating leukocytes and formation of transient attachments reducing velocity and permitting signalling to occur between the endothelium and leukocyte.
2. The triggering and formation of strong adhesive links between the leukocyte and the endothelial cells.
3. The migration of the leukocyte to its point of penetration and diapedesis.

A further important consideration in this process and one that has not been investigated at the specialized vascular barriers, is the secretion of degradative enzymes by the leukocyte that are thought to assist in its penetration of the vascular wall and basal lamina.

The degree of leukocyte migration into different sites is governed by a variety of factors such as the state of activation of the leukocyte and the local endothelia as well as the inherent ability of the endothelia to express the requisite adhesion molecules. The capacity of brain and retinal endothelia to bind lymphocytes *in vitro* has been shown to differ from that of non-CNS endothelium, and is believed to be a consequence of a limited expression of adhesion molecules. Moreover, the patterns of leukocyte migration into the CNS *in vivo* are distinctive with polymorphonuclear cells (neutrophils) being comparatively rare, except in acute infectious diseases and early in the development of EAE (Cross & Raine, 1991) and EAU (McMenamin *et al.*, 1992), compared to T lymphocytes and monocytes. The migration of B cells is also uncommon although they are capable of migrating across brain

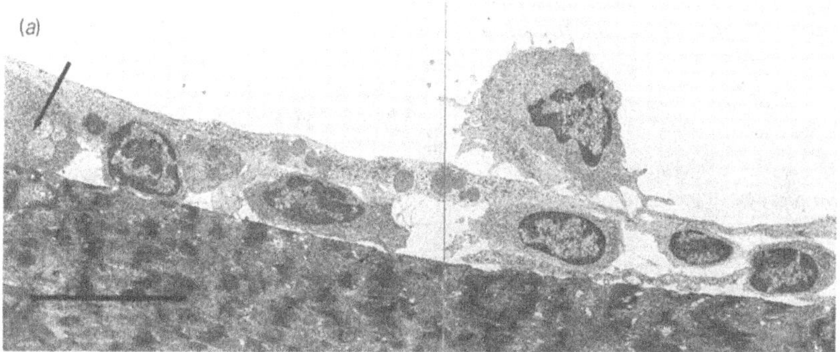

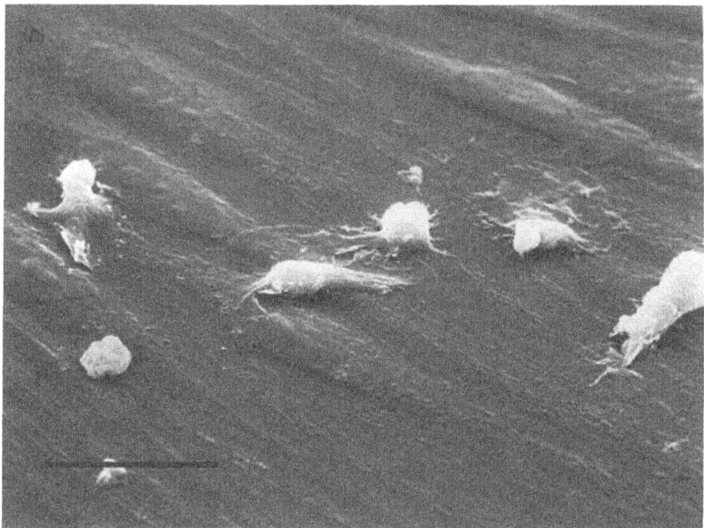

Fig. 5.3. (*a*) Transmission electron micrograph of a peripheral lymph node T lymphocyte adhering to the surface of a rat brain endothelial cell monolayer grown on a solid collagen filter. The endothelial monolayer has been lifted by other lymphocytes that have migrated through the monolayer and are now lying between it and the collagen membrane. Note the B cell (arrow) that has also migrated across the monolayer. Bar = 5 μm. (*b*) Scanning electron micrograph of T cell line lymphocytes adhering to a monolayer of cultured rat retinal vascular endothelial cells. Bar = 20 μm.

endothelial monolayers *in vitro* (Male *et al.*, 1992; Fig. 5.3). In the experimental autoimmune diseases, $CD4^+$ and $CD8^+$ T cells and mononuclear phagocytes appear at later time-points than the few initial neutrophils and in MS plaques and CSF, activated T cells (interleukin-2 receptor$^+$; IL-$2R^+$) and memory cells ($CD29^+$) are over-represented particularly in active

Table 5.1. *Motility and migration of lymphocytes across and through retinal endothelial cell monolayers and the effect of cell activation*

Lymphocyte	Lymphocyte activation	Endothelial cell activation	Motile lymphocytes. % on the monolayer surface	Motile lymphocytes. % under the monolayer (migrated)	Total % of motile lymphocytes
PLN	No	No	2.8 ± 0.9	0.8 ± 0.4	3.6 ± 0.8
PLN	Con A 48–72 h	No	29 ± 3	3.2 ± 1.4	32 ± 3
PLN	Con A 24–48 h	IFN-γ	13 ± 4	2.7 ± 0.7	16 ± 3
PLN	Con A 48–72 h	IFN-γ	44 ± 7	3.8 ± 1.8	48 ± 7
PLN	PHA 48–72 h	IFN-γ	15 ± 2	24 ± 1.0	39 ± 2
BSA T cell line	Antigen	IFN-γ	37 ± 10	50 ± 10	87 ± 4
S-Antigen T cell line	Antigen	No	24 ± 4	51 ± 8	75 ± 6
S-Antigen T cell line	Antigen	IFN-γ	25 ± 4	54 ± 8	79 ± 5

Data taken from Greenwood & Calder, 1993.

disease (Hafler & Weiner, 1987). This accords with the experimental finding that activated T cells preferentially migrate across brain and retinal endothelia both *in vitro* (Table 5.1; Greenwood & Calder, 1993; Male *et al.*, 1990), and *in vivo* in EAE and EAU (Cross *et al.*, 1990; Calder & Lightman, 1992; Greenwood, Howes & Lightman, 1994). At later stages of MS, the proportion of $CD8^+$ T cells is often extremely high and comparative studies *in vitro* have shown that $CD8^+$ cells bind more strongly than $CD4^+$ cells to brain and retinal endothelia (Pryce, Male & Sarkar, 1991; Wang *et al.*, 1993; Fig. 5.3), while $CD4^+$ cells migrate across it in greater numbers (Pryce *et al.*, 1991).

At present it is not yet known whether there are any CNS endothelium-specific adhesion molecules or whether these cells use the same molecules in a distinctive pattern and temporal sequence. There is no evidence for specific homing of lymphocytes to the nervous system unlike that found within the post-capillary venules of the paracortex of the lymph node where the endothelia have evolved specifically to capture circulating leukocytes from the blood. The endothelia that form these vessels are morphologically and functionally distinct from other endothelia and are referred to as high endothelial venules (HEV; see Chapter 4). In particular they express a unique set of adhesion molecules, the addressins, which are largely responsible for the homing of leukocytes to the lymph nodes. Although the expression of these addressins was originally thought to be restricted to HEV, it has recently been reported that enothelia in inflamed tissue, including that of the CNS in EAE, are capable of expressing these adhesion molecules, and that the degree of expression corresponds to the level of inflammatory cell invasion (Cannella, Cross & Raine, 1991; Raine *et al.*, 1990) particularly during the relapsing phase in CREAE (O'Neill *et al.*, 1991).

Our current understanding is that the endothelia of the central and peripheral nervous system utilize many of the adhesion molecules used in extravasation across non-nervous tissue endothelia. The pattern of expression of these molecules, and hence the cells they recruit, depends upon the state and timing of activation. Some molecules such as intercellular adhesion molecule-2 (ICAM-2) are expressed constitutively whereas others like vascular cell adhesion molecule-1 (VCAM-1) require induction. Indeed, following activation there is a distinct sequence of adhesion molecule expression with the selectins, which are responsible for the initial stages of leukocyte recruitment peaking within hours whilst others such as ICAM-1 and VCAM-1 peak after 1–3 days.

Within both the CNS and PNS the role of the selectins, which are responsible for the initial leukocyte/endothelial interactions at other vascular beds (see Chapter 3), have been inadequately investigated although indirect evidence does support a role for these carbohydrates in leukocyte recruitment at the vascular barriers of the nervous system (Simmons & Cattle, 1992). Both ICAM-1 and VCAM-1 expression on neural endothelia, however, have been implicated in leukocyte recruitment during immunologically mediated disease. In EAE, the level of ICAM-1 expression is up-regulated from basal levels during the active stages of disease (Raine *et al.*, 1990; Cannella *et al.*, 1991) and correlates with the induction of addressins during relapse. VCAM-1, however, which is not expressed constitutively, is believed to be induced on nervous tissue endothelia following cytokine activation. It is possible, therefore, that the early up-regulation of ICAM-1 and the induction of VCAM-1 may be responsible for the extravasation of CNS-antigen-specific T cells, and that a subsequent induction of addressins is important in recruiting the naive antigen non-specific cells into the parenchyma.

In adoptive transfer studies donor encephalitogenic T cells cross the BBB but remain in the perivascular space (Cross *et al.*, 1990) whilst other host inflammatory cells migrate deep into the parenchyma. It has been suggested that the perivascular location of the antigen-specific donor cells is long term (Skundric *et al.*, 1993) enabling them to influence the vascular endothelium through the secretion of cytokines and to orchestrate the influx of non-CNS antigen-responsive immune cells. Indeed, recent evidence indicates that non-specific cells play a vital role in the pathogenesis of both EAE (Kawai *et al.*, 1993) and EAU (Caspi *et al.*, 1993). The likely temporal sequence of events at the vascular barriers, therefore, is an initial influx of activated antigen-specific T cells which are known to possess the capacity to migrate across non-activated endothelia irrespective of their antigen specificity (Hickey *et al.*, 1991; Greenwood & Calder, 1993). These cells will cross the vessel wall and enter the perivenular space and once resident within the tissue will release cytokines which will influence the expression of adhesion molecules on the vascular endothelium. This localized increase in the molecules responsible for recruiting leukocytes from the circulation will lead to enhanced leukocyte traffic and the recruitment of naive T cells. This first cohort of cells may also be further stimulated through contact with their antigen in association with MHC class II on resident APCs and lead to clonal expansion within the tissue. The shift in emphasis from the leukocyte to the endothelium in determining recruitment is central to the concept of leukocyte homing to areas of inflammation. One problem associated with this hypothesis, however, is the recruitment of naive T cells into the nervous tissue. Although up-regulation of adhesion molecules on the luminal surface of the endothelial cell will capture naive lymphocytes from the circulation, they do not appear to possess the necessary machinery to migrate across an intact barrier (Greenwood & Calder, 1993). They may overcome this problem, however, if the barrier is sufficiently damaged for them to migrate through disrupted tight junctions in a manner similar to that occurring across the non-specialized vascular beds where diapedesis is less restricted.

It is evident that many of the events described above rely on the secretion of cytokines by lymphocytes within the tissue. Using immunohistochemistry and *in situ* hybridization, many reports have confirmed the presence of cytokines in brain, retina and nerve in inflammatory conditions. The cytokine concentrations normally used *in vitro* to induce lymphocyte adhesion to endothelial monolayers are believed to exceed the assumed physiological range, but highly localized concentractions in the extracellular space *in vivo* may reach such levels. Of recent interest is the role of the chemokines such as interleukin-8 and MIP1β in inducing leukocyte adhesion and migration and in particular the maintenance of high concentrations of these compounds at the site of inflammation. This is thought to be achieved by their binding to cell surface and extracellular matrix glycosaminoglycans (GAGs). This is of particular relevance for chemokines that are secreted from the vascular endothelia where blood flow would both dilute their concentration and rapidly remove them from the desired site of action. By binding to endothelial cell surface proteoglycans they are immobilized and can thus be maintained at high concentrations allowing activation of marginated cells and targeting to the inflammatory site (Tanaka, Adams & Shaw, 1993).

At most vascular beds, the interaction between the integrin LFA-1 on the leukocyte and ICAM-1, a member of the immunoglobulin superfamily, on the endothelia is critical in leukocyte extravasation. In the nervous system,

ICAM-1 levels on endothelia are normally low and correlate with depressed levels of leukocyte migration, but *in vitro* studies have highlighted the importance of this relationship in inflammation. Activation of CNS-derived endothelial monolayers with cytokines such as IFN-γ, TNF-α and IL-1 induce an increased expression of ICAM-1 over 24 h (Wilcox *et al.*, 1990; Wong & Dorovini-Zis, 1992; Fabry *et al.*, 1992), which coincides with an increase in lymphocyte adhesion (Hughes, Male & Lantos, 1988; Male *et al.*, 1990, 1992; Liversidge *et al.*, 1990; Wang *et al.*, 1993; McCarron *et al.*, 1993). This adhesion can be blocked, but only in part, by pre-treatment of the endothelia with antibody to ICAM-1. Antibodies directed against the counter-receptor, LFA-1, however, lead to a greater inhibition of adhesion (Waldschmidt *et al.*, 1991) implying an involvement of receptors other than ICAM-1 in this process. We have found that, following pretreatment of either lymphocytes or endothelium with antibody to LFA-1 or ICAM-1, respectively, the migration of antigen-specific T cells through a monolayer is greatly reduced. This supports the view, derived from studies on non-nervous system endothelia, that the LFA-1/ICAM-1 pathway is more dominant in migration than adhesion. Although it has been established that the cytokine IFN-γ up-regulates both the expression of ICAM-1 on non-nervous system endothelia and lymphocyte migration, it fails to increase migration across cerebral (Male *et al.*, 1992) and retinal (Greenwood & Calder, 1993) endothelia. This is not due to the failure of IFN-γ to induce ICAM-1 on nervous system endothelia as this has been demonstrated (Liversidge *et al.*, 1990; Wilcox *et al.*, 1990; Wong & Dorovini-Zis, 1992; Fabry *et al.*, 1992). This possibly indicates a significant difference between the vascular beds of the nervous system and elsewhere.

In support of the view that ICAM-1 is involved predominantly in diapedesis and VCAM-1 in adhesion is the observation that the former is expressed on both the luminal and abluminal membrane of the endothelia whereas VCAM-1 expression is restricted to the luminal membrane only. However, blocking LFA-1 (Welsh *et al.*, 1993; Cannella, Cross & Raine, 1993) *in vivo* with monoclonal antibodies does not reduce the severity of EAE but instead is found to augment the disease. Studies with non-nervous system vasculature conclude that the pairing of the integrin very late activation antigen-4 (VLA-4) on the leukocyte with VCAM-1 on the endothelia is of equal importance in both adhesion and migration. Despite good evidence that this pathway is influential in lymphocyte migration across non-nervous system endothelia, there is little direct evidence to demonstrate its importance in controlling migration in the CNS and PNS. In support of this pathway being influential in leukocyte recruitment is the report that antibodies directed to VLA-4 ($\alpha 4/\beta 1$ integrin) *in vivo* are capable of blocking the development of EAE lesions (Yednock *et al.*, 1992) and that this adhesion molecule is required for T cell entry into brain parenchyma (Baron *et al.*, 1993).

Moreover, in current studies we have found that antibodies directed against VLA-4 on $CD4^+$ antigen-specific T cell lines lead to a small reduction in their adhesion to resting CNS-derived endothelia but not their subsequent migration through the monolayer, whereas on IL-1 activated endothelia, where presumably VCAM-1 is induced, migration is significantly reduced. However, it is possible to cause an apparent inhibition of the mechanisms of migration by blocking the earlier stage of adhesion.

The possibility that MHC class II plays a part in lymphocyte adhesion, independently of its role in antigen presentation, has been suggested. Treatment of EAE following adoptive transfer of encephalitogenic T cells with anti-Ia antibodies prevents the onset of the disease and is correlated with a decreased infiltration of lymphocytes into the brain (Sriram & Carroll, 1991). Furthermore, the increase in adhesion of lymphocytes brought about by IFN-γ activation of a brain endothelial cell monolayer *in vitro* can be blocked by anti-class II antibody, indicating a role for the MHC class II molecule in adhesion (Goodall, Curtis & Lang, 1992). In another study, however, only a marginal reduction in adhesion was achieved following blocking with anti-Ia antibodies (Hughes *et al.*, 1988).

Most studies investigating adhesion and migration of leukocytes at the vascular barriers of the nervous system have concentrated on lymphocyte entry. This is despite the fact that, in many immunologically mediated diseases of the nervous system, monocytes also play a significant part in the disease process. Although few studies have addressed the issue of monocyte migration across these specialized endothelia, depletion studies have clearly indicated their importance in diseases such as EAE. Macrophage/monocyte depletion in EAE dramatically suppresses the expression of clinical signs and correlates with a marked reduction of infiltrated macrophages in the CNS (Huitinga *et al.*, 1990). Of particular interest is the suppression of EAE in Lewis rats following treatment *in vivo* with antibodies against the monocyte integrin CR3 (CD11b/CD18). Among the numerous ligands for this receptor is ICAM-1 and monocytes are thought to utilize this pathway for adherence and migration across the vascular wall. The attenuation of clinical signs in animals treated with the anti-CR3 antibodies is therefore believed to be due partly to the blockade of macrophage infiltration across the BBB (Huitinga *et al.*, 1993).

The mechanisms of PMN migration across the vascular barriers of the nervous system have similarly lacked concerted investigation. In a recent report, however, the adhesion and migration of PMN across bovine brain endothelia *in vitro* has been studied (Dorovini-Zis, Bowman & Prameya, 1992). Migration of PMN through endothelial cell monolayers is augmented by chemotactic gradients produced by leukotriene B_4 (LTB_4), platelet-activating factor (PAF) and N-formyl-methionyl-leukyl-phenylalanine (fMLP). Although the adhesion molecules involved were not investigated, it was suggested that the CD18 molecule was partly responsible for LTB_4-induced migration as LTB_4 is known to increase PMN adhesiveness via this molecule.

What is now abundantly clear is that the adhesive property of endothelial cells is pivotal in the inflammatory response as they are able to regulate the degree of binding of circulating leukocytes, and hence the level of extravasation. Although it is evident that the state of activation of the leukocyte is paramount in determining its ability to extravasate, the state of activation of the endothelial cell is central in overcoming the shear forces of circulating leukocytes and recruiting them from the blood.

Pathophysiological role of the vascular barriers in immunologically mediated disease

In addition to restricting the passage of cells into the nervous system, an intact barrier will also restrict the movement of molecules. The limiting nature of this barrier confers immunological properties over and above the control of leukocyte migration. The minimal transfer of molecules such as immunoglobulins and complement from the blood to the nervous tissue extracelluar fluid (ECF) and the limited passage of antigen out into the systemic circulation isolates the nervous system from the immune system. The absence of a conventional lymphatic system has previously been thought to hinder the afferent arm of the immune response. Recent work, however, has shown that there is a substantially greater degree of drainage from nervous tissue ECF into the lymphatics and blood than previously believed (Cserr & Knopf, 1992), and that antigens introduced into the intact CNS can cause a systemic antigen-specific antibody response. When damage to the blood–tissue barriers occurs, either through disruption of the tight junctions or vesicular transport, transfer of molecules from the nervous system to the circulation is markedly elevated and can lead to the immune system being exposed to previously masked auto-antigens.

Disruption of the blood–tissue barriers during inflammatory disorders can also lead to the more immediate problem of vasogenic oedema and the well-defined clinical problems related to this condition. In fact, much of the visual dysfunction associated with posterior uveitis is a direct consequence of macular oedema. The mechanisms of barrier disruption in immunologically mediated diseases of the nervous system, however, remain poorly defined despite a considerable effort to resolve this problem. What is becoming clear, however, is that disruption of the barrier is not a static all-or-nothing event but a phenomenon that varies dramatically in its distribution, its degree of permeability and its ability to resolve.

During an inflammatory response there is the release of a vast array of inflammatory agents, many of which have been implicated in disruption of

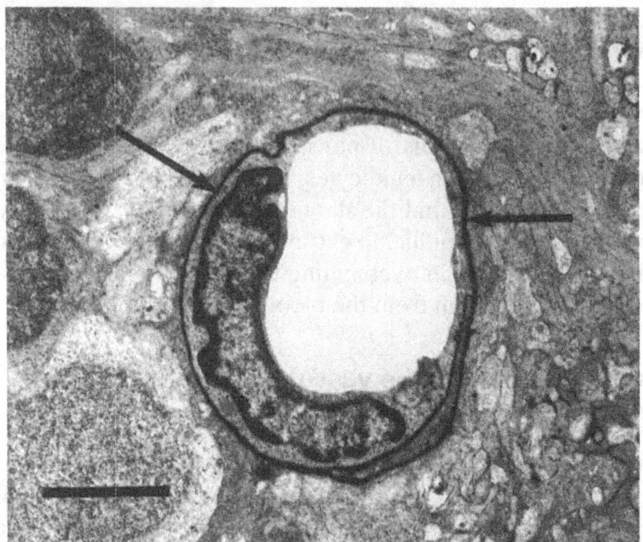

Fig. 5.4. Transmission electron micrograph of a retinal capillary from a rat with EAU showing extravasated horseradish peroxidase filling the basement membrane (arrow) and extending into the extracellular space of the parenchyma. Bar = 5 μm.

the vascular barriers of the nervous system (Greenwood, 1992*a*). The list of compounds associated with barrier breakdown includes the interleukins and other cytokines; products of the arachidonic acid cascade; vasoactive amines (e.g. histamine); components of plasma enzyme systems (e.g. the complement and kinin systems), platelet activating factor (PAF) and the polyamines. Many of these compounds have diverse physiological and pathological roles but their modes of action upon the vascular barriers are mostly unclear. It is likely that only a few of these substances, in particular the classic vasoactive agents such as histamine, bradykinin and the eicosanoids, operate in a direct manner on the endothelial cell causing vessel leakage. They may also function in an indirect way through their chemotactic properties whereby induction of leukocyte extravasation and all the accompanying phenomena may lead to damage of the barriers. This indirect process is the most likely manner in which many of these substances, especially the cytokines, bring about barrier disruption in diseases such as MS, uveitis and GBS and in their experimental analogues (Fig. 5.4). Indeed, breakdown of the barriers appears to occur concomitantly with the appearance of infiltrating immune cells (Lightman & Greenwood, 1992; Greenwood, 1992*b*; Hawkins *et al.*, 1990) although this does not exclude the direct involvement of these compounds.

Histamine, which has been widely studied, has a variety of vasoactive and immunological properties including the induction of increased permeability. Histamine can be released not only from preformed stores in mast cells and basophils, but is also produced *de novo* from T cells. Brain endothelial cells respond to histamine by increasing internal calcium levels (Revest, Abbott & Gillespie, 1991) and reducing vascular permeability from a transvascular resistance of 1500 Ω cm^2 to around 400 Ω cm^2 (Butt & Jones, 1992). This change in permeability is mediated by abluminal H_2 receptors and may result from opening of the tight junctions or induction of vesicular transport. The release of histamine from intraneural mast cells is also thought to contribute to the dysfunction of the BNB and formation of oedema during the development of EAN (Brosnan *et al.*, 1990) although the process may also be mediated by catecholamines. Interestingly, in the retina, histamine does not appear to bring about increases in vascular permeability.

Arachidonic acid and its metabolites, the eicosanoids, have also been widely implicated in the breakdown of the vascular barriers of the nervous system during immune-mediated diseases. Both arachidonic acid (Unterberg *et al.*, 1987) and its metabolites (Bhatterjee *et al.*, 1981; Dorovini-Zis *et al.*, 1992) have been found to promote the penetration of PMN across the vascular barriers of the nervous system by acting as powerful chemotactic agents although their direct action upon barrier permeability is poorly understood.

As has already been demonstrated, endothelial cells are a prime target for cytokine action eliciting a number of diverse cellular responses (reviewed in Chapter 2). The potential role of cytokines in directly affecting barrier permeability has more recently been proposed with IL-1, interleukin-2 (IL-2) and TNF all being implicated in barrier disruption. IL-1 or TNF injected into the vitreous of the rabbit eye causes a transient increase in endothelial cell pinocytosis (Brosnan *et al.*, 1990) and cellular infiltration of neutrophils (Fig. 5.5) and macrophages (Brosnan *et al.*, 1990; Martiney *et al.*, 1990) which we have found to correlate with an increase in barrier permeability. IL-2 has also been reported to induce breakdown of the BBB (Ellison, Kreig & Povlishock, 1990) with alterations in cerebrovascular morphology evident as early as 6 hours after a single dose. In studies conducted in our laboratory, however, we have been unable to elicit any changes in either the BBB or BRB of the rat following IL-2 administration.

Much of the confusion relating to the efficacy of different agents on barrier dysfunction arises from the large number of experimental variables such as dose, species and route of application. However, it is also important to note that large decreases in the ionic permeability of the barrier can occur (i.e. 1500 Ω cm^2 to 500 Ω cm^2) before disruption is of a magnitude to allow the extravasation of even small molecular weight tracers such as mannitol.

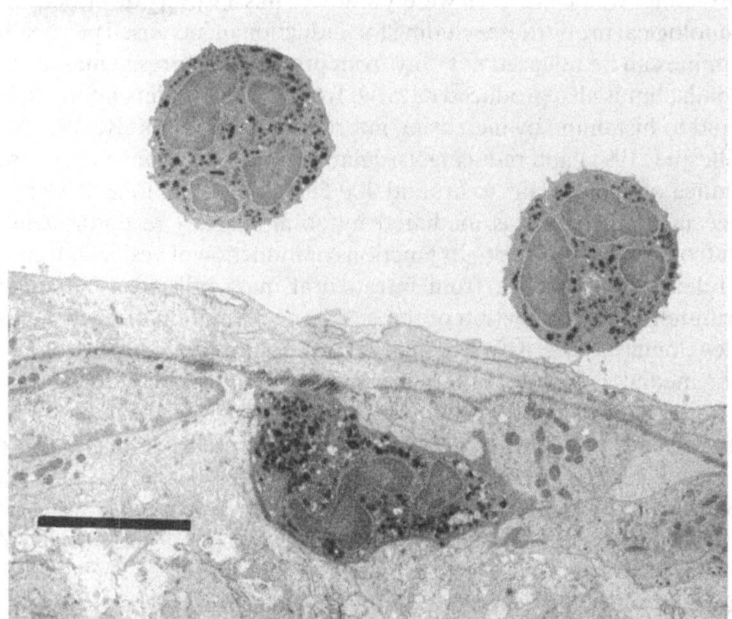

Fig. 5.5. Transmission electron micrograph of a rat retinal blood vessel following an intravitreal injection of IL-1 showing adherent and migrated neutrophils. Bar = 5 μm.

Morphological investigations

In EAE, EAU and EAN, the vascular endothelium remains structurally unchanged until the onset of the active phase of the disease when alterations in endothelial cell morphology become evident. Major structural abnormalities, however, do not occur until there is a substantial inflammatory cell infiltrate. At this point, the vascular endothelia are often thickened with increased levels of luminal surface activity as manifest by a greater number of microvilli. Increased amounts of cytosol and an up-regulation in the levels of cytosolic organelles such as rough endoplasmic reticulum (RER), ribosomes and vesicular-like profiles have also been described. This endothelial activation has been reported in both EAE (Claudio *et al.*, 1989) and EAU (Lin, Essner & Shichi, 1991; Greenwood *et al.*, 1994) and is likely to be a consequence of increased endothelial cell metabolism and protein synthesis. This is consistent with cytokine-induced up-regulation and increased expression of molecules of immunological significance such as ICAM-1 (Wong & Dorovini-Zis, 1992), MHC class II, (Male & Pryce, 1988*a*), IL-1 and IL-6 (Fabry *et al.*, 1993), transforming growth factor (TGF)-β and increased production of extracellular matrix proteins (Mahalak *et al.*, 1991). These structural changes have been shown to correlate with the severity of the disease (McMenamin *et al.*, 1992).

Raised, bulbous endothelia have also been described in EAE (O'Neill *et al.*, 1991; Raine *et al.*, 1990; Cross *et al.*, 1990; Lossinsky *et al.*, 1989), multiple sclerosis (Prineas, 1979), EAU (Lightman & Greenwood, 1992; McMenamin *et al.*, 1992; Greenwood *et al.*, 1994) uveitis (Charteris & Lee, 1990) and EAN (Powell *et al.*, 1991) with the implication that these endothelia resemble the specialized high endothelial venules (HEV). As has been described above, some of these endothelia have also been shown to express addressin adhesion molecules although a raised morphology on its own may also be due to other factors causing structural distortion.

The accumulated data relating to the alteration of structural integrity of the barriers during inflammatory diseases strongly indicates that an increase in barrier permeability occurs concomitantly with leukocyte extravasation in EAU (Lightman & Greenwood, 1992; Greenwood *et al.*, 1994), EAE (Claudio *et al.*, 1990; Hawkins *et al.*, 1990; Butter *et al.*, 1991) and EAN (Hahn, Feasby & Gilbert, 1985). Leakage of tracer is largely restricted to the areas of inflammation and results from the disruption of tight junctions (Lossinsky *et al.*, 1989; Lin *et al.*, 1991; Powell *et al.*, 1991; Greenwood *et al.*, 1994). The differential permeability described for tracers of different molecular weights supports this idea as extravasation via pinocytosis and vesicular transport would not distinguish between different-sized tracers. This does not, of course, exclude the possibility that a limited amount of vesicular transport occurs (Claudio *et al.*, 1989; Hawkins *et al.*, 1992; Greenwood *et al.*, 1994) expecially as vesicular profiles are a common feature of endothelial cells in EAE and EAU particularly in the later stages of disease. Whether these so-called vesicles result from pinocytosis or play a role in net transfer, however, remains a contentious issue.

Many ultrastructural studies have been carried out to assess the route of leukocyte migration through the vascular barriers of the nervous system. In experimental inflammatory diseases mononuclear cells can be readily identified adhering to the vascular endothelium, often by fine tenuous connections, and probing into the endothelial cell at parajunctional sites (Raine *et al.*, 1990; Greenwood *et al.*, 1994). Different populations of leukocytes are thought to extravasate by different routes with PMNs migrating at the junction between endothelial cells (Dorovini-Zis *et al.*, 1992). Lymphocytes, on the other hand, do not appear to penetrate the tight junctions but migrate through the body of the endothelial cell (Lossinsky *et al.*, 1989; Raine *et al.*, 1990; McMennamin *et al.*, 1992; Greenwood *et al.*, 1994). This process seems to involve invagination of the plasma membrane of the endothelial cell at the point of lymphocyte penetration until the cell becomes attenuated and the luminal and abluminal plasma membranes touch. Once this has occurred, pore formation between the two membranes develops allowing the unhindered passage of the leukocyte into the perivascular space and closure of the endothelial aperture after diapedesis is completed. However, this process may cause small transient leaks in barrier integrity as a result of plasma constituents diffusing between the lymphocyte and the endothelia (Lossinsky *et al.*, 1989; Claudio *et al.*, 1990). An advantage of this route would be the increased degree of control over diapedesis afforded by the endothelial cell.

Conclusions

Although the endothelia of the nervous system are highly specialized and shield the cells of the parenchyma from the immune system under normal conditions, they can be activated to recruit leukocytes from the circulation in a manner similar to that described for other vascular beds. To date, no adhesion molecules specific for the endothelia of the nervous system have been described and differences in leukocyte recruitment to nervous tissue are more likely due to distinct temporal patterns of expression of the same molecules utilized elsewhere. The endothelia of the nervous system are also thought to possess the capacity to present antigen in a class II restricted manner leading to T cell proliferation. Their ability to do this, however, is less than for professional APCs and hence the relevance of this *in vivo* is uncertain. Finally, the disruption of the vascular barriers resulting from large scale leukocyte extravasation and release of associated inflammatory compounds remains a major problem related to immunologically mediated diseases of the nervous system and our understanding of the underlying mechanisms of barrier dysfunction remain limited. The recent expansion in this field, however, is providing us with a greater understanding of the mechanisms involved in the pathogenesis of the immunologically mediated diseases of the nervous system and the important role the endothelial cell plays in the disease process.

References

Baron, J. L., Madri, J. A., Ruddle, N. H., Hashim, G. & Janeway, C. A. Jr. (1993). Surface expression of α4 integrin by CD4 T cells is required for their entry into brain parenchyma. *Journal of Experimental Medicine,* **177**, 57–68.

Bellamy, A. S., Calder, V. L., Feldmann, M. & Davison, A. N. (1985). The distribution of interleukin-2 receptor bearing lymphocytes in multiple sclerosis: evidence for a key role of activated lymphocytes. *Clinical and Experimental Immunology,* **61**, 248–56.

Berendt, A. R., Simmons, D. L., Tansey, J., Newbold, C. I. & Marsh, K. (1989). Intercellular adhesion molecule-1 is an endothelial cell adhesion receptor for *Plasmodium falciparum. Nature,* **341**, 57–9.

Bhatterjee, P., Hammond, B., Salmon, J. A., Stepney, R. & Eakins, K. E. (1981). Chemotactic response to some arachidonic acid lipoxygenase products in the rabbit eye. *European Journal of Pharmacology,* **73**, 21–8.

Brosnan, C. F., Claudio, L., Tansey, F. A. & Martiney, J. (1990). Mechanisms of autoimmune neuropathies. *Annals of Neurology,* **27**(Suppl), S75–9.

Butt, A. M. & Jones, H. C. (1992). Effect of histamine and antagonists on electrical resistance across the blood–brain barrier in rat brain surface microvessels. *Brain Research,* **569**, 100–5.

Butter, C., Baker, D., O'Neill, J. K. & Turk, J. L. (1991). Mononuclear cell trafficking and plasma protein extravasation into the CNS during chronic relapsing experimental allergic encephalomyelitis in Biozzi AB/H mice. *Journal of Neurological Science,* **104**, 9–12.

Calder, V. L. & Lightman, S. L. (1992). Experimental autoimmune uveoretinitis (EAU) verses experimental allergic encephalomyelitis (EAE): a comparison of T cell-mediated mechanisms. *Clinical and Experimental Immunology,* **89**, 165–9.

Cannella, B., Cross, A. H. & Raine, C. S. (1991). Adhesion-related molecules in the central nervous system. Upregulation correlates with inflammatory cell influx during relapsing experimental autoimmune encephalomyelitis. *Laboratory Investigation,* **65**, 23–31.

Cannella, B., Cross, A. H. & Raine, C. S. (1993). Anti-adhesion molecule therapy in experimental autoimmune encephalomyelitis. *Journal of Neuroimmunology,* **46**, 43–56.

Caspi, R. R., Chan, C -C., Fujino, Y., Najafian, F., Grover, S., Hansen, C. T. & Wilder, R. L. (1993). Recruitment of antigen-nonspecific cells plays a vital role in the pathogenesis of a T cell-mediated organ-specific autoimmune disease, experimental autoimmune uveoretinitis. *Journal of Neuroimmunology,* **47**, 177–88.

Charteris D. G. & Lee, W. R. (1990). Multifocal posterior uveitis: clinical and pathological findings. *British Journal of Ophthalmology,* **74**, 688–93.

Claudio, L., Kress, Y., Norton, W. T. & Brosnan, C. F. (1989). Increased vesicular transport and decreased mitochondrial content in blood–brain barrier endothelial cells during experimental autoimmune encephalomyelitis. *American Journal of Pathology,* **135**, 1157–68.

Claudio, L., Kress, Y., Factor, J. & Brosnan, C. F. (1990). Mechanisms of edema formation in experimental autoimmune encephalomyelitis. *American Journal of Pathology,* **137**, 1033–45.

Cross, A. H., Cannella, B., Brosnan, C. F. & Raine, C. S. (1990). Homing to central nervous system vasculature by antigen-specific lymphocytes. I. Localization of ^{14}C-labeled cells during acute, chronic and relapsing experimental allergic encephalomyelitis. *Laboratory Investigation,* **63**, 162–70.

Cross, A. H. & Raine, C. S. (1991). Central nervous system endothelial cell-polymorphonuclear cell interactions during autoimmune demyelination. *American Journal of Pathology,* **139**, 1401–9.

Cserr, H. F. & Knopf, P. M. (1992). Cervical lymphatics, the blood–brain barrier and the immunoreactivity of the brain: a new view. *Immunology Today,* **13**, 507–12.

Deschênes J., Char, D. H. & Kaleta, S. (1988). Activated T lymphocytes in uveitis. *British Journal of Ophthalmology,* **72**, 83–7.

Dorovini-Zis, K., Bowman, P. D. & Prameya, R. (1992). Adhesion and migration of polymorphonuclear leukocytes across cultured brain microvessel endothelial cells. *Journal of Neuropathology and Experimental Neurology,* **51**, 194–205.

Ellison, M. D., Krieg, R. J. & Povlishock, J. T. (1990). Differential central nervous sytem responses following single and multiple recombinant interleukin-2 infusions. *Journal of Neuroimmunology,* **28**, 249–60.

Fabry, Z., Waldschmidt, M. M., Moore, S. A. & Hart, M. N. (1990). Antigen presentation by brain microvessel smooth muscle and endothelium. *Journal of Neuroimmunology,* **28**, 63–71.

Fabry, Z., Waldschmidt, M. M., Hendrickson, D. *et al.* (1992). Adhesion molecules on murine brain microvascular endothelial cells: expression and regulation of ICAM-1 and Lgp 55. *Journal of Neuroimmunology,* **36**, 1–11.

Fabry, Z., Fitzsimmons, K. M., Herlein, J. A., Moninger, T. O., Dobbs, M. B. & Hart, M. N. (1993). Production of the cytokines interleukin 1 and 6 by murine brain microvessel endothelium and smooth muscle pericytes. *Journal of Neuroimmunology,* **47**, 23–34.

Fujikawa, L. S. & Haugen, J. P. (1990). Immunopathology of vitreous and retinochoroidal biopsy in posterior uveitis. *Ophthalmology,* **97**, 1644–53.

Goodall, C. A., Curtis, A. S. G. & Lang, S. C. (1992). Modulation of adhesion of lymphocytes to murine brain endothelial cells *in vitro*: relation to class II major histocompatability complex expression. *Journal of Neuroimmunology,* **37**, 9–22.

Greenwood, J. (1991). Astrocytes, cerebral endothelium, and cell culture. The pursuit of an *in vitro* blood–brain barrier. *Annals of the New York Academy of Sciences,* **633**, 426–31.

Greenwood, J. (1992*a*). Experimental manipulation of the blood–brain and blood–retinal barriers. In Bradbury, M. W. B. ed. *Physiology and pharmacology of the blood–brain barrier,* Handbook Exp Pharmacol 103 pp 459–86, New York: Springer-Verlag.

Greenwood, J. (1992*b*). The blood–retinal barrier in experimental autoimmune uveoretinitis (EAU): a review. *Current Eye Research,* **11**(Suppl), 25–32.

Greenwood, J. & Calder, V. (1993). Lymphocyte migration through cultured endothelial cell monolayers derived from the blood–retinal barrier. *Immunology,* **80**, 401–6.

Greenwood, J., Howes, R. & Lightman, S. (1994). The blood–retinal barrier in experimental autoimmune uveoretinitis: leukocyte interactions and functional damage. *Laboratory Investigation,* **70**, 39–52.

Hafler, D. A. & Weiner, H. L. (1987). T cells in multiple sclerosis and inflammatory central nervous system disease. *Immunology Reviews,* **100**, 307–32.

Hahn, A. F., Feasby, T. E. & Gilbert, J. J. (1985). Blood–nerve barrier studies in experimental allergic neuritis. *Acta Neuropathologica (Berl.),* **68**, 101–9.

Hart, M. N., Waldschmidt, M. M., Hanley-Hyde, J. M., Moore, S. A., Kemp, J. D. & Schelper, R. L. (1987). Brain microvascular smooth muscle expresses class II antigens. *Journal of Immunology,* **138**, 2960–3.

Hawkins, C. P., Munro, P. M. G., Landon, D. N. & McDonald, W. I. (1992). Metabolically dependent blood-brain barrier breakdown in chronic relapsing experimental allergic encephalomyelitis. *Acta Neuropathologica (Berl.),* **83**, 630–6.

Hawkins, C. P., Munro, P. M. G., MacKenzie, F., Kesselring, J., Tofts, P. S., du Boulay, E. P. G. H., Landon, D. N. & McDonald, W. I. (1990). Duration and selectivity of blood–brain barrier breakdown in chronic relapsing experimental allergic encephalomyelitis studied by gadolinium-DTPA and protein markers. *Brain,* **113**, 365–78.

Hickey, W. F., Hsu, B. L. & Kimura, H. (1991). T-lymphocyte entry into the central nervous system. *Journal of Neuroscience Research,* **28**, 254–60.

Hughes, C. C. W., Male, D. K. & Lantos, P. L. (1988). Adhesion of lymphocytes to cerebral microvascular cells: effects of interferon-γ tumour necrosis factor and interleukin-1. *Immunology,* **64**, 677–81.

Huitinga, I., van Rooijen, N., de Groot, C. J. A., Uitdehaag, B. M. J. & Dijkstra, C. D. (1990). Suppression of experimental allergic encephalomyelitis in Lewis rats after elimination of macrophages. *Journal of Experimental Medicine,* **172**, 1025–33.

Huitinga, I., Damoiseaux, J. G. M. C., Döpp, E. A. & Dijkstra, C. D. (1993). Treatment with anti-CR3 antibodies ED7 and ED8 suppresses experimental allergic encephalomyelitis in Lewis rats. *European Journal of Immunology,* **23**, 709–15.

Jemison, L. M., Williams, S. K., Lublin, F. D., Knobler, R. L. & Korngold, R. (1993). Interferon-γ-inducible endothelial cell class II major histocompatibility complex expression correlates with strain- and site-specific susceptibility to experimental allergic encephalomyelitis. *Journal of Neuroimmunology,* **47**, 15–22.

Kawai, K., Ito, K., Imamura, K., Hickey, W. F., Zweiman, B. & Takahashi, A. (1993). Enhancing effects of irrelevant lymphocytes on adoptive transferred experimental allergic encephalomyelitis. *Journal of Neuroimmunology,* **42**, 39–46.

Khalili-Shirazi, A., Hughes, R. A., Brostoff, S. W., Linington, C. & Gregson, N. (1992). T cell responses to myelin proteins in Guillain-Barre syndrome. *Journal of Neurological Sciences,* **111**, 200–3.

Lassmann, H., Schmied, M., Vass, K. & Hickey, W. F. (1993). Bone marrow derived elements and resident microglia in brain inflammation. *Glia,* **7**, 19–24.

Lightman, S. & Chan, C -C. (1990). Immune mechanisms in choroido-retinal inflammation in man. *Eye,* **4**, 345–53.

Lightman, S. & Greenwood, J. (1992). Effect of lymphocytic infiltration on the blood–retinal barrier in experimental autoimmune uveoretinitis. *Clinical and Experimental Immunology,* **88**, 473–7.

Lin, W -L., Essner, E. & Shichi, H. (1991). Breakdown of the blood–retinal barrier in S-antigen-induced uveoretinitis in rats. *Graefe's Archive for Clinical and Experimental Ophthalmology,* **229**, 457–63.

Liversidge, J., Sewell, H. F. & Forrester, J. V. (1990). Interactions between lymphocytes and cells of the blood–retina barrier: mechanism of T lymphocyte adhesion to human retinal capillary endothelial cells and retinal pigment epithelial cells *in vitro*. *Immunology,* **71**, 390–6.

Lossinsky, A. S. Badmajew, V., Robson, J. A., Moretz, R. C. & Wisniewski, H. M. (1989). Sites of egress of inflammatory cells and horseradish peroxidase transport across the blood-brain barrier in a murine model of chronic relapsing experimental allergic encephalomyelitis. *Acta Neuropathologica (Berl.),* **78**, 359–71.

McCarron, R. M., Kempski, O., Spatz, M. & McFarlin, D. E. (1985). Presentation of myelin basic protein by murine cerebral vascular endothelial cells. *Journal of Immunology,* **134**, 3100–3.

McCarron, R. M., Racke, M., Spatz, M. & McFarlin, D. E. (1991*a*). Cerebral vascular endothelial cells are effective targets for *in vitro* lysis by encephalitogenic T lymphocytes. *Journal of Immunology,* **147**, 503–8.

McCarron, R. M., Wang, L., Cowan, E. P. & Spatz, M. (1991*b*). Class II MHC antigen expression by cultured human cerebral vascular endothelial cells. *Brain Research,* **566**, 325–8.

McCarron, R. M., Wang, L., Racke, M. K., McFarlin, D. E. & Spatz, M. (1993). Cytokine-regulated adhesion between encephalitogenic T lymphocytes and cerebrovascular endothelial cells. *Journal of Neuroimmunology,* **43**, 23–30.

McMenamin, P. G., Forrester, J. V., Steptoe, R. J. & Dua, H. S. (1992). Ultrastructural pathology of experimental autoimmune uveitis. *Laboratory Investigation,* **67**, 42–55.

Mahalak, S. M., Lin, W-L., Essner, E. & Shichi, H. (1991). Increased immunoreactivity of collagen types I, III, and V, fibronectin and TGF-β in retinal vessels of rats with experimental autoimmune uveoretinitis. *Current Eye Research,* **10**, 1059–63.

Male, D. K., Pryce, G. & Hughes, C. C. W. (1987). Antigen presentation in brain: MHC induction on brain endothelium and astrocytes compared. *Immunology,* **60**, 453–9.

Male, D. K. & Pryce, G. (1988*a*). Kinetics of MHC gene expression and mRNA synthesis in brain endothelium. *Immunology,* **63**, 37–42.

Male, D. K. & Pryce, G. (1988*b*). Synergy between interferons and monokines in MHC induction on brain endothelium. *Immunology Letters,* **17**, 267–72.

Male, D. K. & Pryce, G. (1988*c*). Induction of Ia molecules on brain endothelium is related to susceptibility to experimental allergic encephalomyelitis. *Journal of Neuroimmunology,* **21**, 87–90.

Male, D., Pryce, G., Hughes, C. & Lantos, P. (1990). Lymphocyte migration into brain modelled *in vitro*: control by lymphocyte activation, cytokines and antigen. *Cellular Immunology,* **127**, 1–11.

Male, D., Pryce, G., Linke, A. & Rahman, J. (1992). Lymphocyte migration into the CNS modelled *in vitro*. *Journal of Neuroimmunology,* **40**, 167–72.

Martiney, J. A., Litwak, M., Berman, J. W., Arezzo, J. C. & Brosnan, C. F. (1990). Pathophysiologic effect of interleukin-β in the rabbit retina. *American Journal of Pathology,* **137**, 1411–23.

Myers, K. J., Dougherty, J. P. & Ron, Y. (1993). *In vivo* presentation by both brain parenchymal cells and hematopoietically derived cells during the induction of experimental autoimmune encephalomyelitis. *Journal of Immunology,* **151**, 2252–60.

O'Neill, J. K., Butter, C., Baker, D., Gschmeissner, S. E., Kraal, G., Butcher, E. C. & Turk, J. L. (1991). Expression of vascular addressins and ICAM-1 by endothelial cells in the spinal cord during chronic relapsing experimental allergic encephalomyelitis in the Biozzi AB/H mouse. *Immunology,* **72**, 520–5.

Powell, H. C., Myers, R. R., Mizisin, A. P., Olee, T. & Brostoff, S. W. (1991). Response of the axon and barrier endothelium to experimental allergic neuritis induced by autoreactive T cell lines. *Acta Neuropathologica (Berl.),* **82**, 364–77.

Prineas, J. W. (1979). Multiple sclerosis: presence of lymphatic capillaries and lymphoid tissue in the brain and spinal cord. *Science,* **203**, 1123–5.

Pryce, G., Male, D. & Sedgwick, J. (1989). Antigen presentation in brain: brain endothelial cells are poor stimulators of T cell proliferation. *Immunology,* **66**, 207–12.

Pryce, G., Male, D. & Sarkar, C. (1991). Control of lymphocyte migration into brain: selective interactions of lymphocyte subpopulations with brain endothelium. *Immunology,* **72**, 393–8.

Pryce, G., Santos, W. & Male, D. (1994). An assay for the analysis of lymphocyte migration across cerebral endothelium *in vitro*. *Journal of Immunological Methods,* **167**, 55–63.

Raine, C. S., Cannella, B., Duijvestijn, A. M. & Cross, A. H. (1990). Homing to central nervous system vasculature by antigen-specific lymphocytes. II Lymphocyte/endothelial cell adhesion during the initial stages of autoimmune demyelination. *Laboratory Investigation,* **63**, 476–89.

Revest, P. A., Abbott, N. J. & Gillespie, J. I. (1991). Receptor-mediator changes in intracellular [Ca^{2+}] in cultured rat brain capillary endothelial cells. *Brain Research,* **549**, 159–61.

Risau, W., Engelhardt, B. & Wekerle, H. (1990). Immune function of the blood–brain barrier: incomplete presentation of protein (auto-)antigens by rat brain microvascular endothelium *in vitro*. *Journal of Cell Biology,* **110**, 1751–66.

Rossler, K., Neuchrist, C., Kitz, K., Scheiner, O., Kraft, D. & Lassmann, H. (1992). Expression of leucocyte adhesion molecules at the human blood–brain barrier (BBB). *Journal of Neuroscience Research,* **31**, 365–74.

Rostami, A. M. (1993). Pathogenesis of immune-mediated neuropathies. *Pediatric Research,* **33**(Suppl), S90–4.

Sedgwick, J. D., Hughes, C. C., Male, D. K., MacPhee, I. A. M. & Ter Meulen, V. (1990). Antigen-specific damage to brain vascular endothelial cells mediated by encephalitogenic and nonencephalitogenic $CD4^+$ T cell lines *in vitro*. *Journal of Immunology,* **145**, 2474–81.

Selmaj, K., Raine, C. S., Cannella, B. & Brosnan, C. F. (1991). Identification of lymphotoxin and tumor necrosis factor in multiple sclerosis lesions. *Journal of Clinical Investigations,* **87**, 949–54.

Simmons, R. D. & Cattle, B. A. (1992). Sialyl ligands facilitate lymphocyte accumulation during inflammation of the central nervous system. *Journal of Neuroimmunology,* **41**, 123–30.

Skundric, D. S., Kim, G., Tse, H. Y. & Raine, C. S. (1993). Homing of T cells to the central nervous system throughout the course of relapsing experimental autoimmune encephalomyelitis in Thy-1 congenic mice. *Journal of Neuroimmunology,* **46**, 113–22.

Sobel, R. A., Blanchette, B. W., Bhan, A. K. & Colvin, R. B. (1984). The immunopathology of acute experimental allergic encephalomyelitis. II. Endothelial cell Ia increases prior to inflammatory cell infiltration. *Journal of Immunology,* **132**, 2402–7.

Sobel, R. A., Natale, J. M. & Schneeberger, E. E. (1987). The immunopathology of acute experimental allergic encephalomyelitis. IV. An ultrastructural immunocytochemical study of class II major histocompatability complex molecule (Ia) expression. *Journal of Neuropathology and Experimental Neurology,* **46**, 239–49.

Sriram, S. & Carroll, L. (1991). Haplotype-specific inhibition of homing of radiolabeled lymphocytes in experimental allergic encephalomyelitis following treatment with anti-Ia antibodies. *Cellular Immunology,* **135**, 222–31.

Tanaka, M. & McCarron, R. M. (1990). The inhibitory effect of tumor necrosis factor and interleukin-1 on Ia induction by interferon-γ on endothelial cells from murine central nervous system microvessels. *Journal of Neuroimmunology,* **27**, 209–15.

Tanaka, Y., Adams, D. H. & Shaw, S. (1993). Proteoglycans on endothelial cells present adhesion-inducing cytokines to leukocytes. *Immunology Today,* **14**, 111–15.

Towler, H. M. A., Whiting, P. H. & Forrester, J. V. (1990). Combination low dose cyclosporin A and steroid therapy in chronic intraocular inflammation. *Eye,* **4**, 514–20.

Traugott, U., Scheinberg, L. C. & Raine, C. S. (1985). On the presence of Ia-positive endothelial cells and astrocytes in multiple sclerosis lesions and its relevance to antigen presentation. *Journal of Neuroimmunology,* **8**, 1–14.

Unterberg, A., Wahl, M., Hammersen, F. & Baethmann, A. (1987). Permeability and vasomotor response of cerebral vessels during exposure to arachidonic acid. *Acta Neuropathologica (Berl.),* **73**, 209–19.

Vass, K., Lassmann, H., Wekerle, H. & Wisniewski, H. M. (1986). The distribution of Ia antigens in the lesions of rat acute experimental allergic encephalomyelitis. *Acta Neuropathologica (Berl.),* **70**, 149–60.

Waldschmidt, M. M., Fabry, Z., Keiner, J., Love Homan, L. & Hart, M. N. (1991). Adhesion of splenocytes to brain microvascular endothelium in the BALB/c and SJL/j mouse systems. *Journal of Neuroimmunology,* **35**, 191–200.

Wang, Y., Calder, V., Greenwood, J & Lightman, S. (1993). Lymphocyte adhesion to cultured endothelial cells of the blood–retinal barrier. *Journal of Neuroimmunology,* **48**, 161–8.

Welsh, C. T., Rose, J. W., Hill, K. E. & Townsend, J. J. (1993). Augmentation of adoptively transferred experimental allergic encephalomyelitis by administration of a monoclonal antibody specific for LFA-1α. *Journal of Neuroimmunology,* **43**, 161–8.

Whitcup, S. M., Chan, C. C., Li, Q. & Nussenblatt, R. B. (1992). Expression of cell adhesion molecules in posterior uveitis. *Archives of Ophthalmology,* **110**, 662–6.

Wilcox, C. E., Healy, D. G., Baker, D., Willoughby, D. A. & Turk, J. L. (1989). Presentation of myelin basic protein by normal guinea pig brain endothelial cells and its relevance to experimental allergic encephalomyelitis. *Immunology,* **67**, 435–40.

Wilcox, C. E., Ward, A. M. V., Evans, A., Baker, D., Rothlein, R. & Turk, J. L. (1990). Endothelial cell expression of the intercellular adhesion molecule-1 (ICAM-1) in the central nervous system of guinea pigs during acute and chronic relapsing experimental allergic encephalomyelitis. *Journal of Neuroimmunology,* **30**, 43–51.

Wong, D. & Dorovini-Zis, K. (1992). Upregulation of intercellular adhesion molecule-1 (ICAM-1) expression in primary cultures of human brain microvessel endothelial cells by cytokines and lipopolysaccharide. *Journal of Neuroimmunology,* **39**, 11–21.

Yednock, T. A., Cannon, C., Fritz, L. C., Sanchez-Madrid, F., Steinman, L. & Karin, N. (1992). Prevention of experimental autoimmune encephalomyelitis by antibodies against $\alpha 4\beta 1$ integrin. *Nature,* **356**, 63–6.

Zurbriggen, A. & Fujinami, R. S. (1988). Theiler's virus infection in nude mice: viral RNA in vascular endothelial cells. *Journal of Virology,* **62**, 3589–96.

–6–

The role of the endothelium in systemic lupus erythematosus and Sjögren's syndrome

H. L. C. BEYNON, P. ATHANASSIOU and K. A. DAVIES

Introduction

Systemic lupus erythematosus (SLE) and Sjögren's syndrome form part of a spectrum of rheumatological autoimmune diseases of unknown aetiology. A significant proportion of patients with primary SLE may exhibit clinical features of Sjögren's syndrome (secondary Sjögren's syndrome) and share similar autoantibodies against extractable nuclear antigens.

In this chapter we discuss first systemic lupus erythematosus, referring briefly to the main clinical features of the condition, and then discussing the pathogenesis of the disease in some detail, with specific reference to endothelial activation, the evidence for the role of immune complexes in mediating endothelial damage in SLE, the mechanisms involved in immune complex processing, and the role played by erythrocyte CR1 in protecting the endothelium.

We then discuss the pathogenesis of Sjögren's syndrome, again with particular reference to the endothelium, and finally address the possible role of anti-endothelial cell antibodies in the pathogenesis of SLE and Sjögren's syndrome.

Systemic lupus erythematosus

Clinical features and epidemiology

Systemic lupus erythematosus encompasses a group of multisystem inflammatory diseases characterized by the presence of a variety of autoantibodies directed against both intracellular and extracellular antigens. The clinical features of SLE are varied, and the American College of Rheumatology

Table 6.1. *American College of Rheumatology revised classification criteria for the diagnosis of SLE*

Malar rash
Discoid lupus
Photosensitivity
Aphthous ulcers
Arthritis
Serositis (pleurisy or pericarditis)
Renal disease (persistent proteinuria >0.5 g/day or cellular casts)
Neurological disorder (fits or psychosis)
Haematological disorder (haemolytic anaemia, leukopenia, lymphopenia or thrombocytopenia)
Immunological disorder (LE cells, anti-dsDNA antibody, anti-Sm or false positive VDRL)
Antinuclear antibody

classification criteria (Table 6.1) are widely used in clinical practice because of the heterogeneous nature of the disease.

The prevalence of SLE in the United Kingdom is of the order 1 per 3000 and women are affected more commonly than men (10:1). SLE is commoner in certain parts of the world where the incidence rises to 1 per 400 of the population and in general, more severe disease is seen in black Americans and Asians.

SLE is characterized by the presence of a variety of autoantibodies directed against both intracellular and extracellular antigens. The aetiology of SLE is unknown, though it is likely to be multifactorial and disease expression, which itself is often heterogeneous, is likely to present the final pathway of several environmental factors superimposed upon a genetic susceptibility.

A number of hypotheses have been proposed to explain the pathogenesis of SLE (for review see Walport, 1993). These include: i) failure of the mononuclear phagocytic system to clear immune complexes, leading to stimulation of autoimmunity by autoantigens, ii) autonomous polyclonal B cell activation leading to the production of a range of autoantibodies, iii) breakdown of tolerance to autoantigens by antigenic mimicry by microbial antigens or by interaction of viral antigens with host intracellular molecules, iv) abnormality of idiotypic networks, and v) a specific viral aetiology.

Many workers believe that the formation of immune complexes constitutes the major pro-inflammatory stimulus in SLE, and the role of immune complexes in causing tissue damage in the disease is discussed in detail below, as well as the specific protective mechanisms which exist to prevent immune complex mediated injury.

Endothelial activation in the vasculopathy of SLE

Systemic vasculitis or angiitis may be defined as an inflammatory disorder of blood vessels that usually results in necrosis of the vessel wall with subsequent vascular occlusion. The original view that endothelial cells were damaged as passive targets of inflammation during the vasculitic process has been radically altered by the appreciation that they may play an active role in the pathogenesis of many of the vasculitic illnesses. Endothelial cell activation, in response to stimulation by cytokines, may promote inflammation and allow endothelial cells to influence the immune response (reviewed in Chapters 2 and 3, also see Cotran & Pober, 1988; Pober, 1988). Such changes include: i) stimulated adhesion of leukocytes, promoted by increased expression of endothelial adhesion molecules such as P-selectin, E-selectin ICAM-1, and VCAM-1 (Mason, Kapahi & Haskard 1993); ii) pro-coagulant activity, mediated by increased synthesis of tissue factor and plasminogen activator inhibitor, and decreased thrombomodulin synthesis (Crossman & Tuddenham, 1990); iii) up-regulation of expression of Class I and II HLA molecules, allowing endothelial cells to act as antigen presenting cells and as targets for cytotoxic T lymphocytes (Hirshberg, Bergh & Thorsby, 1980; Gibofsky *et al.*, 1975; Moreas & Stasny, 1977; Teitel *et al.*, 1989); iv) cytokine production, for example membrane-bound IL-1 (Bröker *et al.*, 1988); and v) changes in cell morphology (Kurt Jones, Fiers & Pober, 1987), which may promote increased vascular permeability.

Belmont *et al.* (1994) have demonstrated statistically significant up-regulation of the endothelial adhesion molecules E-selectin, VCAM-1 and ICAM-1 on skin biopsies from non-light exposed skin in patients with active SLE compared with patients with inactive SLE and normal controls, supporting the hypothesis that exacerbations of SLE are characterized by widespread activation of the vascular endothelium. During disease flares circulating neutrophils are also activated as indicated by up-regulation of the surface β_2 integrin CD11b/CD18(CR3). Recent studies *in vitro* have demonstrated that corticosteroids are effective in down-regulating the expression of E-selectin and ICAM-1 on human umbilical vein endothelial cells (Cronstein *et al.*, 1992) and this may be one of the mechanisms which accounts for the efficacy of steroids in the management of SLE. Elevated circulating levels of the endothelial cell adhesion molecule VCAM-1 have been detected in SLE, and the elevated levels have been positively correlated with the ESR (Fig. 6.1). This observation may reflect the degree of endothelial activation seen in SLE and prospective studies are under way to determine the usefulness of VCAM-1 levels in the management of SLE (Mason *et al.*, 1993).

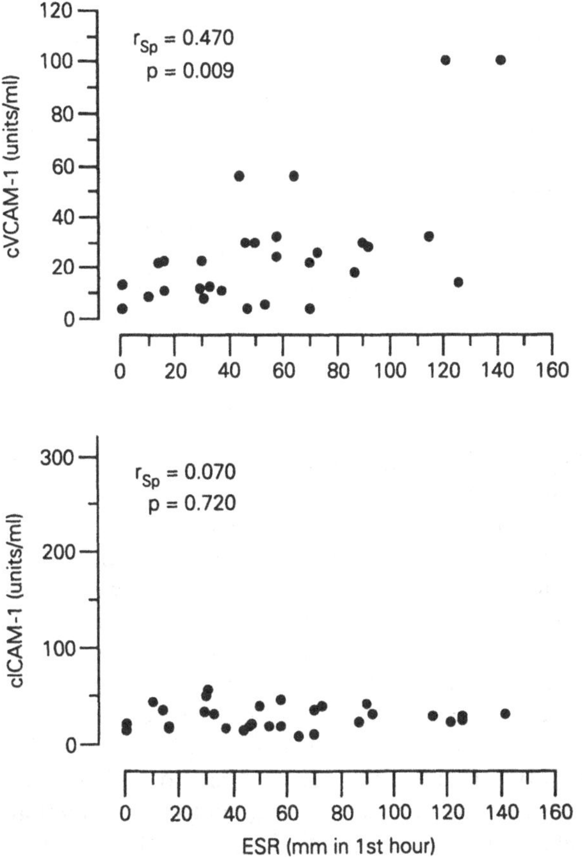

Fig. 6.1. Circulating VCAM and ICAM levels in SLE. cVCAM correlates with the erythrocyte sedimentation rate, whereas no such relationship is seen for cICAM. (Adapted from Mason *et al.*, 1993, with permission.)

Immune complexes and vascular injury

The formation of immune complexes of antibodies with foreign antigens is a central part of adaptive immunity. The mononuclear phagocytic system is an efficient scavenger of such immune complexes. However, in certain circumstances, immune complexes apparently escape this system and deposit in other tissues causing inflammation, tissue injury and release of autoantigens. These autoantigens may stimulate an autoimmune response with formation of more immune complexes and development of a cycle of further tissue injury and autoantigen release, leading to a self-perpetuating process

(Kimberly, 1987; Schifferli, Ng & Peters 1986). Systemic lupus erythematosus is often considered to be the prototype of a disease mediated by immune complexes.

Historically, the first association between immune complex deposition and systemic necrotizing vasculitis in man was decribed in a patient with serum sickness (Clark & Kaplan, 1937). Subsequently animal models of serum sickness, developed during the 1940s and 1950s (for review see Cochrane & Koffler, 1973), have formed the experimental basis of our current understanding of vasculitis mediated by immune complexes, though the relevance of these models to the natural occurrence of vasculitis in humans remains uncertain.

Animal models of immune complex-mediated injury

Acute serum sickness. Rabbits injected with bovine serum albumin developed circulating immune complexes at the time of immune elimination of the antigen, with subsequent deposition in arteries and glomeruli (Cochrane & Koffler, 1973). Electron micrographs implied that immune complexes and colloidal carbon (a tracer macromolecule) entered between endothelial cells (Cochrane, 1963). It was proposed that the increased vascular permeability followed from antigen interaction with IgE-coated basophils which led to the release of platelet-activating factor with subsequent release of vasoactive amines from platelets (Majno, Shea & Leventhal, 1969; Cochrane, 1971). Platelet depletion was associated with diminished immune complex deposition (Cochrane, 1971). There was also evidence of recruitment of neutrophils by complement following deposition of immune complexes, which could be abrogated by depletion of complement using cobra venom factor (Ward, Cochrane & Muller-Eberhard, 1965). Evidence for the pathogenic role of neutrophils in this model of necrotizing vasculitis came from observations that depletion of polymorphonuclear cells prevented the development of vasculitis (Kniker & Cochrane, 1965).

Arthus reaction. Injection of antigen into the skin of sensitized animals was followed by a vasculitis mediated by the local formation of immune complexes. Immune complexes that formed in the walls of blood vessels were rapidly removed by neutrophils with 90% disappearance in 24–48 hours (Cochrane, Weigle & Dixon, 1959). Subsequent experiments *in vitro* showed that neutrophils, activated by immune complexes in vessel walls, released proteases which digested proteins such as fibronectin (Harlan *et al.*, 1981), and generated a respiratory burst with formation of hydrogen peroxide and superoxide anion (Sachs *et al.*, 1978) causing endothelial cell detachment and lysis with vessel wall damage and occlusion.

The role of immune complexes in the pathogenesis of SLE

Several candidate antigens have been implicated in the formation of pathogenic immune complexes in SLE. The best studied complexes are probably those comprising DNA:anti-DNA antibodies. The occurrence of immune complexes containing DNA and anti-dsDNA antibodies in lupus plasma is controversial. Tan *et al.* (1966) identified DNA and anti-dsDNA in sera and plasma, and DNA and anti-dsDNA have been identified as constituents of cryoglobulins in lupus patients (Davis, Godfrey & Winfield, 1978; Adu, Dobson & Williams, 1981). Harbeck *et al.* (1973) reported an increase in the levels of measurable anti-dsDNA antibodies after treating lupus plasma with DNAase. This latter observation is difficult to reconcile with the more recent report that anti-dsDNA antibodies may protect short stretches of complexed DNA from digestion with DNAase (Burdick & Emlen, 1985). Others have failed to detect DNA/anti-dsDNA immune complexes in lupus sera (Izui, Lambert & Meischer, 1977). Difficulty in the demonstration of such immune complexes in the circulation may either reflect their very rapid transit time, which has been demonstrated experimentally in mice (Emlen & Mannik, 1982), or alternatively such immune complexes may form *in situ*.

The overall conclusion that can be drawn from a large number of studies is that small amounts of circulating immune complexes, of largely unknown composition, may be found in patients with SLE. The probable role of anti-DNA antibodies in causing disease has been reviewed (Fournie, 1988). DNA and anti-DNA antibodies were found in renal tissue (Koffler, Schur & Kunkel, 1967; Krishnan & Kaplan, 1967) and in skin (Tan & Kunkel, 1966; Landry & Sams, 1973). Anti-DNA antibodies could be eluted from renal tissue (Krishnan & Kaplan, 1967) and were concentrated compared with their levels in serum (Koffler *et al.*, 1967). Most workers found correlations between the levels in sera of anti-dsDNA antibodies and disease activity, in both cross-sectional and longitudinal studies, though almost everyone identified some patients with very high levels of anti-dsDNA and apparently inactive disease and vice versa (Schur & Sandson, 1968; Bardana *et al.*, 1975; Cameron *et al.*, 1976; Bröker *et al.*, 1988). It remains unclear how anti-dsDNA antibodies localize to tissues and several possibilities have been considered: i) that complexes comprising anti-dsDNA/DNA are deposited from plasma; ii) that dsDNA is deposited in tissues and immune complexes form *in situ* (Izui, Lambert & Miescher, 1976), or that DNA binding to the surface of endothelial cells may contribute to the build up of immune complexes at the vascular surface (Frampton *et al.*, 1991); iii) that anti-dsDNA antibodies bind to other cross-reacting antigens in tissues such as 'lupus associated membrane protein' – LAMP (Jacob *et al.*, 1987), or proteoglycan heparin sulphate, which is a normal constituent of glomerular basement membrane (Faaber *et al.*, 1984).

It is not always possible to demonstrate the presence of immune complexes in blood vessels in SLE even when there is good indirect evidence in the form of low complement levels and circulating cryoglobulins. Histologically, there may be evidence only of complement and fibrin deposition in the vessel walls; this may be related to the age of biopsy material, as illustrated by the Arthus reaction (Cochrane *et al.*, 1959).

The role of the endothelium in immune complex vasculitis

The above scheme of disease mediated by immune complexes portrays the endothelial cell in an essentially passive role. However, there is some evidence that endothelial cells express complement and Fc receptors and hence may have the capacity to bind immune complexes directly. Some authors have detected Fc receptors on unstimulated endothelial cells (Johnson, Trenchev & Faulk, 1975; Matre, 1977; Andrews *et al.*, 1981; Lyss *et al.*, 1989), although these findings have not been confirmed by others (Daha *et al.*, 1988; Cines *et al.*, 1982; Ryan, Schultz & Ryan, 1981).

Receptors for C1q on endothelial cells were first demonstrated by Linder (1981) and this observation has subsequently been confirmed (Andrews *et al.*, 1981; Daha *et al.*, 1988; Zhang, Schultz & Ryan, 1986). Daha and coworkers demonstrated that endothelial C1q receptors bound the collagenous part of C1q and that binding was saturable (Daha *et al.*, 1988). Cultured endothelial cells bound heat aggregated immunoglobulin and thyroglobulin/anti-thyroglobulin immune complexes only after pre-incubation with C1q, evidence against the presence of Fc receptors on unstimulated endothelial cells. The physiological significance of endothelial surface C1q receptors is questionable; intact C1 cannot bind to C1q receptors (Veehuis, Van Es & Daha, 1985), and, although C1 inhibitor rapidly dissociates C1r and C1s from activated C1 (Ziccardi & Cooper, 1979), immune complexes bearing C1q have not been shown to exist in the circulation. If C1q receptors on endothelial cells were able to bind circulating immune complexes this would serve to localize immune complexes to endothelial cells. Alternatively, such receptors might augment the binding of immune complexes to endothelium caused by other mechanisms, for example DNA/anti-DNA immune complexes attached to basement membrane, in the vicinity of endothelium (Izui *et al.*, 1976).

Antibodies against the collagenous part of C1q may also have a role in this context. These were first described in hypocomplementaemic urticarial vasculitis by McDuffie *et al.* (1973), and they have subsequently been detected in around 30% of patients with SLE (Wisnieski & Naff, 1989). They are directed against neo-epitopes on the collagenous part of the molecule (Uwatoko, Gauthier & Mannik, 1991), and are strongly associated with hypocomplementaemia in SLE (Davies *et al.*, 1994*a*), possibly as a consequence of direct activation of the classical pathway by the antibodies. It is also possible that they may play a pathogenic role in the genesis of endothelial cell damage, either by forming immune complexes directly with C1q, which can then bind to C1q receptors on the endothelial cell surface, or by targeting immune complexes comprising other antigens to the cell surface.

There is some evidence that viruses may play an indirect role in mediating endothelial damage in SLE and Sjögren's syndrome (discussed in detail below). Herpes viruses possess genes for Fc and complement receptors which may be expressed on the surface of infected cells. Herpes simplex virus 1 infection of cultured human umbilical vein endothelial cells is followed by expression of Fc and C3b receptors within 4 hours (Cines *et al.*, 1982). Likewise, Herpes simplex virus 2, Cytomegalovirus and Herpes zoster virus have been shown to induce Fc receptors on endothelial cells (Ryan *et al.*, 1981; Para, Goldstein & Speak, 1982; Smiley, Hoxie & Friedman, 1985). The Fc receptor of Herpes simplex virus 1 appears to be glycoprotein E (Baucke & Spear, 1979) and the C3b receptor is glycoprotein C (Friedman *et al.*, 1984). Expression of these receptors is thought to be a mechanism for the protection of infected cells from destruction by specific antibody and complement. However, such receptors might also serve to localize immune complexes to infected endothelium and cause injury.

Immune complex processing in SLE

The pathophysiology of immune complex processing in SLE

Immune complexes are normally cleared by the fixed mononuclear phagocytes of the liver and spleen. Opsonized immune complexes bind to red cells via complement receptor type 1 (CR1), and this process facilitates the transport of complexes within the circulation (Davies, Schifferli & Walport, 1994*b*). This preferential binding of C3b-opsonized complexes to red cells may facilitate endothelial protection in two possible ways: i) by delivering complexes safely to the fixed macrophages of the reticuloendothelial system, and ii) by keeping them in the central jet stream of the vessel, away from the endothelial lining (Schifferli & Ng, 1988) (Fig. 6.2).

Tissue macrophages in the liver and spleen bear both Fc and complement receptors – CR3 and CR4, and opsonized complexes can interact with both groups of receptors. It has long been mooted that there may be a primary or acquired defect in mononuclear phagocytic function in SLE which predisposes to the development of disease by impairment of complex clearance. This idea that abnormal function of the reticuloendothelial system might result in failure of immune complex processing stems from early experimental work in animals by Biozzi and colleagues using colloidal carbon particles

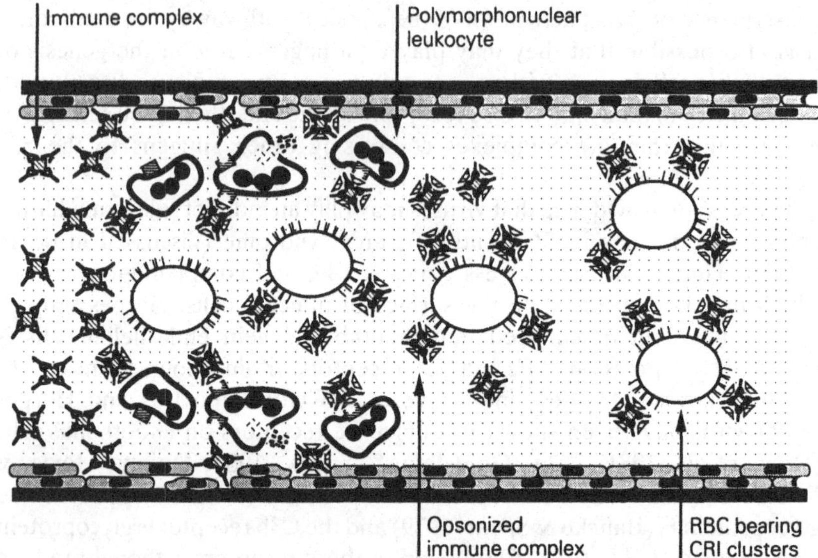

Fig. 6.2. The proposed role of erythrocyte CR1 in endothelial protection. Immune complexes are opsonised with C3b and bind preferentially to clustered erythrocyte CR1 in the jet stream of the vessel, whence they are delivered to the fixed macrophages of the liver and spleen.

(Biozzi, Benacerraf & Halpern, 1953), and by Haakenstaad & Mannik (1974), who demonstrated that immune complex injection into rabbits resulted in saturable hepatic uptake, followed by spillover into other organs.

Whether or not this so-called 'reticuloendothelial saturation' occurs in humans, and is a contributory factor in the development of disease is not clear. Much experimental effort has been devoted to addressing the question of whether there is indeed a fundamental abnormality of mononuclear phagocytic system function in SLE, related primarily to immune complex clearance mediated by Fc receptors, or whether the primary problem is one of defective immune complex delivery to the mononuclear phagocytic system secondary to hypocomplementaemia and/or low levels of erythrocyte CR1.

A number of different model systems have been employed to address these questions. Early studies used erythrocytes coated with IgG or IgM, and more recent studies have employed either aggregated immunoglobulin, or soluble immune complexes (Frank *et al.*, 1983; Lobatto *et al.*, 1987, 1988; Schifferli *et al.*, 1989). Erythrocytes coated with IgG are cleared in the spleen (Fc-receptor dependent) (Frank *et al.*, 1983; Kimberly & Ralph, 1983), while IgM-coated cells show transient retention in the liver mediated by reversible binding to complement receptors (Atkinson & Frank, 1974).

The clearance of IgG-coated erythrocytes has been specifically studied in SLE patients. Frank and colleagues demonstrated a correlation between clearance rate, disease activity, and levels of circulating immune complexes (Frank *et al.*, 1979; Hamburger *et al.*, 1982) in patients with SLE, but a number of other similar studies have failed to show any such direct correlations (Kimberly *et al.*, 1983; Parris *et al.*, 1982; Valentijn *et al.*, 1985). Splenic blood flow is an important factor affecting the clearance of IgG-coated red cells (Walport *et al.*, 1985*a*), and this may influence disease-associated clearance of these cells.

More recently Lobatto and colleagues have assessed mononuclear phagocyte function in different diseases, using radiolabelled soluble aggregates of IgG (Lobatto *et al.*, 1988). These aggregates were predominantly cleared from the circulation in the liver and spleen. Significant differences were seen between normal subjects and patients with SLE. In particular, the liver/spleen uptake ratios were higher in the patients, owing to reduced splenic uptake of the aggregates. Halma *et al.* (1989) analysed clearance of aggregated IgG in 22 patients with SLE and 12 normal volunteers, demonstrating reduced binding of aggregates to red cell CR1 in the patient group, with a faster initial elimination rate. In this study the major factor influencing the aggregate clearance rate was the serum IgG concentration.

Soluble immune complex clearance has been studied using [^{125}I]-labelled tetanus-toxoid/anti-tetanus toxoid complexes (Schifferli *et al.*, 1989). Either native complexes, or complexes pre-opsonized *in vitro* with autologous serum, were injected into normal volunteers and into 15 patients with immune complex disease or hypocomplementaemia. Immune complexes bound to erythrocyte CR1 receptors in a complement-dependent manner, with CR1 number correlated with the level of uptake. Two phases of clearance were seen. In subjects with low CR1 numbers and hypocomplementaemia there was a very rapid initial disappearance of immune complexes, which was attributed at that time to deposition of complexes outside the reticuloendothelial system, although our subsequent studies using hepatitis B surface antigen (HBsAg)/anti-HBsAg immune complexes indicated that this explanation was incorrect, and that this initial rapid phase of clearance is, in fact, due to hepatic uptake of the complexes (Davies *et al.*, 1992, 1993). The second phase of clearance was approximately monoexponential, and the observed elimination rate correlated inversely with CR1 numbers and red cell complex binding. It was also observed that the fast initial phase of clearance in the complement deficient patients (who had normal CR1 numbers) was abolished when immune complexes, pre-opsonized and bound to autologous erythrocytes *in vitro*, were injected.

Imaging studies performed with HBsAg/anti-HBsAg immune complexes provided the most direct evidence that a reduction in plasma complement levels and erythrocyte CR1 profoundly affects *in vivo* processing of immune complexes. Hypocomplementaemia was associated with more rapid uptake of complexes into the liver, with subsequent release into the circulation of immune complexes of intermediate size (Davies *et al.*, 1992, 1993). As discussed above, it had been noted in previous studies using [^{125}I]-labelled tetanus-toxoid/anti-tetanus toxoid complexes (Schifferli *et al.*, 1989) that there was more rapid initial clearance of immune complexes from the circulation in patients with SLE, or C1q-deficiency. This was attributed to 'trapping' of complexes outside the reticuloendothelial system, but in these earlier studies direct imaging was not available. In the HBsAg/anti-HBsAg studies we saw no evidence of 'trapping' outside the liver and spleen. The markedly increased rapidity of initial clearance from the circulation was due to more rapid hepatic uptake, both in the profoundly hypocomplementaemic SLE patients and in a C2-deficient subject before treatment with fresh–frozen plasma. In both cases there was release of immune complexes from the liver following this initial uptake phase. We do not know the true significance of this observation, but clearly material of this sort could have phlogistic potential in itself, or serve to modulate autoantibody production.

There was markedly reduced uptake and retention of complexes in the spleen in the SLE patients, and the pre- and post-treatment studies in the C2-deficient patient demonstrated for the first time in man that uptake of immune complexes in the spleen is a complement-dependent phenomenon (Davies *et al.*, 1993). Similar observations were made in mice in the 1970s, and complement has been demonstrated in a number of model systems to be important for the localization of certain antigens to follicular dendritic cells and within splenic lymphoid follicles (Pepys, 1974; Pryjma & Humphrey, 1975; Klaus & Humphrey, 1977). In guinea-pigs, the spleen has also been shown to be of major importance for the clearance of complement-opsonized bacteria (Hosea *et al.*, 1981). These observations relating to the complement-dependent nature of splenic immune complex processing in humans have both immunopathological and clinical implications. Failure to localize immune complexes and their antigens in the spleen in SLE may have a bearing on the production of antibodies in this condition, either to self- or exogenous antigens. Efficient and safe processing of certain bacterial or viral antigens, or auto-antigens derived, for example, from apoptotic leukocytes, may depend on their uptake in the spleen, localization to the appropriate antigen-presenting cells, and the rapid production of antibody. It is tempting to speculate that persistence of either exogenous or auto-antigens as a result of impaired clearance in the reticuloendothelial system might result in the presentation of antigen to 'non-professional' antigen-presenting cells elsewhere in the immune system, resulting in an abnormal cellular or humoral immune response. Alternatively, the 'planting' of a persistent antigen, for example in the kidney, might then result in the *in situ* formation of potentially harmful immune complexes, as has been demonstrated in various experimental models of glomerulonephritis (Couser & Salant, 1980).

One of the criticisms of the studies of immune complex processing described above is that they were all performed using large immune complexes prepared *in vitro*, in the absence of complement, and may not therefore be physiological. There is conflicting evidence regarding the binding of immune complexes formed in the presence of complement to erythrocyte CR1. Varga, Thiry & Furst (1988) demonstrated that BSA–anti-BSA complexes formed in the presence of serum failed to bind to erythrocytes. However, others have shown that the successive infusion of human dsDNA antibodies and dsDNA into monkeys and rabbits leads to rapid formation of immune complexes capable of binding to red cell CR1 (Edberg, Kujala & Taylor, 1987). Immune complexes formed *in vivo* in man have been shown to bind erythrocyte CR1, in a model system using radiolabelled mouse antibodies to human milk fat globule-1 (HMFG-1) and a polyclonal affinity-purified anti-mouse antibody (Davies *et al.*, 1990). Complexes thus formed are removed by mechanisms which involve CR1 on erythrocytes, but non-erythrocyte bound complexes could clearly also be eliminated in the liver.

The role of erythrocyte CR1 in endothelial protection

As described above, an alteration in endothelial monolayer integrity is believed to be a pre-requisite for the deposition of circulating immune complexes (Cochrane, 1963). We have recently developed a model system which provides a reliable method for assessing endothelial monolayer integrity by measuring the access of a radiolabelled anti-FITC antibody to its target antigen fixed on a fibronectin matrix, upon which the endothelial cells were cultured in monolayers. We have previously reported the effects of selected inflammatory mediators which may play a part *in vivo* in disrupting the endothelial barrier, thereby facilitating the deposition of immune reactants (Beynon *et al.*, 1993). More recently, we have explored the interaction between HBsAg/anti-HBsAg immune complexes, neutrophils and the endothelium using this model system (Beynon *et al.*, 1994).

In initial experiments we demonstrated that HBsAg/anti-HBsAg immune complexes did not bind to either resting or cytokine-stimulated endothelial cells, confirming the observation than an increase in endothelial monolayer permeability is a prerequisite for the deposition of circulating immune complexes.

Cochrane and colleagues first demonstrated the importance of neutrophils in rabbit models of small vessel vasculitis (Cochrane, 1968, 1971). In the rabbit experimental serum sickness model, coronary arteritis was characterized by a neutrophil influx, fibrinoid necrosis and destruction of the internal elastic lamina. Neutrophil depletion was shown to completely abrogate the inflammatory reaction (Cochrane *et al.*, 1959, Cochrane, 1968). Flingiel *et al.* (1984) demonstrated that neutrophil proteases were primarily responsible for the destruction of the internal elastic lamina but that oxygen radicals released from activated neutrophils also played a role in vascular injury. Endothelial damage by neutrophils *in vitro* has been demonstrated by several authors in response to various stimuli including immune complexes (Harlan *et al.*, 1981; Breedveld *et al.*, 1988; Hashimoto, Tanimoto & Miyamoto, 1987), chemotactic factors (Sachs *et al.*, 1978) and chemicals (Weiss *et al.*, 1981). Hashimoto *et al.* (1992) demonstrated that sera from SLE patients is capable of activating PMN to induce endothelial cell damage, as measured by ^{51}Cr release, and the degree of toxicity was shown to be related to circulating immune complex levels. Harlan *et al.* (1981) demonstrated that heat aggregated IgG was effective in inducing neutrophil damage to endothelial cells and the effect was dependent on immune complex size, with large 13–22S complexes being more efficient than smaller 7S complexes. Immune complexes have been shown to activate neutrophils via Fcγ-receptors type II and III (Brunkhorst *et al.*, 1992) and signal transduction was shown to be a G protein dependent process (Dougherty *et al.*, 1984; Gierschik *et al.*, 1986; Brunkhorst *et al.*, 1992; Hashimoto *et al.*, 1992). We have demonstrated that HBsAg/anti-HBsAg immune complexes will directly activate neutrophils to increase endothelial monolayer permeability, and the degree of permeability was potentiated by prestimulation of the endothelial cells with IL-1β (Beynon *et al.*, 1994). A combination of endothelium expressing adhesion molecules and activated neutrophils may thus provide a protected microenvironment on the endothelial cell surface for activated neutrophils to release oxygen radicals and proteases, with the end result of increasing monolayer permeability.

In vivo, the binding of immune complexes to erythrocyte CR1 is thought to play an important protective role in preventing peripheral immune complex deposition by transporting immune complexes to the mononuclear phagocytic system where the immune complex–CR1 is removed (Cornacoff *et al.*, 1983; Schifferli & Taylor, 1989). Acquired CR1 deficiency is a feature of active disease in patients with SLE (Walport *et al.*, 1985*b*) and the *in vivo* studies of radiolabelled immune complexes, which we discussed above, demonstrated abnormal clearance patterns in SLE patients with active disease and low CR1 numbers (Davies *et al.*, 1992), supporting the hypothesis that, in health, the binding of immune complexes to erythrocyte CR1 plays a protective role in abrogating immune complex-mediated vasculitis. Using our *in vitro* model we have demonstrated that erythrocytes with normal CR1 status may play a protective role in abrogating HBsAg/anti-HBsAg immune complex mediated neutrophil-induced increases in endothelial monolayer permeability. This protective effect was CR1-dependent,

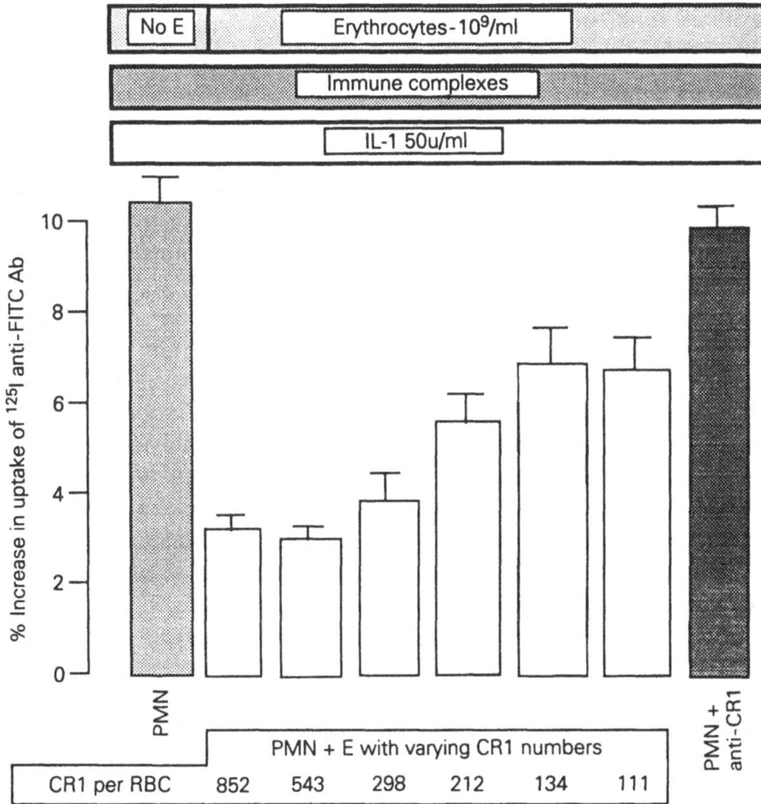

Fig. 6.3. The protective effect exerted by erythrocytes [E] with varying CR1 number per cell on endothelial permeability induced by HBsAg/anti-HBsAg immune-complex activated neutrophils (1×10^6/ml). The degree of protection offered by erythrocytes was seen to vary with CR1 molecule expression. Thus, erythrocytes with 852 CR1 per cell reduced the increased endothelial monolayer permeability from 9.5% to 3.1% compared with erythrocytes with 101 CR1 numbers per cell which only reduced the permeability increase from 9.5% to 6.7%. Values are plotted as the mean + 1s.d. of three different experiments (adapted from Beynon *et al.*, 1994, with permission).

as it was lost when erythrocyte CR1 was specifically blocked by pre-incubation of erythrocytes with an anti-CR1 antibody but not by an irrelevant antibody. Using erythrocytes prepared from four SLE patients and two normal controls we were able to show that the protective effect was directly dependent on the number of erythrocyte CR1 receptors (Fig. 6.3).

Sjögren's syndrome

Clinical features and pathogenesis

Sjögren's syndrome is a chronic autoimmune disease characterized by a lymphocytic infiltrate and destruction of epithelial exocrine glands. Sjögren's syndrome may occur as a separate disease entity (primary Sjögren's syndrome) or in association with another autoimmune disease such SLE (secondary Sjögren's syndrome). The cardinal features are dry eyes (keratoconjunctivitis sicca) and dry mouth (xerostomia). Clinical features seen in Sjögren's syndrome are summarized in Table 6.2. The diagnosis of primary Sjögren's syndrome is based on the presence of xerostomia, keratoconjunctivitis sicca and/or parotid gland enlargement and the finding of focal lymphocytic infiltrates on minor salivary gland biopsy. The presence of antibodies to the extractable nuclear antigens Ro and La provide confirmatory evidence of the diagnosis. Table 6.3 summarizes the range of autoantibodies seen in SLE and Sjögen's syndrome. The prevalence of primary Sjögren's syndrome is unknown though it is probably common and like SLE is commoner in females than males (9:1). Secondary Sjögren's syndrome occurs in approximately 50% of patients with rheumatoid arthritis and up to 20% of patients with SLE.

Recent advances in our understanding of Sjögren's syndrome suggest that an environmental agent may be instrumental in initiating an autoimmune reaction in a genetically susceptible host leading to a chronic disease which results in exocrine gland destruction. Viral infections have been implicated in both animal and human models and candidate viruses include members of the herpes and retrovirus families. Epstein–Barr and cytomegalovirus have been shown to replicate in salivary glands during primary infection (Hudson *et al.*, 1979; Wolf, Haus & Wilmes, 1984) and Fox, Pearson & Vaughan (1986*b*) demonstrated the presence of Epstein–Barr associated antigen in salivary gland biopsies and Epstein–Barr DNA in saliva, but these findings although suggestive, do not confirm a causal role in the aetiopathogenesis. Recent evidence to support a role for Epstein–Barr virus infection has come from studies which demonstrate increased expression of the *c-myc* protooncogene in both peripheral monocytes (Boumpas *et al.*, 1990) and salivary gland acinar epithelial cells (Skopouli *et al.*, 1992) in patients with Sjögren's syndrome. This oncogene has previously been demonstrated to be involved in Epstein–Barr-associated Burkitt's lymphoma. In animal models, transgenic mice bearing the *tax* gene of the human T-lymphotropic virus type 1 develop an autoimmune exocrinopathy leading to acinar destruction and a surrounding lymphocytic infiltration (Green *et al.*, 1989). The human T-lymphotropic virus type I *tax* gene has also recently been detected in salivary gland epithelium from two patients with Sjögren's syndrome – the diffuse lymphocytic infiltration syndrome (Miyasaka *et al.*, 1986).

Table 6.2. *Clinical features of Sjögren's syndrome*

Glandular manifestations
Xerostomia
Keratoconjunctivitis sicca
Salivary gland enlargement
Dyspareunia
Extraglandular manifestations
Arthralgias/arthritis
Raynaud's phenomenon
Lymphadenopathy
Vasculitis
Kidney involvement
Renal tubular acidosis
Interstitial nephritis
Glomerulonephritis
Other features
Hepatitis
Splenomegaly
Peripheral neuropathy
Myositis
B cell lymphoma

Sjögren's syndrome – pathology at the cellular level

B cell hyperactivity

Hypergammaglobulinaemia, and the production of autoantibodies directed both against non-organ specific antigens such as immunoglobulin (rheumatoid factors), extractable nuclear antigens – anti-Ro and anti-La, and specific cell-associated antigens, e.g. against determinants expressed on salivary ductal epithelial cells (Harley, 1987), are characteristic of the condition.

High circulating levels of IgA-containing immune complexes have also been reported in Sjögren's syndrome (Bendaoud *et al.*, 1991). Antibodies against Ro (SSA) and La (SSB), two ribonucleoproteins, are detected by immunofluorescence in approximately 45% and 20% respectively of patients for Sjögren's but the incidence rises to 95% and 85% using the more sensitive enzyme linked immunoabsorbent method (Moutsopoulos & Talal,

Table 6.3. *Incidence of non-organ specific autoantibodies in SLE and Sjögren's syndrome*

SLE
- Antinuclear antibodies 95%
- Antibodies to double-stranded DNA 75%
- Antibodies to RNP
- Antibodies to Sm
- Antibodies to Ro (SSA)
- Antibodies to La (SSB)

Sjögren's syndrome
- Anti-nuclear antibodies 80%
- Rheumatoid factors 80%
- Antibodies to Ro (SSA) 60%
- Antibodies to La (SSB) 40%
- Anti-mitochondrial antibodies 7%
- Cryoglobulins 20%

1987). These antibodies are also found in SLE but differ in their fine specificity (Bey-Chetrit, Fox & Tay, 1990). The presence of antibodies to Ro and La correlates with earlier onset, prolonged duration, vasculitis, hepatosplenomegaly, recurrent salivary gland enlargement and the intensity of salivary gland lymphocytic infiltrate (Manoussakis *et al.*, 1986).

There is evidence that, quite early on in the natural history of primary Sjögren's, patients have detectable levels of monoclonal proteins. Moutsopolos *et al.* (1983) have demonstrated that 80% of patients with primary Sjögren's with extraglandular involvement can be shown to have monoclonal light chains or immunoglobulins in the serum, compared with 25% of patients with disease limited to the salivary glands. Analysis of circulating cryoglobulins from patients with primary Sjögren's demonstrates that these are type II cryoglobulins containing an IgM monoclonal rheumatoid factor (Tzioufas *et al.*, 1986). It is well established that there is an increased risk of lymphoproliferative disease particularly in patients with extraglandular Sjögren's syndrome and as can be seen, monoclonality is commonest in these patients. Moutsopoulos *et al.* (1990) demonstrated specific monoclonal B cell expansion in patients with circulating monoclonal immunoglobulins. Seven of twelve patients with Sjögren's syndrome with IgMκ cryoprecipitable monoclonal proteins had a predominance of κ plasma cells in their minor salivary glands compared to equal numbers of κ and λ positive plasma cells in patients without cryoblobulins or with polyclonal cryoglobulins. It is hoped that future studies will determine the utility of these monoclonal markers in predicting the onset of lymphoma.

Lymphocyte studies

Pathological examination of the major salivary glands classically shows a benign lymphoepithelial lesion with lymphocytic infiltrate of the salivary epithelium and the presence of keratin containing epithelial cells, so-called 'epimyoepithelial islands'. The biopsy of minor labial salivary glands has become an established test in the diagnosis of Sjögren's syndrome, and characteristically shows focal aggregates of 50 or more lymphocytes, and macrophages adjacent to, and replacing, normal acini throughout the biopsy specimen. Various diagnostic scoring criteria based on the density and size of the lymphocytic infiltrate have been proposed to aid in the diagnosis as the histological appearance appears to be the best single criterion for the diagnosis of Sjögren's syndrome (Chisholm & Mason, 1968; Greenspan *et al.*, 1974). The progressive lymphocytic infiltrate eventually leads to salivary gland acinar destruction.

Evidence suggests that the increased levels of circulating immunoglobulin seen in Sjögren's syndrome arise from lymphocytes infiltrating the salivary glands as neither blood nor bone marrow lymphocytes can be shown to secrete increased quantities of immunoglobulin (Fauci & Moutsopoulos, 1981). The advent of monoclonal antibody technology has facilitated characterization of the salivary gland lymphocytic infiltrate. A predominantly helper/inducer T cell ($CD4^+$) lymphocytic infiltration which starts around the ductal epithelium is seen initially (Skopouli *et al.*, 1991), and although the T cells were shown to express HLA-DR, implying activation, IL-2 receptors were not detected on the infiltrating cells (Fox *et al.*, 1986*a*; Dalavanga, Drosos & Montsopoulos, 1986). These class II-restricted $CD4^+$ cytotoxic T cells may be involved in the destruction of the salivary epithelium. Despite the predominant T cell infiltrate, evidence to date suggests that the B cell activation may be autonomous. This hypothesis is supported by the findings that i) blood lymphocytes isolated from patients with Sjögren's will spontaneously develop into B cell lines expressing EBV (Miyasaka *et al.*, 1986) and ii) B cells isolated from Sjögren's patients will spontaneously secrete autocrine B cell growth fractors and interleukins 1, 2 and 3 (Miyasaka *et al.*, 1986; Moutsopoulos & Manoussakis, 1989). An increase in the CD5 population of lymphocytes in both peripheral blood and salivary gland infiltrates has also been demonstrated and numbers were significantly greater in individuals with circulating monoclonal rheumatoid factors (Dauphinee, Tovar & Talal, 1988). Mononuclear cells isolated from patients with chronic lymphatic leukaemia, which interestingly is characterized by expansion of the CD5 subpopulation, can be induced to produce a range of autoantibodies (Bröker *et al.*, 1988), supporting the hypothesis of a link between CD5 B cell proliferation and non-organ specific autoimmunity.

Gentric, Lydyard & Youinou (1990) have demonstrated that a significant proportion of monoclonal IgM may exhibit autoantibody activity.

Aberrant HLA-expression and endothelial activation

The triggering factor for the focal exocrine gland cell-mediated reaction is unknown. Recent studies on salivary gland biopsies from patients with Sjögren's syndrome have demonstrated strong expression of VCAM-1 and ICAM-1 on the endothelial cells which have the appearance of high endothelial cell venules. The venules are surrounded by $CD4^+$ $CD45RO^+$ T cells suggesting that cytokine mediated up-regulation of endothelial adhesion molecules might facilitate the accumulation of VLA-4 and LFA-1 expressing T cells (Aziz *et al.*, 1992; Saito *et al.*, 1993). The enhanced expression of HLA-DR molecules on endothelial cells, ductal and acinar epithelial cells and monocytes may have a role in the immunopathogenesis of Sjögren's syndrome (Dalavanga *et al.*, 1986; Aziz *et al.*, 1992).

Anti-endothelial antibodies

There have been many studies suggesting a role for antibodies directed against endothelium in the aetiology of SLE. Some of these studies require critical appraisal, as there are important methodological difficulties in the identification of true anti-endothelial cell antibodies. In particular, endothelium is bathed *in vivo* in plasma containing antibodies. It should therefore be very difficult to detect anti-endothelial antibodies of high binding constant, unless these are present in gross antibody excess. Many of the assays for anti-endothelial antibodies have measured binding to endothelial cells fixed in microtitre plates. These assays may measure binding of immunoglobulins of relatively low binding constant, which may be of little pathophysiological significance.

Anti-endothelial cell antibodies were found in sera from patients with active SLE (Cines *et al.*, 1984), which bound saturably via the $F(ab')_2$ domain to endothelial cells, deposited complement on endothelial surfaces, induced prostacyclin release, caused platelets to adhere and disrupted the endothelial monolayer. Others (Shingu & Hurd, 1981; Rosenbaum *et al.*, 1988), have shown circulating anti-endothelial cell antibodies in a variety of connective tissue diseases including SLE and rheumatoid arthritis, but these antibodies have not been shown to be in any way pathogenic.

It is possible that anti-endothelial cell antibodies require co-factors to induce vascular damage. The addition of peripheral blood mononuclear cells was shown to induce endothelial cell cytoxicity in combination with anti-endothelial cell antibodies from some patients with active SLE (Penning *et al.*, 1985). Cytokine stimulation of endothelium may be necessary for mediation of the pathogenic affects of anti-endothelial cell antibodies (as discussed above); there is evidence for increased cytokine production in SLE (Ramirez *et al.*, 1986). Studies have identified antibodies in sera from patients with systemic lupus erythematosus which react with cultured endothelial cells and increase production of a pro-coagulant tissue factor (Tannenbaum, Finko & Cines, 1986), which could promote vascular thrombosis. More recently, IgG isolated from patients with SLE has been shown to stimulate the release of von Willebrand factor from cultured endothelial cells and this may contribute to a pro-thrombotic tendency *in vivo* (Lindsey *et al.*, 1993).

The question as to whether anti-endothelial cell antibodies are a cause or consequence of vascular damage has not been answered. That such antibodies are only detected with low frequency in sera from patients with diabetes and atherosclerosis, argues against them developing as a general consequence of vascular damage (Rosenbaum *et al.*, 1988). If pathogenic anti-endothelial cell antibodies are present in patients with SLE, a question that needs to be resolved is: what determines binding of such antibodies *in vivo*? In a flare of SLE not all organs are involved at the same time. One explanation for the restriction of diseases to particular organ-specific vascular beds could be variation in the type and density of surface endothelial cell antigens from organ to organ. There is some evidence in support of this hypothesis. The monoclonal antibody, OKM5 showed differential binding to endothelial cells present in different parts of the kidney; the antibody was reactive with renal medullary endothelial cells but not glomerular or cortical small vessel endothelium (Knowles *et al.*, 1984).

Concluding remarks

The endothelium clearly constitutes a major potential target for immune-mediated injury in SLE. It may be damaged by neutrophils and/or immune complexes as discussed above, or may be a target for specific autoantibodies. There is a range of protective mechanisms which are particularly designed to protect the endothelium from immune complex-mediated damage. The preferential binding of C3b-opsonized complexes facilitates their carriage in the circulation to the fixed macrophage system, and by preventing potentially phlogistic interactions with neutrophils. Soluble CR1 (sCR1) has been used therapeutically in a number of model systems (Kalli, Hsu & Fearon, 1994), and clearly has exciting potential as a therapeutic agent for the prevention or amelioration of endothelial damage in conditions such as SLE. It remains to be clarified whether the endothelium constitutes a target for specific cell-mediated or humoral auto-immune attack in vasculitis. There is no doubt that the development of a fuller understanding of the role of the endothelium in diseases such as SLE and Sjögren's syndrome will lead ultimately to novel, and more precisely targeted therapeutic approaches in these diseases.

Acknowledgements

Dr Davies is an Arthritis and Rheumatism Council Senior Fellow. Dr Athanassiou is supported by a fellowship from the Hellenic Society for Rheumatology. The experimental work in this chapter performed by Dr Beynon was performed while he was an MRC training fellow in the Rheumatology Unit, Hammersmith Hospital.

References

Adu, D., Dobson, J. & William, D. G. (1981). Effects of soluble aggregates of IgG on the binding, uptake and degradation of the C1q subcomponent by adherent guinea pig macrophages. *Clinical Experimental Immunology*, **43**, 605.

Andrews, B. S., Shadford, M., Cunningham, P. & Davis, J. S. (1981). Demonstration of a C1q receptor on the surface of human endothelial cells. *Journal of Immunology*, **127**, 1075–80.

Atkinson, J. P. & Frank, M. M. (1974). Studies on the *in vivo* effects of antibody. Interaction of IgM antibody and complement in the immune clearance and destruction of erythrocytes in man. *Journal Clinical Investigation*, **54**, 339–48.

Aziz, K. E., McCluskey, P. J., Montanaro, A. & Wakefield, D. (1992). Vascular endothelium and lymphocyte adhesion molecules in minor salivary glands of patients with Sjögren's syndrome. *Journal of Clinical Laboratory Immunology*, **37**, 39–49.

Bardana, E. J., Harbeck, R. J., Hoffman, A. A., Pirofsky, B. & Carr, R. (1975). The prognostic and therapeutic implications of DNA–anti-DNA complexes in systemic lupus erythematosus. *American Journal of Medicine*, **59**, 515–22.

Baucke, R. B. & Spear, P. G. (1979). Membrane proteins specified by herpes simplex virus on cultured human endothelial cells. *Journal of Virology*, **32**, 779.

Belmont, H. M., Buyon, J., Giorno, R. & Abramson, S. (1994). Up-regulation of endothelial cell adhesion molecules characterizes disease activity in systemic lupus erythematosus. *Arthritis Rheumatism*, **37**(3), 376–83.

Bendaoud, B., Pennec, Y. L., Lelong, A. *et al.* (1991). IgA-containing immune complexes in the circulation of patients with primary Sjögren's syndrome. *Journal of Autoimmunity*, **4**, 177–84.

Bey-Chetrit, E., Fox, R. I. & Tay, E. M. (1990). Dissociation of immune responses to the SSA(Ro) 52 kd and 60 kd polypeptides in systemic lupus erythematosus and Sjögren's syndrome. *Arthritis Rheumatism*, **33**, 3449–55.

Beynon, H. L. C., Haskard, D. O., Davies, K. A., Haroutanian, R. & Walport, M. J. (1993). Combinations of low concentrations of cytokines and acute agonists synergize in increasing the permeability of endothelial monolayers. *Clinical and Experimental Immunology*, **91**, 314–19.

Beynon, H. L. C., Davies, K. A., Haskard, D. O. & Walport, M. J. (1994). Erythrocyte complement receptor type 1 and interactions between immune complexes, neutrophils and endothelium. *Journal of Immunology*, **153**, 3160–7.

Biozzi, G., Benacerraf, B. & Halpern, B. N. (1953). Quantitative study of the granulopoietic activity of the reticuloendothelial system II. *British Journal of Experimental Pathology*, **34**, 441–57.

Boumpas, D. T., Eleftheriades, E. G., Molina, R. *et al.* (1990). C-myc proto-oncogene expression in peripheral blood mononuclear cells from patients with primary Sjögren's syndrome. *Arthritis Rheumatism*, **33**, 49–56.

Breedveld, F. C., Heurkens, H. M., Lafber, G. J. M., Van Hinsbergh, M. & Cats, A. (1988). Immune complexes in sera from patients with rheumatoid vasculitis induce polymorphonuclear cell mediated injury to endothelial cells. *Clinical Immunology and Immunopathology*, **48**, 202.

Bröker, B. M., Klajman, A., Youinou, P. *et al.* (1988). Chronic lymphocytic leukemic cells secrete multispecific autoantibodies. *Journal of Autoimmunity*, **1**, 469–81.

Brunkhorst, B. A., Strohmeir, G., Lazzari, K. *et al.* (1992). Differential role of FcγRII and FcγRIII in immune complex stimulation of human neutrophils. *Journal of Biological Chemistry*, **267**, 20659–66.

Burdick, G. & Emlen, W. (1985). Effect of antibody excess on the size, stoichiometry and DNAase resistance of DNA–anti-DNA immune complexes. *Journal of Immunology*, **135**, 2593–7.

Cameron, J. S., Lessof, M. H., Ogg, C. S., Williams, B. D. & Williams, D. G. (1976). Disease activity in the nephritis of systemic lupus erythematosus in relation to serum complement concentrations. DNA-binding capacity and precipitating anti-DNA antibody. *Clinical and Experimental Immunology*, **25**, 417–27.

Chisholm, D. M. & Mason, D. K. (1968). Labial salivary gland biopsy in Sjögren's syndrome. *Journal of Clinical Pathology*, **21**, 656–60.

Cines, D. B., Lyss, A. P., Bina, M., Corkey, R., Kefalides, N. A. & Friedman, H. M. (1982). Fc and C3 receptors induced by herpes simplex virus on cultured human endothelial cells. *Journal of Clinical Investigation*, **69**, 123–8.

Cines, D. B., Lyss, A. P., Reeber, M. B. & DeHoratius, R. J. (1984). Presence of complement-fixing anti-endothelial cell antibodies in systemic lupus erythematosus. *Journal of Clinical Investigation*, **73**, 611–25.

Clark, E. & Kaplan, B. J. (1937). Endocardial, arterial and other mesenchymal alterations associated with serum sickness disease in man. *Archives in Pathology*, **24**, 458.

Cochrane, C. G., Weigle, W. O. & Dixon, F. J. (1959). The role of polymorphonuclear leucocytes in the initiation and cessation of the Arthus reaction. *Journal of Experimental Medicine*, **110**, 481.

Cochrane, C. G. (1963). Studies on localisation of antigen–antibody complexes and other macromolecules in vessels. *Journal of Experimental Medicine*, **142**, 242.

Cochrane, G. C. (1968). Immunologic tissue injury mediated by neutrophil leucocytes. *Advances in Immunology*, **9**, 97.

Cochrane, G. C. (1971). Mechanisms involved in deposition of immune complexes in tissues. *Journal of Experimental Medicine*, **134**, 75–89.

Cochrane, C. G. & Koffler, D. (1973). Immune complex disease in experimental animals and man. *Advances in Immunology*, **16**, 185.

Cornacoff, J. B., Hebert, L. A., Smead, W. L., Van Aman, M. E., Birmingham, D. J. & Waxman, F. J. (1983). Primate erythrocyte–immune complex-clearing mechanism. *Journal of Clinical Investigation*, **71**, 236–7.

Cotran, R. S. & Pober, J. S. (1988). Endothelial activation: Its role in inflammatory and immune reactions. In Simionescu, N. & Simionescu, M. eds, *Endothelial Cell Biology*, pp. 335–44, New York, London: Plenum Press.

Couser, W. G. & Salant, D. J. (1980). *In-situ* immune complex formation and glomerular injury. *Kidney International*, **17**, 1–13.

Cronstein, B. N., Kimmel, S. C., Levin, R. L. *et al.* (1992). A mechanism for the anti-inflammatory effects of corticosteroids: the glucocorticoid receptor-regulates leukocyte adhesion to endothelial cells and expression of endothelial leukocyte adhesion molecule 1 and intercellular adhesion molecule 1. *Proceedings of the National Academy of Sciences* USA, **89**, 9991–5.

Crossman, D. C. & Tuddenham, E. G. D. (1990). Procoagulant function of endothelium. In Warren, J. B. ed, *The Endothelium. An Introduction to current Research,* pp. 119–28, New York, London: Wiley-Liss.

Daha, M. R., Miltenburg, A. M. M., Hiemstra, P. S., Klar-Mohamad, N., van Es, L. A. & van Hinsbergh, V. W. M. (1988). The complement subcomponent C1q mediates binding of immune complexes and aggregates to endothelial cells *in vitro. European Journal of Immunology,* **18**, 783–7.

Dalavanga, Y. A., Drosos, A. A. & Moutsopoulos, H. M. (1986). Labial minor salivary gland immunopathology in Sjögren's syndrome. *Scandinavian Journal of Rheumatology,* **61**(suppl), 67–70.

Dauphinee, M., Tovar, Z. & Talal, N. (1988). B-cells expressing CD5 are increased in Sjögren's syndrome. *Arthritis Rheumatism,* **31**, 642–7.

Davies, K. A., Hird, V., Stewart, S. *et al.* (1990). A study of *in vivo* immune complex formation and clearance in man. *Journal of Immunology,* **144**, 4613–20.

Davies, K. A., Peters, A. M., Beynon, H. L. C. & Walport, M. J. (1992). Immune complex processing in patients with systemic lupus erythematosus – *in vivo* imaging and clearance studies. *Journal of Clinical Investigation,* **90**, 2075–83.

Davies, K. A., Erlendsson, K., Beynon, H. L. C. *et al.* (1993). Splenic uptake of immune complexes in man is complement-dependent. *Journal of Immunology,* **151**, 3866–73.

Davies, K. A., Norsworthy, P. A., Athanassiou, P., Mason, P. D., Loizou, S. & Walport, M. J. (1994*a*). Anti-C1q antibodies in SLE. *British Journal of Rheumatology,* **33**(abstr suppl 1), 96. (Abstract)

Davies, K. A., Schifferli, J. A. & Walport, M. J. (1994*b*). Complement deficiency and immune complex disease. *Springer Seminars in Immunopathology,* **15**, 397–416.

Davis, J. S., Godfrey, S. M. & Winfield, J. B. (1978). Direct evidence for circulating DNA/anti-DNA complexes in systemic lupus erythematosus. *Arthritis and Rheumatism,* **21**, 17–22.

Dougherty, R. W., Godfrey, P. P., Hoyle, P. C., Putney, J. W. J. & Freer, R. J. (1984). Secretagogue-induced phosphoinositide metabolism in human neutrophils. *Biochemical Journal,* **222**, 307.

Edberg, J. C., Kujala, G. A. & Taylor, R. P. (1987). Rapid immune adherence reactivity of nascent, soluble antibody/DNA immune complexes in the circulation. *Journal of Immunology,* **139**, 1240–4.

Emlen, W. & Mannik, M. (1982). Clearance of circulating DNA–anti-DNA immune complexes. *Journal of Experimental Medicine,* **155**, 1210–15.

Faaber, P., Capel, P. J. A., Rijke, G. S. M. *et al.* (1984). Cross reactivity of anti-DNA antibodies with proteoglycan. *Clinical and Experimental Immunology,* **55**, 502–8.

Fauci, A. S. & Moutsopoulos, H. M. (1981). Polyclonally triggered B-cells in the peripheral blood of normal individuals and in patients with SLE and primary Sjögren's syndrome. *Arthritis Rheumatism,* **24**, 577–84.

Flingiel, S. E. G., Waro, P. A., Johnson, K. J. & Till, G. O. (1984). Evidence for a role of hydroxyl radicals in immune-complex-induced vasculitis. *American Journal of Pathology,* **115**, 375.

Fournie, G. J. (1988). Circulating DNA and lupus nephritis. *Kidney International,* **33**, 487–97.

Fox, R. I., Bumol, T., Fantozzi, R., Bone, R. & Schreiber, R. (1986*a*). Expression of histocompatibility antigen HLA-DR by salivary gland epithelial cells in Sjögren's syndrome. *Arthritis and Rheumatology,* **29**, 1105–11.

Fox, R. I., Pearson, G. & Vaughan, J. H. (1986*b*). Detection of Epstein–Barr virus-associated antigens and DNA in salivary gland biopsies from patients with Sjögren's syndrome. *Journal of Immunology,* **137**, 3162–7.

Frampton, G., Hobby, P., Morgan, A., Staines, N. A. & Cameron, J. S. (1991). A role for DNA in anti-DNA antibodies binding to endothelial cells. *Journal of Autoimmunity,* **4**, 463–78.

Frank, M. M., Hamburger, M. I., Lawley, T. J., Kimberly, R. P. & Plotz, P. H. (1979). Defective reticuloendothelial system Fc-receptor function in systemic lupus erythematosus. *New England Journal of Medicine,* **300**, 518–23.

Frank, M. M., Lawley, T. J., Hamburger, M. I. & Brown, E. J. (1983). Immunoglobulin G Fc receptor-mediated clearance in autoimmune diseases. *Annals of Internal Medicine,* **98**, 206–18.

Friedman, H. M., Cohen, G. H., Eisenberg, R. J., Seidel, C. A. & Cines, D. B. (1984). Glycoprotein C of herpes simplex virus 1 acts as a receptor for the C3b complement component on infected cells. *Nature,* **309**, 644–5.

Gentric, A., Lydyard, P. & Youinou, P. (1990). Multispecific autoantibody reactivity of human monoclonal immunoglobulins. *European Journal of Internal Medicine,* **1**, 277–84.

Gibofsky, A., Jaffe, E. A., Fotino, M. & Becker, C. G. (1975). The identification of HLA antigens on fresh and cultured human endothelial cells. *Journal of Immunology,* **115**, 730–3.

Gierschik, P., Falloon, J., Milligan, G., Pines, M., Gallin, J. I. & Speigel, A. (1986). Immunochemical evidence for a novel pertussis toxin substance in human neutrophils. *Journal of Biological Chemistry,* **261**, 8058–62.

Green, J. E., Hinricks, S. H., Vogel, J. & Jay G. (1989). Exocrinopathy resembling Sjögren's syndrome in HTLB-1 tax transgenic mice. *Nature,* **341**, 72–4.

Greenspan, J. S., Daniels, T. E., Talal, N. & Sylvester, R. A. (1974). The histopathology of Sjögren's syndrome in labial salivary gland biopsies. *Oral Surgery Oral Medicine Oral Pathology,* **37**, 217–29.

Haakenstaad, A. E. & Mannik, M. (1974). Saturation of the reticuloendothelial system with soluble immune complexes. *Journal of Immunology,* **112**, 1939–48.

Halma, C., Daha, M. R., van Furth, R., Camps, J. A. J., Evers-Schouten, J. H., Pauwels, E. K. K., Lobatto, S. & van Es, L. A. (1989). Elimination of soluble ^{123}I-labelled aggregates of human immunoglobulin G in humans: the effect of splenectomy. *Clinical Experimental Immunology,* **77**, 62–6.

Hamburger, M. I., Lawley, T. J., Kimberly, R. P., Plotz, P. H. & Frank, M. M. (1982). A serial study of splenic reticuloendothelial system Fc-receptor functional activity in systemic lupus erythematosus. *Arthritis and Rheumatism,* **25**, 48–54.

Harbeck, R. J., Bardana, E. J., Kohler, P. F. & Carr, R. I. (1973). DNA: antiDNA complexes: their detection in systemic lupus erythematosus sera. *Journal of Clinical Investigation,* **52**, 789–95.

Harlan, J. M., Killen, P. D., Henker, L. A., Striker, G. E. & Wright, D. G. (1981). Neutrophil mediated injury: *in vitro* mechanism of cell detachment. *Journal of Clinical Investigation,* **68**, 1394.

Harley, J. B. (1987). Autoantibodies in Sjögren's syndrome. In Talal, N., Moutsopoulos, H. M. & Kassan, S. S. eds, *Sjögren's Syndrome: Clinical and Immunological Aspects,* pp. 218–34, Berlin: Springer-Verlag.

Hashimoto, Y., Tanimoto, K. & Miyamoto, T. (1987). Destruction of red blood cells and cultured vascular endothelial cells by immune activated polymorphonuclear leukocytes. *Inflammation,* **11**, 201.

Hashimoto, Y., Nakano, K., Yoshinoya, S., Tanimoto, K. & Itoh, K. (1992). Endothelial cell destruction by polymorphonuclear leukocytes incubated with sera from systemic lupus erythematosus. *Scandinavian Journal of Rheumatology,* **21**, 209.

Hirshberg, H., Bergh, O. J. & Thorsby, E. (1980). Antigen-presenting properties of human vascular endothelial cells. *Journal of Experimental Medicine,* **152**, 249s–55s.

Hosea, S. W., Brown, E. J., Hamburger, M. I. & Frank, M. M. (1981). Opsonic requirements for intravascular clearance after splenectomy. *New England Journal of Medicine,* **304**, 245–50.

Hudson, J., Chantler, J., Lok, L., Misra, V. & Muller, M. (1979). Model systems for analysis of latent CMV infections. *Canadian Journal of Microbiology,* **25**, 245–50.

Izui, S., Lambert, P. H. & Miescher, P. A. (1976). *In vitro* demonstration of a particular affinity of glomerular basement membrane and collagen for DNA. A possible basis for a local formation of DNA–anti-DNA complexes in systemic lupus erythematosus. *Journal of Experimental Medicine,* **144**, 428–43.

Izui, S., Lambert, P. H. & Miescher, P. A. (1977). Failure to detect circulating DNA–anti DNA complexes by four radioimmunological methods in patients with systemic lupus erythematosus. *Clinical and Experimental Immunology,* **30**, 384.

Jacob, L., Lety, M. A., Louvard, D. & Bach, J. F. (1985). Binding of a monoclonal anti-DNA autoantibody to identical protein(s) present at the surface of several human cell types involved in lupus pathogenesis. *Journal of Clinical Investigation,* **75**, 315–7.

Jacob, L., Lety, M. A., Choquette, D. *et al.* (1987). Presence of antibodies against a cell-surface protein, cross-reactive with DNA in systemic lupus erythematosus: a marker of the disease. *Proceedings of the National Accadamy of Sciences USA,* **84,** 2956–9.

Johnson, P. M., Trenchev, P. & Faulk, W. P. (1975). Immunological studies of human placentae. Binding of complexed immunoglobulin by stromal endothelial cells. *Clinical and Experimental Immunology,* **22**, 133.

Kalli, K. R., Hsu, P. & Fearon, D. T. (1994). Therapeutic uses of recombinant complement protein inhibitors. *Springer Seminars in Immunopathology,* **15**, 417–31.

Kimberly, R. P., Parris, T. M., Inman, R. D. & McDougal, J. S. (1983). Dynamics of mononuclear phagocyte system Fc receptor function in systemic lupus erythematosus. Relation to disease activity and circulating immune complexes. *Clinical and Experimental Immunology,* **51**, 261–8.

Kimberly, R. P. & Ralph, P. (1983) Endocytosis by the mononuclear phagocyte system and autoimmune disease. *American Journal of Medicine,* **74**, 481–93.

Kimberley, R. P. (1987). Immune complexes in the rheumatic diseases. *Rheumatic Disease Clinics North America,* **13**, 583–96.

Klaus, G. G. B. & Humphrey, J. H. (1977). The generation of memory cells. I. The role of C3 in the generation of B memory cells. *Immunology,* **33**, 31–40.

Kniker, W. & Cochrane, C. G. (1965). Pathogenic factors in vascular lesions of experimental serum sickness. *Journal of Experimental Medicine,* **122**, 83–98.

Knowles, D. M., Tolidjian, B., Marboe, C., D'Agati, B., Grimes, M. & Chess, I. (1984). Monoclonal antibodies OKM1 and OKM5 possess distinctive tissue distributions including differential reactivity with vascular endothelium. *Journal of Immunology,* **132**, 2170–3.

Koffler, D., Schur, P. H. & Kunkel, H. G. (1967). Immunological studies concerning the nephritis of systemic lupus erythematosus. *Journal of Experimental Medicine,* **126**, 607–24.

Krishnan, C. & Kaplan, M. H. (1967). Immunopathologic studies of systemic lupus erythematosus. II. Anti-nuclear reaction of gamma-globulin eluted from homogenates and isolated glomeruli of kidneys from patients with lupus nephritis. *Journal of Clinical Investigation,* **46**, 569.

Kurt Jones, E. A., Fiers, W. & Pober, J. S. (1987). Membrane bound IL 1 induction on human endothelial cells and dermal fibroblasts. *Journal of Immunology,* **139**, 2317–24.

Landry, M. & Sams, W. M. (1973). Systemic lupus erythematosus: studies of the antibodies bound to skin. *Journal of Clinical Investigation,* **52**, 1871–80.

Linder, E. (1981). Binding of C1q and complement activation by vascular endothelium. *Journal of Immunology,* **126**, 648–57.

Lindsey, N. J., Dawson, R. A., Henderson, F. I., Greaves, M. & Highes, P. (1993). Stimulation of von Willebrand factor antigen release by immunoglobulin from thrombosis prone patients with systemic lupus erythematosus and the anti-phospholipid syndrome. *British Journal of Rheumatology,* **32**, 123–6.

Lobatto, S., Daha, M. R., Voetman, A. A., Evers-Schouten, J. H., Van Es, A. A., Pauwels, E. K. J. & Van Es, L. A. (1987). Clearance of soluble aggregates of immunoglobulin G in healthy volunteers and chimpanzees. *Clinical and Experimental Immunology,* **69**, 133–41.

Lobatto, S., Daha, M. R., Breedveld, F. C., Panwels, E. K. J., Evers-Schouten, J. H., Voetman, A. A., Cats, A & Van Es, L. A. (1988). Abnormal clearance of soluble aggregates of human immunoglobulin G in patients with systemic lupus erythematosus. *Clinical and Experimental Immunology,* **72**, 55–9.

Lyss, A. P., Finko, R., Knight, K., Bina, M., Reeber, M. & Cines, D. B. (1989). Interaction of IgC with human endothelial cells. *Clinical Research,* **30**, 323A.

McDuffie, F. C., Sams, W. M. Jr., Maldonado, J. E., Adreini, P. H., Conn, D. L. & Samoya, E. A. (1973). Hypocomplementaemia with cutaneous vasculitis and arthritis: possible immune complex syndrome. *Mayo Clinical Proceedings,* **48**, 340–8.

Majno, G., Shea, S. M. & Leventhal, M. (1969). Endothelial contraction induced by histamine type mediators. *Journal of Biological Chemistry,* **42**, 647–73.

Manoussakis, M. N., Tzioufas, A. G., Pange, P. J. E. & Moutsopoulos, H. M. (1986). Serological profiles in subgroups of patients with Sjögren's syndrome. *Scandinavian Journal of Rheumatology,* **61**(suppl), 89–92.

Mariette, X., Agbalika, F., Daniel, M. T. *et al.* (1993). Detection of human T lymphotropic virus type I tax gene in salivary gland epithelium from two patients with Sjögren's syndrome. *Arthritis and Rheumatism,* **36**, 1423–8.

Mason, J. C., Kapahi, P. & Haskard, D. O. (1993). Detection of increased levels of circulating intercellular adhesion molecule 1 in some patients with rheumatoid arthritis but not in patients with systemic lupus erythematosus. *Arthritis and Rheumatism,* **36**, 519–27.

Matre, R. (1977). Similarities of Fcγ receptors on trophoblasts and placental endothelial cells. *Scandinavian Journal of Immunology,* **6**, 953–8.

Miyasaka, N., Yamaoka, K., Sato, K. *et al.* (1986). An analysis of polyclonal B-cell activation in Sjögren's syndrome: characterization of B-cell lines spontaneously established from the peripheral blood. *Journal of Rheumatism,* **61**(suppl), 123–6.

Moreas, J. R. & Stasny, P. (1977). A new antigen system expressed in human endothelial cells. *Journal of Clinical Investigation,* **66**, 449–54.

Moutsopoulos, H. M., Steinberg, A. D., Fauci, A. S., Lane, H. C. & Papadopoulos, N. M. (1983). High incidence of free monoclonal light chains in the sera of patients with Sjögren's syndrome. *Journal of Immunology,* **130**, 2263–5.

Moutsopoulos, H. M. & Talal, N. (1987). Immunologic abnormalities in Sjögren's syndrome. In Talal, N., Moutsopoulos, H. M. & Kassan, S. S. eds, *Sjögren's Syndrome: Clinical and Immunological Aspects,* pp. 258–65, Berlin: Springer-Verlag.

Moutsopoulos, H. M. & Manoussakis, M. N. (1989). Immunopathogenesis of Sjögren's syndrome: facts and fancy. *Autoimmunity,* **5**, 17–24.

Moutsopoulos, H. M., Tzioufas, A. G., Bai, M. K., Papadopoulos, N. M. & Papadimitriou, C. S. (1990). Serum IgMk monoclonicity in patients with Sjögren's syndrome is associated with an increased proportion of k-positive plasma-cells infiltrating the labial minor salivary glands. *Annals of Rheumatic Disease,* **49**, 929–31.

Para, M. F., Goldstein, L. & Speak, P. G. (1982). Similarities and differences in the Fc binding glycoprotein of herpes simplex virus types 1 and 2 and tentative mapping of the viral genome for this glycoprotein. *Journal of Virology,* **41**, 137–44.

Parris, T. M., Kimberly, R. P., Inman, R. D., McDougal, S., Gibofsky, A. & Christian, C. (1982). Defective Fc-receptor mediated function of the mononuclear phagocyte system in lupus nephritis. *Annals of Internal Medicine,* **97**, 526.

Penning, C. A., French, M. A. H., Rowell, N. R. & Hughes, P. (1985). Antibody-dependent cellular toxicity of human vascular endothelium in systemic lupus erythematosus. *Journal of Clinical Laboratory Immunology,* **17**, 125–30.

Pepys, M. B. (1974). Role of complement in induction of antibody production *in vivo*. Effect of cobra factor and other C3-reactive agents on thymus-dependent and thymus-independent antibody responses. *Journal of Experimental Medicine,* **140**, 126–45.

Pober, J. S. (1988). Cytokine-mediated activation of vascular endothelium. *American Journal of Pathology,* **133**, 426–33.

Pryjma, J. & Humphrey, J. H. (1975). Prolonged C3 depletion by cobra venom factor in thymus-deprived mice and its implication for the role of C3 as an essential second signal for B-cell triggering. *Immunology,* **28**, 569–76.

Ramirez, F., Williams, R. C., Sibbitt, W. L. & Searles, R. P. (1986). Immunoglobulin from systemic lupus erythematosus serum induces interferon release by normal mononuclear cells. *Arthritis and Rheumatism,* **29**, 326–36.

Rosenbaum, J., Pottinger, B. E., Woo, P. *et al.* (1988). Measurement and characterisation of circulating anti-endothelial cell IgG in connective tissue disease. *Clinical and Experimental Immunology,* **72**, 450–6.

Ryan, U. S., Schultz, D. R. & Ryan, J. W. (1981). Fc and C3b receptors on pulmonary endothelial cells: induction by injury. *Science,* **214**, 557–9.

Sachs, T., Moldow, C. F., Craddock, P. R., Bowers, T. K. & Jacob, H. S. (1978). Oxygen radicals mediate endothelial damage by complement stimulated granulocytes. *Journal of Clinical Investigation,* **61**, 1161–7.

Saito, I., Terauchi, K., Shimuta, M. *et al.* (1993). Expression of cell adhesion molecules in the salivary and lacrimal glands of Sjögren's syndrome. *Journal of Clinical Laboratory Analysis,* **7**, 180–7.

Schifferli, J. A., Ng, Y. C. & Peters, D. K. (1986). The role of complement and its receptor in the elimination of immune complexes. *New England Journal of Medicine,* **315**, 488–95.

Schifferli, J. A. & Ng, Y. C. (1988). The role of complement in the processing of immune complexes. *Baillière's Clinical Immunology Allergy,* **2**(2), 319–34.

Schifferli, J. A., Ng, Y. C., Paccaud, J. P. & Walport, M. J. (1989). The role of hypocomplementaemia and low erythrocyte complement receptor type 1 numbers in determining abnormal immune complex clearance in humans. *Clinical and Experimental Immunology,* **75**, 329–35.

Schifferli, J. A. & Taylor, R. P. (1989). Physiological and pathological aspects of circulating immune complexes. *Kidney International,* **35**, 993.

Schur, P. H. & Sandson, J. (1968). Immunologic factors and clinical activity in systemic lupus erythematosus. *New England Journal of Medicine,* **278**, 533–8.

Shingu, M. & Hurd, E. R. (1981). Sera from patients with systemic lupus erythematosus reactive with human endothelial cells. *Journal of Rheumatology,* **8**, 581–6.

Skopouli, F. N., Fox, P. C., Galanopoulou, V., Atkinson, J. C., Jaffe, E. C. & Moutsopoulos, H. M. (1991). T-cell subpopulation in the labial minor salivary gland histopathologic lesion of Sjögren's syndrome. *Journal of Rheumatology,* **18**, 210–14.

Skopouli, F. N., Kousvelari, E. E., Mertz, P., Jaffe, E. S., Fox, P. C. & Moutsopoulos, H. M. (1992). C-myc mRNA in labial salivary glands of patients with Sjögren's syndrome. *Journal of Rheumatology,* **19**(5), 693–9.

Smiley, M. L., Hoxie, J. A. & Friedman, H. M. (1985). Herpes simplex virus type 1 infection of endothelial, epithelial, and fibroblast cells induces a receptor for C3b. *Journal of Immunology,* **134**, 2673–8.

Tan, E. M. & Kunkel, H. G. (1966). An immunofluorescent study of skin lesions in systemic lupus erythermatosus. *Arthritis and Rheumatology,* **9**, 37–46.

Tan, E. M., Schur, P. H., Carr, R. I. & Kunkel, H. G. (1966). Deoxyribonucleic acid (DNA) and antibodies to DNA in serum of patients with systemic lupus erythematosus. *Journal of Clinical Investigation,* **45**, 1732–40.

Tannenbaum, S. H., Finko, R. & Cines, D. B. (1986). Antibody and immune complexes induce tissue factor production by human endothelial cells. *Journal of Immunology,* **137**, 1532–7.

Teitel, J. M., Shore, A., McBarron, J. & Schiavone, A. (1989). Enhanced T cell activation due to combined stimulation by both endothelial cells and monocytes. *Scandinavian Journal of Immunology,* **29**, 165–73.

Tzioufas, A. G., Manoussakis, M. N., Costello, R., Silis, M., Papadopoulos, N. M. & Moutsopoulos, H. M. (1986). Cryoglobulinemia in autoimmune rheumatic diseases: Evidence of circulating monoclonal cryoglobulins in patients with primary Sjögren's syndrome. *Arthritis and Rheumatology,* **29**, 1098–104.

Uwatoko, S., Gauthier, V. J. & Mannik, M. (1991). Autoantibodies to the collagen-like region of C1q deposit in glomeruli via C1q in immune deposits. *Clinical Immunology and Immunopathology,* **61**, 268–73.

Valentijn, R. M., van Overhagen, H., Hazevoet, H. M. *et al.* (1985). The value of complement and immune complex determinations in monitoring disease activity in patients with systemic lupus erythematosus. *Arthritis and Rheumatology,* **28**, 904–13.

Varga, L., Thiry, E. & Furst, G. (1988). BSA-anti-BSA immune complexes formed in the presence of serum do not bind to autologous red cells. *Immunology,* **64**, 381–6.

Veerhuis, R., van Es, L. A. & Daha, M. R. (1985). Effects of soluble aggregates of IgG on the binding, uptake and degradation of the C1q subcomponent by adherent guinea pig macrophages. *European Journal of Immunology,* **15**, 881–7.

Walport, M. J., Peters, A. M., Elkon, K. B., Pusey, C., Lavender, J. P. & Hughes, G. R. V. (1985*a*). The splenic extraction ratio of antibody-coated erythrocytes and its response to plasma exchange and pulse methylprednisolone. *Clinical and Experimental Immunology,* **60**, 465–73.

Walport, M. J., Ross, G. D., Mackworth-Young, C., Watson, J. V., Hogg, N. & Lachmann, P. J. (1985*b*). Family studies of erythrocyte complement receptor type 1 levels: reduced levels in patients with SLE are acquired, not inherited. *Clinical and Experimental Immunology,* **59**, 547–54.

Walport, M. J. (1993). Systemic lupus erythematosus. In Lachmann, P. J., Peters, D. K., Rosen, F. S. & Walport, M. J. eds, *Clinical Aspects of Immunology,* 5th edn, pp. 1161–1204, Boston, Oxford, London, Edinburgh, Melbourne, Paris, Berlin, Vienna: Blackwell Scientific Publications.

Ward, P. A., Cochrane, C. G. & Muller-Eberhard, H. J. (1965). The role of serum complement in chemotaxis of leukocytes *in vitro. Journal of Experimental Medicine,* **122**, 327–46.

Weiss, S. J., Young, J., LoBuglio, A. F., Slivka, A. & Nimeh, N. F. (1981). Role of hydrogen peroxide in neutrophil-mediated destruction of cultured endothelial cells. *Journal of Clinical Investigation,* **68**, 714–21.

Wisnieski, J. J. & Naff, G. B. (1989). Serum IgG antibodies to C1q in hypocomplementemic urticarial vasculitis syndrome. *Arthritis and Rheumatism,* **32**, 1119–27.

Wolf, H., Haus, M. & Wilmes, E. (1984). Persistence of Epstein–Barr virus in the parotid gland. *Journal of Virology,* **51**, 795–8.

Zhang, S. C., Schultz, D. R. & Ryan, U. S. (1986). Receptor-mediated binding of C1q on pulmonary endothelial cells. *Tissue Cell*, **18**, 13–18.
Ziccardi, R. J. & Cooper, N. R. (1979). Active disassembly of the first complement component C1 by C1 inactivator. *Journal of Immunology*, **123**, 788–92.

–7–
The role of the endothelium in rheumatoid arthritis and scleroderma

R. J. MOOTS and P. EMERY

Scleroderma (systemic sclerosis)

Introduction

Scleroderma is a multisystem disorder with a high morbidity and mortality predominantly affecting females. The term 'scleroderma' was first coined by Gintrac in 1857, although the first written description of a case may have been as early as 1753. It is derived from the Greek for 'hard skin' which aptly describes the cutaneous manifestations dominating the patient's appearance. The other name for this disorder, 'systemic sclerosis', reflects the widespread organ involvement that determines the patient's survival. It is characterized pathologically by the overproduction of connective tissue, notably collagen, together with widespread vascular disease (see Fig. 7.1). Clinically, there is a spectrum of disease, ranging from widespread skin thickening (diffuse systemic sclerosis) and multiple internal organ involvement, to localized skin thickening limited to the face and extremities (limited systemic sclerosis). There is still a need for a good classification system. Once established in its full-blown form, systemic sclerosis is a disease process that is difficult to stem and often impossible to reverse. It still results in an unacceptably high mortality as well as significant morbidity.

The exact pathogenesis of scleroderma remains unknown, although various hypotheses to explain the underlying mechanisms have been proposed, including autoimmunity, innate fibroblast defects and primary angiopathy. There is a growing and compelling body of evidence to suggest that the earliest pathological changes lie in the endothelium and this will be reviewed here.

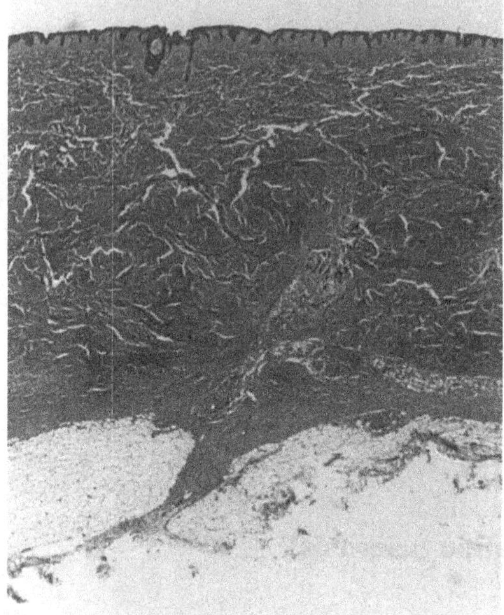

Fig. 7.1. Low power view of skin from a patient with scleroderma (haematoxylin and eosin stain). There is a marked thickening and fibrosis.

The vascular lesion

Scleroderma is histologically a disease of the small arteries. Whilst large- and medium-sized arteries are generally unremarkable on histological examination, small arteries of less than 150–500 μm in diameter are profoundly abnormal (Campbell & LeRoy, 1975). The intima enlarges concentrically with proliferation and swelling of the endothelial cells, a mucoid ground substance with staining properties of glycoprotein and mucopolysaccharide develops, and there is an appearance of fine collagen fibrils. The internal elastic lamina remains intact and the media is either normal or slightly thin. The adventitia possesses a characteristic fibrous cuff around the artery, which frequently obliterates the periarterial capillaries and lymphatics (see Fig. 7.2). Although inflammatory cells do not infiltrate the arterial wall (possibly because they have been obliterated by atrophy and fibrosis), mononuclear cells may be present in the periarterial cuff. Downstream from this small artery lesion, the smaller arteries (50–150 μm in diameter) may undergo intimal sclerosis, fibrinoid change and necrosis, particularly in the kidney. Capillaries are affected in a distinctive but non-

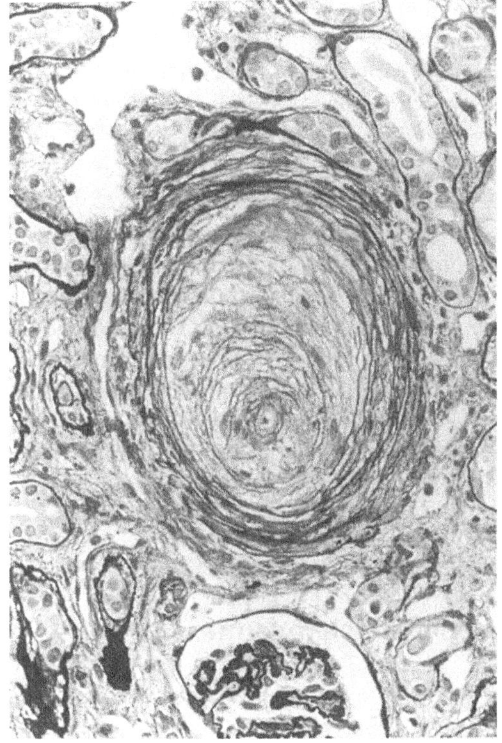

Fig. 7.2. Periodic acid methanerium silver stain of a small artery from the renal biopsy of a patient with scleroderma. The fibrous cuff around the artery causing obliteration is clearly seen.

specific manner and these changes will be discussed below. Electron microscope studies of affected skeletal muscles from patients with scleroderma have shown thickening and reduplication of the capillary basement membranes, with swelling of the endothelial cells and a marked decrease in a number of capillaries (Norton *et al.*, 1968).

The endothelium and Raynaud's phenomenon

Episodic digital vasospasm in response to stimuli such as cold exposure, often followed by excessive reactive hyperaemia, is known as Raynaud's phenomenon. This is defined as primary when it occurs idiopathically, and secondary when it is related to another, usually connective tissue, disorder. Although only a minority of patients with Raynaud's phenomenon will go on to develop scleroderma (predictable by a combination of history and immunological picture), greater than 90% of patients with established scleroderma suffer from it, and symptoms may precede the skin tightness by a number of years. This progression to full-blown disease demonstrates graphically the consequences of the vascular lesions described above. Clues to the pathogenesis of secondary Raynaud's phenomenon and scleroderma come from nailfold capillary microscopy where the patterns and morphology of small capillaries around nail beds are directly examined using a low-power stereo-microscope. There are two main patterns of abnormalities associated with scleroderma: first, capillary enlargements to form tortuous, mega-capillary loops with dramatically increased density, and second, loss of capillaries, forming bare areas (Lee *et al.*, 1983). The blood flow within such capillaries is altered, with often a sluggish flow and sometimes stasis, especially on cold challenge. The endothelium also appears to be more permeable to tracer molecules. Such appearances are strongly predictive of developing scleroderma, and are commonly found in patients, with established scleroderma (Zufferey *et al.*, 1992). As yet it is not clear whether these microvascular changes are primary or occur as a consequence of the various arteriolar changes.

Endothelial cell dysfunction in scleroderma

Vascular dysfunction, especially of the microvasculature, is a cardinal sign in the development of scleroderma. Nearly 20 years ago Campbell & LeRoy (1975) compared clinical and histological features from a large series of affected patients and concluded that the primary cause of scleroderma involved endothelial damage or dysfunction. Since then, our ability to isolate, maintain and characterize endothelial cells in culture has developed and with it has come a greater understanding of the physiology and pathophysiology of endothelial cells in this condition. Evidence from this area has provided support for the central hypothesis, directly and indirectly.

Indirect evidence for endothelial cell dysfunction

There is much circumstantial evidence to suggest that endothelial dysfunction may be the underlying defect in scleroderma. Mast cells have been implicated in the pathogenesis of scleroderma (Claman, 1989) by playing a role in the stimulation of neo-angiogenesis (Folkman, 1986) and there is evidence for increased endothelial replication in scleroderma lesions (Kazandjian *et al.*, 1982). In addition to the possible effects of mast cell products on fibroblast growth and collagen synthesis, it is possible that histamine released by these cells could contribute to the leakiness of vessels observed in scleroderma.

Powerful support for a primary involvement of the vasculature comes from the clinical observation that Raynaud's phenomenon, with hyperreactivity of small vessels, may be the first manifestation of disease, preceding the development of cutaneous symptoms by many years. This phenomenon used to be considered the benign manifestation of an underlying disorder. However it is possible that the ischaemia and reperfusion produced as consequence of the phenomenon may, in fact, contribute to the vicious cycle of escalating disease. Support for this comes from the anecdotal evidence that patients in whom Raynaud's is abolished have a reversal of their end organ damage as measured by lung function test and digital ischaemia.

Other indirect evidence for endothelial dysfunction comes from consideration of clinical trials that were undertaken to assess the response of patients with scleroderma and Raynaud's syndrome to drugs known to affect the endothelium. Drugs studied included both vasodilators and antagonists of vasoconstrictors, in each case acting directly on the endothelium. Based on the hypothesis that endothelial damage caused platelet dysfunction and increased reactivity with serotonin secretion, the antagonist ketanserin was used clinically with some success (Longstaff *et al.*, 1985). Another study employed the vasodilator prostaglandin E_1, where an improved capillary blood flow and increased transcapillary pressure in patients with scleroderma was observed (Martin & Tooke, 1982). Prostacyclin (PGI_2) and analogues have been used successfully in the treatment of acute, severe Raynaud's syndrome (Lau *et al.*, 1993). PGI_2 is also used in established scleroderma, for example in the healing of skin ulcers as well as Raynaud's phenomenon in this group.

Basal release of nitric oxide (endothelium-derived relaxing factor) by endothelial cells is known to be critical for maintaining active relaxation of the vasculature. It may therefore follow that, if there is endothelial dysfunction or damage in scleroderma, the concentration of nitric oxide falls and produces symptoms, such as Raynaud's phenomenon. Based on this premise, we have used intravenous nitrates in the therapy of acute Raynaud's syndrome successfully when conventional prostacyclin treatment has failed.

Although clinical observations suggest a role for the endothelium in the pathological process of scleroderma, studies reporting direct observations on the effects of imbalance of the above mediators in patients with scleroderma are lacking and will not be possible to perform until endothelial and organ culture techniques have improved further.

Direct evidence for endothelial cell dysfunction or damage

More direct evidence for endothelial dysfunction comes from measurement of circulating markers of endothelial cells in the blood. The potent vasoconstrictor peptide, endothelin-1 is synthesized by endothelial cells (Yanagisawa *et al.*, 1988). This peptide has been measured in the plasma of patients with scleroderma and Raynaud's phenomenon. In both conditions it has been found to be elevated compared to matched normal controls, the levels correlating with the clinical extent of the disease (Yamane *et al.*, 1991; Zamora *et al.*, 1990). Endothelin-1 binding sites in the skin have been measured by autoradiographic techniques in a study by Knock *et al.* (1993). Endothelin-binding density was found to be significantly higher in microvessels of skin from patients with either systemic sclerosis or Raynaud's phenomenon compared to normal controls. They proposed that a lack of down-regulation of endothelin receptors in Raynaud's phenomenon and systemic sclerosis may contribute to the pathogenesis of vasospasm in these diseases.

Basal tissue plasminogen activator (t-PA) concentrations in the plasma of patients with scleroderma have been found to be raised, unlike in patients with primary Raynaud's phenomenon or with peripheral atheromatous vascular disease (Marasini *et al.*, 1992). Plasma concentrations of von Willebrand factor have also been raised in patients with scleroderma (Kahaleh, Osborn & LeRoy, 1981; Gordon *et al.*, 1987; Drenk & Deicher, 1988) and in fact high levels have been shown to correlate with a poor prognosis. Raised von Willebrand factor concentrations are also found in patients with other diseases with endothelial damage. Paradoxically, other authors have reported that the release of t-PA appears to be deficient in patients with Raynaud's syndrome and scleroderma (Holland *et al.*, 1983). Such reciprocal changes, that alter endothelial cell properties towards procoagulant and prothrombotic directions, can be reproduced *in vitro* by treatment with appropriate cytokines such as interleukin 1 and tumour necrosis factor (Schleef *et al.*, 1988; Nawroth & Stern, 1986; Bevilacqua *et al.*, 1984; also see Chapter 2).

Finally, autoantibodies that bind to endothelial cells *in vitro* have been detected in a number of patients with scleroderma (Hashemi, Smith & Izaguirre, 1987; Rosenbaum *et al.*, 1988). These autoantibodies are not totally specific to the endothelium and exhibit cross-reactivity with fibroblasts. Whilst they are not directly cytotoxic to the endothelium *in vitro* (Rosenbaum *et al.*, 1988), some anti-endothelial antibodies were able to mediate damage by antibody-dependent cellular cytotoxicity (ADCC) (Penning *et al.*, 1984; Marks *et al.*, 1988; Holt *et al.*, 1989).

Mechanisms for endothelial cell damage

It is possible that autoantibodies are responsible directly for some of the damage in scleroderma, though there may be a requirement for prior activation of the endothelial cells with cytokines to allow exposure of appropriate parts of the epitope, as is the case in Kawasaki's syndrome (Leung *et al.*, 1986). There is as yet no experimental evidence to support this hypothesis in scleroderma.

If the humoral immune response alone is not responsible, what of cellular immunity? Certainly mononuclear cell infiltrates are typically observed in scleroderma lesions, and ADCC is able to mediate endothelial damage *in vitro*. Two groups have studied cell mediated immune toxicity in scleroderma (Marks *et al.*, 1988; Holt *et al.*, 1989). Both have found that mononuclear cells from a proportion (but not all) of scleroderma patients were able to kill endothelial cells when they were co-cultured in the presence of serum from affected patients. The serum component responsible was found to lie in the immunoglobulin fraction. Apart from ADCC mentioned above, there are other possible mechanisms underlying this observation. Interferons produced from activated white cells would result in up regulation and expression of major histocompatibility complex (MHC)-class II molecules in the endothelium (see Chapter 2). Expression of class II MHC may then allow the endothelial cell to present antigen to CD4 positive T lymphocytes which may result in T lymphocyte proliferation and production of the cytokine interleukin 2 (IL-2) (see Chapter 11). IL-2, amongst its other actions in augmenting an immune response, has been shown to increase the binding of cytotoxic lymphocytes to endothelium *in vitro* (Aronsson *et al.*, 1988). Such an increase of IL-2 production has been documented in patients with scleroderma (Umehara *et al.*, 1988; Kahaleh & LeRoy, 1989*a*) and bears some correlation with the extent of skin changes.

Although immune mechanisms are often thought to mediate endothelial damage in scleroderma, various other mechanisms are possible. Serum samples from patients with scleroderma with direct cytotoxic effects have been found to be functionally deficient in plasma antiproteinase activity, suggesting that damage may be mediated by a protease (Kahaleh, Sherer & LeRoy, 1979; Kahalen & LeRoy, 1983). A serum factor of similar molecular weight to albumin which is cytotoxic to a variety of cells and sensitive to proteolysis by trypsin has also been reported (Cohen, Johnson & Hurd, 1983; Meyer *et al.*, 1993), but many other groups have not been able to confirm this (Summers, Weiss & Jayson, 1984; Penning *et al.*, 1984; Hashemi *et al.*, 1987; Marks *et al.*, 1988; Rosenbaum *et al.*, 1988). Indeed it has been suggested that such activity is merely an artefact due to prolonged storage and a resultant increase in peroxidation (Blake *et al.*, 1985). Other workers have purified a substance of molecular weight less than 5 kD from the sera of patients with scleroderma, which has cytotoxic activity *in vitro*, and leads to raised von Willebrand factor concentrations, capillary dilatation and intimal hyperplasia of arteries and arterioles when injected into rabbits (Drenk & Deicher, 1988).

Endothelium/immune cell interactions

A variety of immunological abnormalities have been found in scleroderma, and have been implicated in the pathogenesis of the disease (Kahaleh & LeRoy, 1989*b*). It is well known that most of the cutaneous cellular perivascular and interstitial infiltrates are T lymphocytes and it is intriguing to postulate that these may be the mediators of this condition, perhaps by direct autoreactivity to components of the endothelium. Some of these lymphocytes do appear to be reactive to endothelial products such as the basement membrane component laminin (Huffstutter, DeLustro & LeRoy, 1985), although others are reactive to retroviral proteins (Maul *et al.*, 1989) or type I collagen (Hawrylko *et al.*, 1991).

Whatever the reactivity of the infiltrating lymphocytes, the first step in the inflammatory process is the exit from the blood pool of peripheral blood mononuclear cells (PBMC) via the vascular endothelium. One study has shown an enhanced interaction between endothelial cells and PBMC in patients with scleroderma which may be responsible for amplifying any possible autoreactivity (Kahaleh & Yin, 1990). A more recent study showed that there is a decreased adhesion of PBMC as a whole to vascular endothelium *in vitro*. However, when the subfraction of theophylline-resistant active rosette-forming cell population was studied (consisting mainly of activated cytotoxic and helper T lymphocytes, and natural killer (NK) cells), there was a pronounced increase in adhesion (Rudnicka *et al.*, 1992). This may be interpreted to suggest that activation of sub-populations of PBMC in scleroderma leads to their enhanced adhesion to vascular endothelium *in vivo*, and hence migration into the extravascular space, resulting in the elimination from the peripheral blood of those PBMC with an increased ability to adhere to the endothelium.

The endothelium itself may play a role in immune cell adhesion in scleroderma. The major alterations in structure and function of the endothelium observed in scleroderma are very likely to produce micro-environments that allow the expression of extracellular matrix epitopes that can interact with T lymphocytes via the $\beta1$ integrins on T cells. Such binding of T cell integrins by the matrix may provide powerful co-stimulatory signals to lower the threshold for T cell activation (Matsuyama *et al.*, 1989) and hence cause tissue damage. The endothelial adhesion molecules responsible for interactions with immune cells are reviewed in Chapter 4. ICAM-1 and E-selectin is expressed by the endothelium in patients with acute scleroderma (Claman, Giorno & Seibold, 1991; Gruschwitz *et al.*, 1992).

The cytokine TGFβ has recently been implicated in the pathogenesis of scleroderma, owing to its effects on activation of fibroblasts (LeRoy *et al.*, 1989), and modulation of cellular adhesion molecules (see Chapter 2). Gabrielli *et al.* (1993) investigated the tissue distribution of this cytokine in full-thickness biopsies of patients with scleroderma, Raynaud's, systemic lupus erythematosus and normals. They found intracellular TGFβ in almost all patients with scleroderma and both intra- and extra-cellular TGFβ in patients with primary Raynaud's. All other control biopsies were negative. It is possible that TGFβ may be one of the cytokines involved in the early pathogenesis of scleroderma, with endothelial cells a source of, or a target for, TGFβ.

Endothelial abnormalities are present in clinically uninvolved skin

The importance of the endothelium is highlighted by consideration of the appearance of so called 'uninvolved' skin in patients with scleroderma. Prescott *et al.* (1992) studied vascular abnormalities quantitatively, qualitatively, and sequentially in patients with scleroderma. They reported changes in endothelial cell function as assessed by a decrease in adenosine uptake, diminished stores of immunodetectable von Willebrand factor and ultrastructural abnormalities, before any overt clinical or histological evidence of tissue fibrosis. It is postulated that the recruitment of mononuclear cells into the dermis to cause the characteristic lesions seen in 'involved' skin may occur as a result of the preceding endothelial cell dysfunction.

Claman *et al.* (1991) studied the immunohistochemistry of paired biopsy samples from clinically 'affected' and 'uninvolved' skin from patients with scleroderma. There was increased expression of E-selectin, suggesting endothelial activation, and of procollagen-I in sclerodermatous skin compared to normal controls, but no difference between clinically affected or non-affected skin samples from patients with known disease. Thus, what appears to be 'normal' skin in scleroderma is already abnormal, with evidence of endothelial cell dysfunction, which is likely to represent the earliest change in the condition.

Conclusions

Scleroderma remains an enigmatic disorder, although there have been undoubted advances that strongly implicate endothelium as the site of the underlying and earliest lesion. The complex nature of this disease, however, suggests that the aetiology is very likely to be multifactorial; not least because the presence of Raynaud's phenomenon is strongly associated with, but not fully predictive for, the development of scleroderma.

There are two main areas where specific endothelial cell dysfunction may be intimately involved in scleroderma. First, loss of endothelial cell control of vascular tone and permeability. Secondly, a possible role of endothelial cells in initiating and maintaining an immune response directed against antigens in small blood vessels, perhaps modulated by the increased production of a variety of cytokines observed in scleroderma.

Whilst a number of studies have provided a glimpse at the answer, definitive reports are lacking and future studies are needed to fully address these intriguing questions. With the recent advances in understanding of endothelial cell function, it is possible that the answers are not too far away.

Rheumatoid arthritis

Introduction

Rheumatoid arthritis (RA) is a chronic, debilitating systemic disorder, characterized by persistent inflammation associated with T lymphocyte infiltration, especially in synovial joints. Proliferation of the synovial membrane leads to the formation of a pannus, which can erode articular cartilage and bone. These processes are associated with an uncontrolled endothelial cell migration and proliferation (angiogenesis). Synovial endothelial cells have been further implicated in the erosive process by their ability to generate pro-inflammatory reactive oxygen species (Blake *et al.*, 1989). The cellular infiltrate composition of affected joints in RA varies with disease activity, from acutely, a predominance of neutrophils, to chronically, a predominance of lymphocytes. The endothelium appears to have a major role in this disease by directing the trafficking of inflammatory cells inducing angiogenesis and by direct toxicity. These features of RA will now be discussed in more detail.

The lymphocyte in rheumatoid arthritis

The lymphocyte appears to play a key role in RA. The strong genetic association between development (and severity) of RA and MHC class II genes suggests that the MHC has a critical role in developing the T cell antigen receptor repertoire during thymic development, or in presenting peptide antigens to mature T lymphocytes. Moreover T lymphocytes are found in abundance in joints involved in the rheumatoid process. At present, despite much effort at investigation, the putative 'arthritogenic' peptide that acts as target for the immune response when presented by the susceptibility-producing MHC molecule remains elusive and the aetiology of RA is unknown (see Chapter 1).

Lymphocyte/endothelium interactions in rheumatoid arthritis

Although the underlying antigenic stimulus for T cell activation in RA is not yet known, it is certain that the interaction between T cells and endothelium is one of the early events in the disease, whereby the T cells gain access into the synovium (Schumacher & Kirtridou, 1972). Trafficking of lymphocytes through lymphoid organs occurs largely at specialized high endothelial venules (HEV), as described in Chapter 4. Fitzgerald *et al.* (1990) have reported that a significant proportion of endothelial cells in rheumatoid synovium from patients with inflamed joints show morphological changes that resemble HEV. There was no corresponding change in appearance in endothelial cells from non-inflamed joints. Such morphological changes are worst in patients who require drug therapy or arthroplasty, and appear to be associated with IL-1β and IL-6 (Yanni *et al.*, 1993).

Thus the endothelial cell can control chemotaxis, adhesion and emigration of T cells into the joint, dependent upon the states of activation of both T cells and endothelial cells (Pearson, Paulus & Machleder, 1975). Activated T lymphocytes in the joints of patients with RA display upregulated expression of VLA-4 (fibronectin receptor) that is a ligand for VCAM-1 on activated endothelial cells (Laffon *et al.*, 1991; and see Chapter 4). Blood monocytes from patients with RA display greater binding to monolayers of human umbilical cord vein endothelial cells than do monocytes from control subjects (Mazure *et al.*, 1993). The patterns of leukocyte immigration into, and their persistence at, these sites may therefore depend upon the selective induction and/or suppression of cellular adhesion molecules, of which those on endothelium appear to play a prime part.

Consideration of the endothelium/lymphocyte interaction also provides clues to the aetiology of RA. The well-recognized association between seronegative arthritis and chronic inflammatory bowel disease/acute dysentery has prompted the hypothesis that there may be abnormal trafficking of cells in these conditions, and by implication in RA also. This could lead to inappropriate migration to synovial membrane by lymphocytes: the iteropathy concept. Kadioglu & Sheldon (1992) have isolated mononuclear cells from paired peripheral blood and synovial fluid from seven patients with RA. A significantly greater proportion of synovial fluid mononuclear cells showed cytoadherence to porcine Peyer's patch high endothelial venules. It would appear that these cells share adherence characteristics with cells known to be of gut mucosa origin and such gut derived cells may migrate to joints. Such a phenomenon, if found to occur in the human system, may provide an intriguing clue to our understanding of the aetiology of RA.

Endothelial adhesion molecules in rheumatoid arthritis

Early investigations into the principles underlying these processes have used endothelial cells isolated from large blood vessels of various species, including man (Yu *et al.*, 1985). However, over recent years it has become recognized that there is heterogeneity not only between endothelial cells from different species but also between those from different sites within a species. This observation implies that there is only limited information that may be gained from modelling the synovial microvasculature using endothelial cells of non-synovial origin. We will therefore limit our discussion to studies using endothelial cells derived from synovial tissue.

Useful observations into the characteristics of rheumatoid synovial endothelial cells are dependent upon the isolation and culture of sufficient numbers of such cells, first achieved by Jackson *et al.* (1990). Veale *et al.* (1993) defined immunohistochemical features of synovial membrane in patients with RA and psoriatic arthritis (PA). They found that, although the synovial membrane is more vascular in PA, E-selectin expression is much more intense in RA. Abbot *et al.* (1992) isolated endothelial cells from the synovium of rheumatoid hip and knee joints by the use of lectin-coated magnetic beads, and compared the characteristics of these cells with human umbilical vein endothelial cells (HUVEC). The synovial cells had characteristic endothelial morphology and function, which were stable in culture. Similar basal patterns of expression of ICAM-1 and E-selectin were observed in both synovial cells and HUVEC. However E-selectin expression was significantly enhanced in the synovial endothelial cells in response to a range of concentrations of IL-1 whereas there was no comparable effect on the HUVEC. Although it is possible that this represents an artefactual effect from the isolation and culture techniques used, it is intriguing to note that raised cytokine levels including IL-1 have been found in active rheumatoid joints. Such an alteration in cytokine levels may then lead to up-regulation of adhesion molecules such as E-selectin (see Chapter 2) and therefore potentiate the chronic inflammation found in the rheumatoid joint. ICAM-1 is also up-regulated in a cytokine-dependent manner, with a synergistic effect between interferon γ and tumour necrosis factor (TNF) (Gerritsen *et al.*, 1993). Monoclonal antibodies directed against ICAM-1 are currently under evaluation as a possible therapy in resistant RA. They have been found clinically to be both effective and also well tolerated (Kavanaugh *et al.*, 1993), although these observations require confirmation in larger groups of patients. Anti-ICAM-1 antibodies appear to have a paradoxical effect *in vitro*, however, where they may result in upregulation of other adhesion molecules and class II MHC (Shingu *et al.*, 1993).

The potential involvement in RA of the adhesion molecules P-selectin and L-selectin has also been studied (Kohnson *et al.*, 1993). In contrast to E-selectin there was no significant difference in expression of P-selectin in the patients studied with RA compared to others and only minimal expression of L-selectin in the synovium of the RA patient group. More recently, circulating forms of vascular cell adhesion molecules have been described and elevated concentrations of soluble VCAM-1 have been found in patients with RA (and SLE) compared to normal individuals (Wellicome *et al.*, 1993; see also Chapter 6). Interestingly in vasculitis and SLE they appear to be of predictive value (Janssen, submitted 1994).

Intramuscular sodium aurothiomalate (gold) therapy is one of the most frequently used so-called 'disease modifying' or 'second line' anti-rheumatic drugs (Thompson, Kirwan & Barnes, 1985). In an interesting study, Corkill *et al.* (1988) investigated endothelial adhesion molecules in sequential synovial biopsies from patients with RA started on gold injections. They found a decrease in expression of E-selectin at weeks 2 and 12 after starting the treatment. The overall vascularity of the synovium did not change over this period. The absolute numbers of neutrophils in the synovial membrane also decreased, although not significantly. These data suggest that one of the early effects of gold therapy may be a down-regulation of the endothelial expression of a neutrophil adhesion receptor and subsequent decreased recruitment of neutrophils into the joint. Further work is needed to determine whether this also occurs for other adhesion molecules.

Angiogenesis and rheumatoid arthritis

The development of new blood vessels, angiogenesis, is a normal physiological process, albeit uncommon in most adult tissues. However, in diseases such as RA, angiogenesis appears to play a part in the pathological process. One of the earliest and most striking histological changes in the rheumatoid synovium occurs in the microvasculature which proliferates to support the massive expansion of the pannus (Fassbender & Simmling-Annefield, 1983). Such angiogenic activity correlates with clinical activity, synovial hyperplasia, and infiltration of inflammatory cells (Rooney *et al.*, 1988). It is interesting to note that the leading edge of encroaching pannus has a relatively decreased microvascular content. This may be due to a cartilage-derived factor that has been demonstrated to block angiogenesis (Moses, Sudhalter & Langer, 1990). Although there is such obvious angiogenic activity in the rheumatoid joint, it is not yet clear whether this is the prime event, driving the rest of the cellular proliferation, or is merely secondary to synovial activation (although this may not matter for the development of novel therapeutic strategies).

Searches for angiogenic factors within the rheumatoid joint have proven fruitful. Within synovial fluid, inflammatory mediators such as IL-1, interferon α and TGFβ may be found (Arend & Dayer, 1990) all of which can exert influence on the angiogenic process. A further endothelial cell specific growth factor 'endothelial-cell stimulating angiogenic factor', similar to a tumour-derived angiogenic factor, has been detected in synovial fluid from a proportion of patients with RA (Brown *et al.*, 1983). Angiogenesis in the pannus is believed to be under the control of cytokines such as TNFα, produced particularly from the monocyte–macrophage lineage. Macrophages from rheumatoid synovium are able to stimulate angiogenesis in rabbit and rat cornea and to stimulate endothelial cell migration *in vitro* although the substance causing this has yet to be fully characterized (Koch, Polverini & Leibovich, 1986). Epidermal and platelet-driven growth factors associated with areas of new vessel growth have been localized immunohistochemically within the pannus (Shiozawa *et al.*, 1989). Induction of platelet-driven growth factor receptors has been demonstrated on cells in pannus tissue of chronically inflamed synovium (Rubin *et al.*, 1988).

Direct toxic effects of the endothelium in RA

The endothelium itself may produce damage within a rheumatoid joint. Blake *et al.* (1989) have suggested that synovitis may be perpetuated by oxidatively driven reperfusion injury. This depends on the intra-articular pressure during exercise rising above the synovial pressure, resulting in temporary ischaemia. Following this episode, reperfusion injury may follow, driven by reactive oxygen species (ROS). This phenomenon may well explain the beneficial response of RA patients with active disease to bed-rest, where production of ROS would be suppressed, and worsening of synovitis with exercise. Support for this hypothesis comes from the observation that there is a significant exercise-induced release of von Willebrand factor in patients with RA and synovitis compared to normal controls (Farrell *et al.*, 1992*b*). The same group have measured nitrite concentrations in patients with RA, as an indirect measurement of nitric oxide produced by endothelial cells (Farrell *et al.*, 1992*a*). They found an increase in nitrite concentration in synovial fluid of patients with both RA and osteoarthritis (OA) compared to controls. The concentration of nitrite was significantly higher in the RA group than the OA group. This observation may suggest that nitric oxide also has a role as inflammatory mediator in RA, however it is perhaps more likely to be produced by the inducible nitric oxide synthase enzyme found mainly in monocytes and macrophages rather than vascular endothelium (see Chapter 2).

Therapeutic implications of endothelial involvement in RA

Therapeutic advances in rheumatoid arthritis have been somewhat slow in arriving until recently. With a greater understanding of the pathogenesis of this condition has come exciting prospects for rational treatment. The drive towards new vessel growth in the rheumatoid synovium prompts the question: does blockage of angiogenesis result in clinical improvement? Studies to test anti-angiogenic agents are now underway in both mouse and human and preliminary data show promise. Anti-adhesion molecule and soluble adhesion molecule therapies are also in the early stages of development. Results from the trials of these agents are eagerly awaited.

Conclusions

The evidence discussed above suggests that the endothelium plays a major role in mediation of the inflammatory response in RA for a number of reasons. T lymphocytes may originate from gut mucosa, perhaps in response to a microbial or food antigen, and after appropriate interaction with the endothelium of Peyer's patches HEV reach the systemic circulation. Once near the joint, they can gain entry into the joint by interaction with synovial vessel endothelium. It is apparent that synovial endothelium is in a suitably activated state in RA to express adhesion molecules to allow such an interaction, and it is likely that the many cytokines present in the rheumatoid joint cause such activation. Thus although endothelium has not yet been ascribed a role in the initiation of inflammatory synovitis, it is likely to be intimately involved in the regulation of disease activity and progression, and may exert its influence on lymphocyte trafficking at two sites, the gut and the joint. The endothelium is further involved by virtue of its effects on the stimulation and control of angiogenesis, and perhaps by production of directly toxic reactive oxygen species. Such a model for the rheumatic disease process is leading naturally to the development of novel therapeutic agents such as anti-endothelial adhesion molecule therapy, anti-angiogenesis therapy and soluble adhesion molecules in treating established RA. This promises much for the future.

Acknowledgement

We acknowledge the help of Dr A. J. Howie (Department of Pathology, University of Birmingham) for providing photographs of histological preparations.

References

Abbot, S. E., Kaul, A., Stevens, C. R. & Blake, D. R. (1992). Isolation and characterisation of synovial microvascular cells. Characterisation and assessment of adhesion molecule expression. *Arthritis and Rheumatism*, **35**, 401–6.

Arend, W. P. & Dayer, J. M. (1990). Cytokines and cytokine inhibitors or antagonists in rheumatoid arthritis. *Arthritis and Rheumatism*, **33**, 305–15.

Aronsson, F. R., Libby, P., Brandon, E. P., Janika, M. W. & Mier, J. W. (1988). IL-2 rapidly induces natural killer cell adhesion to human endothelial cells. A potential mechanism for endothelial injury. *Journal of Immunology*, **141**, 158–63.

Bevilacqua, M. P., Pober, J. S., Majeau, G., Cotran, R. S. & Gimbrone M. A. (1984). Interleukin I induces biosynthesis and cell expression of procoagulant activity in human vascular endothelial cells. *Journal of Experimental Medicine*, **150**, 618–21.

Blake, D. R., Winyard, P., Scott, D. G. I., Brailsford, S., Blann, A & Lunec, J. (1985). Endothelial cell cytotoxicity in inflammatory vascular diseases—the possible role of oxidised lipoproteins. *Annals in Rheumatic Diseases*, **44**, 176–82.

Blake, D. R., Merry, P., Unsworth, J., Kidd, B. L., Outhwaite, J. M., Ballard, R., Morris, C. J., Gray, L. & Lunec, J. (1989). Hypoxic-reperfusion injury in the inflamed human joint. *Lancet*, **i**, 289–93.

Brown, R. A., Tomlinson, I. W., Hill, C. R. R., Weiss, J. B., Phillips, P. & Kumar, S. (1983). Relationship of angiogenesis factor in synovial fluid to various joint diseases. *Annals in Rheumatic Disease*, **42**, 301–7.

Campbell, P. & LeRoy, E. C. (1975) Pathogenesis of systemic sclerosis: a vascular hypothesis. *Seminars in Arthritis and Rheumatism*, **4**, 351–67.

Claman, H. N. (1989). On scleroderma. Mast cells, endothelial cells and fibroblasts. *Journal of the American Medical Association*, **262**, 1206–9.

Claman, H. N., Giorno, R. C. & Seibold, J. R. (1991). Endothelial and fibroblastic activation in scleroderma. The myth of the 'uninvolved skin'. *Arthritis and Rheumatology*, **34**, 1495–501.

Cohen, S., Johnson, A. R. & Hurd, E. (1983) Cytotoxicity of sera from patients with scleroderma: effects on human endothelial cells and fibroblasts in culture. *Arthritis and Rheumatology*, **26**, 170–8.

Corkill, M. M., Kirkham, B. W., Haskard, D. O., Barbitas, C., Gibson, T. & Panayi, G. S. (1988). Gold treatment of rheumatoid arthritis decreases synovial expression of the endothelial leukocyte adhesion receptor ELAM-1. *Journal of Rheumatology*, **18**, 1453–60.

Drenk, F. & Deicher, H. R. G. (1988) Pathophysiological effects of endothelial cytotoxic activity derived from sera of patients with progressive systemic sclerosis. *Journal of Rheumatology*, **15**, 468–74.

Farrell, A. J., Blake, D. R., Palmer, R. M. J. & Moncada, S. (1992*a*). Increased concentrations of nitrite in synovial fluid and serum suggest increased nitric oxide synthesis in rheumatic diseases. *Annals of Rheumatic Diseases*, **51**, 1219–22.

Farrell, A. J., Williams, R. B., Stevens, C. R., Lawrie, A. S., Cox, N. L. & Blake, D. R. (1992*b*). Exercise induced release of von Willebrand factor: evidence for hypoxic reperfusion injury in rheumatoid arthritis. *Annals in Rheumatic Diseases*, **51**, 1117–22.

Fassbender, H. G. & Simmling-Annefield, A. (1983). The potential aggressiveness of synovial tissue in rheumatoid arthritis. *Journal of Pathology*, **139**, 399–406.

Fitzgerald, O., Soden, M., Yanni, G., Robinson, R. & Bresnihan, B. (1990). Morphometric analysis of blood vessels in synovial membranes obtained from clinically affected and unaffected knee joints of patients with rheumatoid arthritis. *Annals of Rheumatic Diseases*, **50**, 792–6.

Folkman, J. (1986) How is blood vessel growth regulated in normal and neoplastic tissue? *Cancer Research*, **46**, 467–73.

Gabrielli, A., Di Loreto, C., Taborro, R., Candela, M., Sambo, P., Nitti, C., Danieli, M. G., De Lustro, F., Dasch, J. R. & Danieli, G. (1993). Immunohistochemical localisation of intracellular and extracellular associated TGF beta in the skin of patients with systemic sclerosis (scleroderma) and primary Raynaud's phenomenon. *Clinical Immunology and Immunopathology*, **68**, 340–9.

Gerritsen, M. E., Kelley, K. A., Ligon, G., Perry, C. A., Shen, C. P., Szczepanski, A. & Carley, W. W. (1993). Regulation of the expression of intracellular adhesion molecule 1 in cultured human endothelial cells derived from rheumatoid synovium. *Arthritis and Rheumatology*, **36**, 593–602.

Gordon, J. L., Pottinger, B. E., Woo, P., Rosenbaum, J. & Black, C. M. (1987) Plasma von Willebrand factor in connective tissue disease. *Annals of Rheumatic Diseases*, **46**, 491–2.

Gruschwitz, M., von den Driesh, P., Kellner, I., Hornstein, O. P. & Sterry, W. (1992). Expression of adhesion proteins involved in the cell–cell and cell–matrix interactions in the skin of patients with progressive systemic sclerosis. *Journal of the American Academy of Dermatology*, **27**, 169–77.

Hashemi, S., Smith, C. D. & Izaguirre, C. A. (1987). Anti-endothelial cell antibodies: detection and characterisation using a cellular enzyme-linked immunosorbant assay. *Journal of Laboratory Clinical Medicine*, **109**, 434–40.

Hawrylko, E., Spertus, A., Mele, C. A., Oster, N. & Frieri, M. (1991). Increased interleukin 2 production in response to human type I collagen stimulation in patients with systemic sclerosis. *Arthritis and Rheumatology*, **34**, 580–7.

Holland, C. D., Keegan, A. L. & Wood, K. (1983). The fibrinolytic response to DDAVP in systemic sclerosis and controls. *Progress in Fibrinolysis*, **6**, 107–10.

Holt, C. M., Lindsey, N., Moult, J., Malia, R. G., Greaves, M., Hume, A., Rowell, R. & Hughes, P. (1989). Antibody-dependent cellular cytotoxicity of vascular endothelium. Characterization and pathogenic associations in systemic sclerosis. *Clinical and Experimental Immunology*, **78**, 359–65.

Huffstutter, J. E., DeLustro, F. A. & LeRoy, E. C. (1985). Cellular immunity to collagen and laminin in scleroderma. *Arthritis and Rheumatology*, **28**, 775–80.

Jackson, C. J., Garbett, P. K., Nissen, B. & Scrieber, L. (1990). Binding of human endothelium to Ulex Europaeus I-coated Dynabeads: application to the isolation of microvascular endothelium. *Journal of Cell Science*, **96**, 257–62.

Kadioglu, A. & Sheldon, P. (1992). Adhesion of rheumatoid peripheral blood and synovial fluid mononuclear cells to high endothelial venules of gut mucosa. *Annals of Rheumatic Diseases*, **51**, 126–7.

Kahaleh, M. B., Sherer, G. K. & LeRoy, E. C. (1979). Endothelial injury in scleroderma. *Journal of Experimental Medicine*, **149**, 1326–35.

Kahaleh, M. B., Osborn, I. & LeRoy, E. C. (1981). Increased factor VII/von Willebrand factor antigen and von Willebrand factor activity in scleroderma and Raynaud's phenomenon. *Annals in Internal Medicine*, **94**, 482–4.

Kahaleh, M. B. & LeRoy, E. C. (1983). Endothelial injury in scleroderma. A protease mechanism. *Journal of Clinical Investigations*, **101**, 553–60.

Kahaleh, M. B. & LeRoy, E. C. (1989*a*). Interleukin-2 in scleroderma: correlation of serum level with extent of skin involvement, and disease duration. *Annals of Internal Medicine*, **110**, 446–50.

Kahaleh, M. B. & LeRoy, E. C. (1989*b*). The immune basis for human fibrotic disease, especially scleroderma (systemic sclerosis). *Clinical Aspects of Immunology*, **3**, 19–28.

Kahaleh, M. B. & Yin, T. (1990). Enhanced lymphocyte-endothelial cell interaction in scleroderma (SSc). *Arthritis and Rheumatism*, **33**(s), A129.

Kavanaugh, A., Nichols, L., Davis, I., Rothlein, R. & Lipsky, P. (1993). Anti-CD54 (intercellular adhesion molecule-1: ICAM-1) monoclonal antibody therapy in refractory rheumatoid arthritis. *Arthritis and Rheumatism*, **36**(S9), 40.

Kazandjian, S., Fessinger, J.-N., Camilleri, J. P., Dadonne, J. P. & Housset, E. (1982). Endothelial cell renewal in skin of patients with progressive systemic sclerosis: an *in vitro* autoradiographic study. *Acta Dermatologia Venereologia (Stockh.)*, **62**, 425–9.

Knock, G. A., Terenghi, G., Bunker, C. B., Bull, H. A., Dowd, P. M. & Polak, J. M. (1993). Characterization of endothelin-binding sites in human skin and their regulation in primary Raynaud's phenomenon and systemic sclerosis. *Journal of Investigative Dermatology*, **101**, 73–8.

Koch, A., Polverini, P. J. & Leibovich, S. J. (1986). Stimulation of neovascularisation by human rheumatoid synovial tissue macrophages. *Arthritis and Rheumatism*, **29**, 471–9.

Kohnson, B. A., Haines, G. K., Harlow, L. A. & Koch, A. E. (1993). Adhesion molecule expression in human synovial tissue. *Arthritis and Rheumatism*, **36**, 137–47.

Laffon, A., Garcia-Vicuna, Humbria, A., Postigo, A. A., Corbi, A. L., de Landazuri, M. O. & Sanchez-Madrid, F. (1991). Upregulated expression and function of VLA-4 fibronectin receptors on human activated T cells in rheumatoid arthritis. *Journal of Clinical Investigations*, **88**, 546–52.

Lau, C. S., Belch, J. J., Madhok, R., Cappell, H., Herrick, A., Jayson, M. & Thompson, J. M. (1993). A randomized, double-blind study of cicaprost, an oral prostacyclin analog, in the treatment of Raynaud's phenomenon secondary to systemic sclerosis. *Clinical and Experimental Rheumatology*, **11**(1), 35–40.

Lee, P,. Leung, F. Y.-K., Alderdice, C. & Armstrong, S. K. (1983). Nailfold capillary microscopy in the connective tissue diseases: a semiquantitative assessment. *Journal of Rheumatology*, **10**, 930–938.

LeRoy, E. C., Smith, E. A., Kahaleh, M. B., Trojanowska, M. & Silver, R. M. (1989). A strategy for determining the pathogenesis of systemic sclerosis: is transforming growth factor β the answer? *Arthritis and Rheumatism*, **32**, 817–25.

Leung, D. Y. M., Geha, R. F., Newburger, J. W., Burns, J. C., Fiers, W., Lapierre, L. A. & Pober, J. S. (1986). Two monokines, interleukin 1 and tumor necrosis factor, render cultured vascular endothelial cells susceptible to lysis by antibodies circulating during Kawasaki syndrome. *Journal of Experimental Medicine*, **164**, 1958–72.

Longstaff, J., Gush, R., Williams, E. H. & Jayson, M. I. (1985) Effects of ketanserin on peripheral blood flow, haemorheology and platelet function in patients with Raynaud's phenomenon. *Journal of Cardiovascular Pharmacology*, **7**, S99–S101.

Marasini, B., Cugno, M., Bassini, C., Stazani, M., Bottasso, B. & Agostini, A. (1992). Tissue-type plasminogen activator and Von Willebrand factor plasma levels as markers of endothelial involvement in patients with Raynaud's phenomenon. *International Journal of Microcirculation and Clinical Experimentation*, **11**(4), 375–82.

Marks, R. M., Czerniecki, M., Andrews, B. S. & Penny, P. (1988). The effects of scleroderma serum on human microvascular endothelial cells. Induction of antibody-dependent cellular cytotoxicity. *Arthritis and Rheumatology*, **31**, 1524–34.

Martin, M. F. R. & Tooke, J. E. (1982). Effects of prostaglandin E_1 on microvascular haemodynamics in progressive systemic sclerosis. *British Medical Journal*, **285**, 1688–90.

Matsuyama, T., Yamada, A., Kay, J., Yamada, K. M., Akiyama, S. K., Schlossman, S. F. & Morimoto, C. (1989). Activation of CD4 cells by fibronectin receptor complex and anti-CD3 antibody, A synergistic effect mediated by the VLA-5 fibronectin receptor complex and anti-CD3 antibody. *Journal of Experimental Medicine*, **170**, 1133–48.

Maul, G. G., Jiminez, S. A., Riggs, E. & Ziemnicka-Kotula, D. (1989). Determination of an epitope of the diffuse systemic sclerosis marker antigen DNA topoisomerase-I: sequence similarity with retroviral p30 gag protein suggests a possible cause for autoimmunity in systemic sclerosis. *Proceedings of the National Academy of Sciences, USA*, **86**, 8492–6.

Mazure, G., Jayawardene, S. A., Perry, J. D., McCarthy, D., Macey, M. G., Dumonde, D. C. & Brown, K. A. (1993). Abnormal binding properties of blood monocytes in rheumatoid arthritis. *Agents Actions*, **38**, C41–C43.

Meyer, D., Haim, T., Dryll, A., Lansaman, J. & Ryckewaert, A. (1983). Vascular endothelial cell injury in progressive systemic sclerosis and other connective tissue disease. *Clinical and Experimental Immunology*, **1**, 29–34.

Moses, M. A., Sudhalter, I. & Langer, R. (1990) Identification of an inhibitor of neovascularisation from cartilage. *Science*, **248**, 1408–10.

Nawroth, P. P. & Stern, D. M. (1986) Modulation of endothelial cell hemostatic properties by tumour necrosis factor. *Journal of Experimental Medicine*, **163**, 740–5.

Norton, W. L., Hurd, E., Lewis, D. & Ziff, M. (1968). Evidence of microvascular injury in scleroderma and systemic lupus erythematosus: quantitative study of the microvascular bed. *Journal of Laboratory and Clinical Medicine*, **71**, 919–23.

Pearson, C. M., Paulus, H. E. & Machleder, H. I. (1975). The role of the lymphocyte and its products in the propagation of joint disease. *Annals of NY Academy of Science*, **256**, 150–7.

Penning, C. A., Cunningham, J., French, M. A. H., Harrison, G., Rowell, N. R. & Hughes, P. (1984). Antibody-dependent cytotoxicity of human vascular endothelium in systemic sclerosis. *Clinical and Experimental Immunology*, **57**, 548–56.

Prescott, R. J., Freemont, A. J., Jones, C. J. P., Hoyland, J. & Fielding, P. (1992) Sequential dermal microvascular and perivascular changes in the development of scleroderma. *Journal of Pathology*, **166**, 155–263.

Rooney, M., Condell, D., Quinlan, W., Daly, L., Whelan, A., Feighery, C. & Bresnihan, B. (1988) Analysis of the histologic variation in rheumatoid arthritis. *Arthritis and Rheumatism*, **3**, 956–63.

Rosenbaum, J. R., Pottinger, B. E., Woo, P., Black, C. M., Byron, M. A. & Pearson, J. (1988). Measurement and characterisation of circulating anti-endothelial cell IgG in connective tissue diseases. *Clinical and Experimental Immunology*, **72**, 450–6.

Rubin, K., Terracio, L., Ronnstrand, L., Heldin, C. H. & Klareskog, L. (1988). Expression of platelet-derived growth factor receptors is included on connective tissue cells during chronic synovial inflammation. *Scandinavian Journal of Immunology*, **27**, 285–94.

Rudnicka, L., Slawomir, M., Blaszczyk, M., Skiendzielewska, A., Makiela, B., Skopinska, M. & Janonska, S. (1992). Adhesion of peripheral blood mononuclear cells to vascular endothelium in patients with systemic sclerosis (scleroderma). *Arthritis and Rheumatism*, **35**, 771–5.

Schleef, R. R., Bevilacqua, M. P., Sawdey, M., Gimbrone, M. A. & Loskutoff, D. J. (1988). Cytokine activation of vascular endothelium. Effects on tissue-type plasminogen activator and type I plasminogen activator inhibitor. *Journal of Biological Chemistry*, **263**, 5797–803.

Schumacher, H. R. & Kirtridou, R. C. (1972). Synovitis of recent onset: a clinicopathologic study during the first month of disease. *Arthritis and Rheumatism*, **15**, 467–85.

Shingu, M., Michi, H., Nobunaga, M. & Yasutake, C. (1993). The effects of intercellular adhesion molecule-1 (ICAM-1) monoclonal antibody (MAB) on the expression of adhesion molecules in synovial cells (SC). *Arthritis and Rheumatism*, **36**(s), 155.

Shiozawa, S., Shiozawa, K., Tanaka, Y, Morimoto, I., Uchihashi, M., Fujita, T., Hirohata, K., Hitata, Y. & Imura, S. (1989). Human epidermal growth factor for the stratification of synovial lining layer and neovascularisation in rheumatoid arthritis. *Annals of Rheumatic Diseases*, **48**, 820–8.

Summers, G. D., Weiss, J. B. & Jayson, M. I. V. (1984) Failure of serum from patients with scleroderma to exhibit cytotoxicity towards human umbilical vein endothelial cells. *Rheumatology International*, **5**, 9–13.

Thompson, P. W., Kirwan, J. R. & Barnes, C. G. (1985). Practical results of treatment with disease-modifying anti rheumatoid drugs. *British Journal of Rheumatology*, **24**, 167–75.

Umehara, H., Kumagai, S., Ishida, H., Suginoshita, T., Maeda, M. & Imura, H. (1988). Enhanced production of interleukin-2 in patients with progressive systemic sclerosis. *Arthritis and Rheumatism*, **31**, 401–7.

Veale, D., Yanni, G., Rogers, S., Barnes, L., Bresnihan, B. & Fitzgerald, O. (1993). Reduced synovial membrane macrophage numbers, ELAM-1 expression, and lining layer hyperplasia in psoriatic arthritis as compared to rheumatoid arthritis. *Arthritis and Rheumatism*, **36**, 893–90.

Wellicome, S. M., Kapahi, P., Mason, J. C., Lebranchu, Y., Yarwood, H. & Haskard, D. O. (1993). Detection of a circulatory form of vascular cell adhesion molecule-1: raised levels in rheumatoid arthritis and systemic lupus. *Clinical and Experimental Immunology*, **92**, 412–18.

Yamane, K., Kashigwagi, H., Suzuki, N, Miyauchi, T., Yanagisawa, M., Goto, K. & Masaki, T. (1991). Elevated plasma levels of endothelin-1 systemic sclerosis. *Arthritis and Rheumatism*, **34**, 243–4.

Yanagisawa, M., Kurihara, H., Kimura, S., Tomobe, V., Kobayashi, M., Matsui, Y., Goto, K., Masaki, T. & Yazaki, Y. (1988). A novel potent vasoconstrictor peptide produced by endothelial cells. *Nature*, **332**, 411–15.

Yanni, G., Whelan, A., Feighery, C., Fitzgerald, O. & Bresnihan, B. (1993). Morphometric analysis of synovial membrane blood vessels in rheumatoid arthritis: associations with the immunohistologic features, synovial fluid cytokine levels and the clinical course. *Journal of Rheumatology*, **20**, 634–8.

Yu, C. L., Haskard, D. O., Cavender, D. & Johnson, A. R. (1985) Human γ interferon increases the binding of lymphocytes to endothelium. *Clinical and Experimental Immunology*, **62**, 554–60.

Zamora, M. R., O'Brien, R. F., Rutherford, R. B. & Weil, J. V. (1990). Serum endothelin-1 concentrations and cold provocation in primary Raynaud's phenomenon. *Lancet*, **336**, 1144–7.

Zufferey, P., Depairn, M., Chamot, A. M. & Monti, M. (1992) Prognostic significance of nailfold capillary microscopy in patients with Raynaud's phenomenon and scleroderma-pattern abnormalities: a six year follow-up study. *Clinical Rheumatology*, **11**, 536–41.

–8–
The role of the endothelium in systemic vasculitis

ABEED A. PALL and CAROLINE O. S. SAVAGE

Introduction

The primary (idiopathic) systemic vasculitides constitute a heterogeneous group of diseases characterized by inflammation of blood vessels. These are typically multisystem disorders although isolated (confined to a single organ) vasculitis is well recognized (Carrington & Liebow, 1966; Borrie, 1972; Orbo & Bostad, 1989; Warfield *et al.*, 1994). The aetiology has yet to be defined but is likely to be multifactorial involving an initiating trigger, possibly infection (Davies *et al.*, 1982; Pinching *et al.*, 1984; DeRemee, McDonald & Weiland, 1985; Savage *et al.*, 1991; Barrett *et al.*, 1993; Stegeman *et al.*, 1994), in genetically susceptible individuals (Katz *et al.*, 1979; Elkon *et al.*, 1983; Hay *et al.*, 1991; Spencer *et al.*, 1992). Further, because there is considerable clinical and histological overlap within the group, this has made advances in the classification difficult and has also led to confusion in terminology. The most clinically useful classification remains that based on the size of blood vessels involved (Adu, Luqmani & Bacon, 1993; Scott, 1993). The problem of nomenclature has been specifically addressed by the Chapel Hill international consensus (Jennette *et al.*, 1994).

In this chapter we will focus on the small vessel, necrotizing systemic vasculitides, Wegener's granulomatosis and microscopic polyarteritis. It is clear from histological studies in this group that the vascular endothelium is a likely target for initial injury, preceding the development of vessel wall or extravascular inflammation. We shall discuss the proposed mechanisms of this endothelial injury and inflammation in vasculitis. We shall describe our current understanding of the role of inflammatory mediators, the cell adhesion molecules and cytokines, the immune effector cells and discuss the evidence for a pathogenic role of anti-neutrophil cytoplasmic (ANCA) and anti-endothelial cell (AECA) autoantibodies.

There is growing evidence that systemic vasculitis has an autoimmune basis involving autoantibodies especially ANCA and probably autoreactive T cells directed against the lysosomal enzymes, proteinase 3 (PR3) and myeloperoxidase (MPO), of neutrophils and monocytes. In common with other autoimmune diseases the mechanism leading to loss of self-tolerance is not known. However, the endothelium acting as a semi-professional antigen-presenting cell may be implicated in the maintenance of the autoimmune response. In this respect and in the localization and acceleration of the inflammation that ensues in vasculitis, there is evidence to support the view that the endothelium is not just an innocent bystander but, in fact, plays an active role in the processes that ultimately bring about its own injury.

Histopathology

Histological findings by light microscopy

Wegener's granulomatosis and microscopic polyarteritis are characterized by a necrotizing vasculitis of small arteries and veins, arterioles, venules and capillaries. There is therefore the potential to involve any organ system in the body but commonly the most life-threatening is inflammation of the respiratory tract and the kidneys.

Within the kidney there are no specific histological features that allow a distinction between these two diseases to be made (Novak, Christianson & Sorensen, 1982; Weiss & Crissman, 1984; D'Agati *et al.*, 1986; Adu *et al.*, 1987; Antonovych *et al.*, 1989). The characteristic glomerular lesion is a focal, segmental, necrotizing and thrombotic glomerulonephritis. Also there is usually a variable degree of interstitial inflammatory infiltrate, sometimes with a severe periglomerulitis. Tubular atrophy, secondary to small vessel vasculitis and ischaemia, correlates more closely with the degree of renal impairment than the glomerular inflammation. Necrotizing arteritis of extraglomerular renal vessels has been reported to be more common in microscopic polyarteritis (Antonovych *et al.*, 1989).

At a cellular level, neutrophils, eosinophils, monocytes, macrophages, giant cells and lymphocytes are seen in varying degrees and combinations in the glomerular and interstitial inflammatory infiltrate. Granulomatous lesions containing mononuclear phagocytes and giant cells may be associated with extensive glomerular destruction, but this feature is not specific to Wegener's granulomatosis. However, when such granulomatous inflammation occurs in the respiratory tract, it is more characteristic of Wegener's granulomatosis (Carrington & Liebow, 1966; Donald, Edwards & McEvoy, 1976; Mark *et al.*, 1988), whilst microscopic polyarteritis commonly causes a pulmonary capillaritis (Savage *et al.*, 1985; Adu *et al.*, 1993).

Indirect immunofluorescence studies

The kidney in Wegener's granulomatosis and microscopic polyarteritis shows scanty or no evidence of immune deposits. This has led to the misleading description 'pauci-immune glomerulonephritis' (Novak *et al.*, 1982; Weiss & Crissman, 1984; Savage *et al.*, 1985; D'Agati *et al.*, 1986; Adu *et al.*, 1987; Antonovych *et al.*, 1989). Rarely, however, subendothelial deposits of IgG, IgA or granular C3 are seen in glomerular capillary walls and mesangium (Brouwer *et al.*, 1994). Staining with ANCA-containing sera has failed to show binding of immunoglobulin or complement to renal biopsies from patients with Wegener's granulomatosis (Antonovych *et al.*, 1989). Infrequently ANCA have been eluted from glomeruli isolated at post-mortem from patients with severe vasculitis but in some instances there has been unusually strong immunoglobulin deposition detectable by direct immunofluorescence (Jayne *et al.*, 1990). There have been conflicting reports of the incidence of circulating immune complexes in systemic vasculitis (Fauci *et al.*, 1983; Ronco *et al.*, 1993; Savage *et al.*, 1985). However, there is no convincing evidence for immune complex-mediated endothelial injury in necrotizing, small vessel, ANCA-associated vasculitis. It remains a possibility that immune complexes are transiently deposited on the endothelium and rapidly cleared by phagocytes. This has been described in the acute serum sickness model in rabbits (Cochrane & Koffler, 1973) and in histamine-induced leukocytoclastic skin vasculitis in humans (Braverman & Yen, 1975; Gower *et al.*, 1977).

Ultrastructural studies

Only a few studies have focused on the early histological lesions in vasculitis, and these are of crucial importance in our understanding of the mechanisms of endothelial injury. Ultrastructural renal biopsy studies have shown that the earliest changes affect the vascular endothelium with endothelial cell swelling and alterations in the numbers of cytoplasmic organelles (Novak *et al.*, 1982; Weiss & Crissman, 1984; D'Agati *et al.*, 1986; Antonovych *et al.*, 1989). In addition, endothelial cells may become necrotic or separate from the basement membrane.

These studies have in addition highlighted the fact that thrombosis may develop prior to any inflammatory infiltrate and be associated with intraluminal and subendothelial platelet aggregation and fibrin deposition. The pathological significance of this has yet to be evaluated fully, but at the very least may reflect intense early endothelial activation by cytokines or other inflammatory mediators towards a procoagulant state. Donald *et al.*, (1976) reported lysis of leukocytes with release of free organelles into the capillary lumen as early features in the lung biopsies of patients with limited Wegener's granulomatosis. In their discussion of these findings, the authors made the interesting and prescient suggestion of a cytophilic antibody to leukocytes.

Animal models in systemic vasculitis

There are no satisfactory models of ANCA-associated small vessel necrotizing systemic vasculitis (Reinisch & Moyer, 1991; Mathieson *et al.*, 1993). This has hindered both the understanding of pathogenesis and the ability to test new treatment modalities in vasculitis. Recently two models of necrotizing vasculitis associated with anti-MPO antibodies have been described. Brouwer *et al.* (1993) have described a rat model of human anti-MPO-associated small vessel necrotizing vasculitis and crescentic glomerulonephritis mediated by the MPO-H_2O_2-halide system and anti-MPO antibodies. In this model, the characteristic lesions developed in MPO-immunized Brown-Norway rats (with detectable circulating anti-MPO antibodies) after unilateral kidney perfusion with neutrophil lysosomal enzyme extract (consisting primarily of MPO) and H_2O_2 but not with MPO or H_2O_2 alone nor in control-immunized rats. The lack of immune deposits seen in this model is consistent with human microscopic polyarteritis. However, Yang *et al.* (1993) in their attempt to reproduce this model did find significant immune complex deposition.

Mercuric chloride is a polyclonal B cell activator, which in Brown-Norway rats produces an autoimmune syndrome associated with a number of autoantibodies including anti-glomerular basement membrane and anti-MPO antibodies. There is widespread tissue injury including a necrotizing leukocytoclastic vasculitis of the gut and lung (Esnault *et al.*, 1992; Mathieson *et al.*, 1993). Of note, however, is the absence of glomerulonephritis and the lack of correlation of anti-MPO levels with the extent of the vasculitic lesions.

Later in this chapter we will discuss the pathogenic role of T cells in systemic vasculitis and the fact that a significant number of patients particularly with microscopic polyarteritis are ANCA negative. In this respect, animal models of cell-mediated necrotizing vasculitis may prove useful.

Mechanisms of endothelial cell injury in systemic vasculitis

Role of antineutrophil cytoplasmic antibodies

Davies *et al.* (1982) first reported ANCA in eight patients with Ross river arbovirus infection and idiopathic segmental necrotizing glomerulonephritis. Subsequently, a number of studies have established the association of ANCA with Wegener's granulomatosis and microscopic polyarteritis (van der Woude *et al.*, 1985; Savage *et al.*, 1987; Falk & Jennette, 1988; Cohen Tervaert *et al.*, 1989; Jennette, Wilkman & Falk, 1989). Immunofluorescence studies on ethanol-fixed normal neutrophils have identified two main patterns of binding of ANCA, granular cytoplasmic (c-ANCA) and perinuclear (p-ANCA). It is now recognized that the predominant antigen for c-ANCA is PR3 (Goldschmeding *et al.*, 1989; Niles *et al.*, 1989; Jenne *et al.*, 1990; Jennette, Hoidal & Falk, 1990), while that for p-ANCA is MPO (Falk & Jennette, 1988; Lee, Adu & Thompson, 1990). The different staining patterns are artefacts of ethanol fixation of the neutrophils, which may result in MPO migrating towards the nucleus (Falk & Jennette, 1988; Segelmark, Baslund & Wieslander, 1994). PR3 and MPO are lysosomal enzymes found in the primary azurophil granules of neutrophils and monocytes (Calafat *et al.*, 1990; Csernok *et al.*, 1990). c-ANCA or anti-PR3 antibodies are associated with Wegener's granulomatosis, while p-ANCA or anti-MPO antibodies are predominantly seen in association with microscopic polyarteritis (van der Woude, 1985; Savage *et al.*, 1987; Falk & Jennette, 1988; Cohen Tervaert *et al.*, 1989; Jennette *et al.*, 1989; Lee *et al.*, 1990; Gaskin *et al.*, 1991*a*). However, there is some overlap, partly as a result of the difficulty in some cases of establishing a diagnosis on the basis of the available clinical and histological evidence. In addition, although there is a high level of specificity of ANCA, particularly c-ANCA for Wegener's granulomatosis, there is an increasing number of reports of ANCA, often p-ANCA, in association with other diseases (Koderisch *et al.*, 1990; Saxon, Shanahan & Landers, 1990; Gallichio & Savige, 1991; Savige *et al.*, 1991; Pudifin *et al.*, 1994).

ANCA pathogenicity

The pathogenic potential of ANCA has been the focus of a large number of studies. ANCA titres correlate with disease activity in Wegener's granulomatosis and microscopic polyarteritis particularly at presentation and at times of relapse (van der Woude, 1985; Cohen Tervaert *et al.*, 1989; Cohen Tervaert *et al.*, 1990; Egner & Chapel, 1990; Gaskin *et al.*, 1991*b*; Pettersson & Heigl, 1992). However, ANCA may remain persistently positive in some patients despite apparent clinical remission (Egner & Chapel, 1990; Gaskin *et al.*, 1991*b*).

ANCA transfer experiments, designed to show direct pathogenicity, have been problematic. Such experiments have been hindered, first by the fact that PR3 is not conserved in non-primates and, secondly, by the fact that infusion of the antibody generates a serum sickness reaction making it impossible to ascribe any induced lesions directly to ANCA (Mathieson *et al.*, 1993).

ANCA-neutrophil interaction. *In vitro* studies using normal human neutrophils and/or monolayers of cultured human umbilical vein endothelial cells (HUVEC) have provided evidence in support of a pathogenic role of

ANCA. Cytokines induce the expression of the autoantigens MPO and PR3 on the surface of normal human neutrophils *in vitro* (Charles, Falk & Jennette, 1992; Csernok *et al.*, 1994) and PR3 has been shown to be expressed on the surface of *ex-vivo* neutrophils from patients with ANCA-associated systemic vasculitis (Csernok *et al.*, 1994). MPO and PR3 on the surface of activated neutrophils are therefore accessible for binding to circulating ANCA *in vivo*.

ANCA can activate primed neutrophils and mononuclear phagocytes to undergo a respiratory burst with the release of oxygen products (H_2O_2 and free oxygen radicals) as well as to degranulate and release enzymes from the primary granules (Falk *et al.*, 1990; Charles *et al.*, 1992). ANCA probably activate the neutrophils by a mechanism that involves both binding to their surface antigens and to their Fc receptors (Mulder *et al.*, 1993). The signal transduction process involved is not known but has been suggested to be dependent upon phospholipase D and calmodulin rather than phospholipase C or protein kinase C (Ewert *et al.*, 1992*a*). Following f-Met–Leu–Phe and PMA stimulation of neutrophils, Lai & Lockwood (1991) in fact found that ANCA resulted in a decrease in inositol phosphates and reduced translocation of protein kinase C.

There is now good evidence *in vivo* to support the role of neutrophil activation in vasculitis. Renal biopsies from patients with active Wegener's granulomatosis can be stained positively for activated neutrophils (chemical staining for H_2O_2) and for extracellular lysosomal enzymes PR3, MPO and human leukocyte elastase (Brouwer *et al.*, 1994). *In vitro* studies using ANCA from the same patients confirmed their capacity to activate primed normal neutrophils to undergo a respiratory burst and to degranulate. The numbers of activated neutrophils correlated with the degree of renal impairment as assessed by the serum creatinine. There was, however, no correlation between the capacity of ANCA to stimulate normal neutrophils *in vitro* and the numbers of activated neutrophils (in renal biopsies) or with renal function. Thus ANCA alone cannot be incriminated in the activation of neutrophils and renal injury in vasculitis. Macconi *et al.* (1993) recently measured the basal release of superoxide anion from *ex-vivo* neutrophils of patients with active ANCA-positive systemic vasculitis and necrotizing glomerulonephritis prior to treatment, and found significantly higher levels compared to normal neutrophils. Interestingly, these levels fell to normal following treatment with high dose intravenous methylprednisolone.

ANCA–neutrophil–endothelial cell interaction. Cytotoxicity assays on cultured HUVEC have demonstrated that ANCA-mediated neutrophil activation can result in endothelial cell lysis (Ewert, Jennette & Falk, 1992*b*; Savage *et al.*, 1992). This requires priming of neutrophils by tumour necrosis factor (TNF) or other agents such as ionomycin or phorbol 12-myristate 13-

acetate (PMA), and in the study by Savage *et al.*, it was also found necessary to make HUVEC susceptible to injury by pre-treatment with 1,3-*bis*-{2-chloroethyl}-1-nitrosurea (BCNU), which inhibits glutathione reductase thus preventing degradation of reactive oxygen species. In this study, cytotoxicity was enhanced when the endothelial cells were themselves stimulated with TNF (Savage *et al.*, 1992).

If neutrophil-mediated endothelial injury is an important mechanism *in vivo* in vasculitis, it is likely that the neutrophils need to be brought into close contact with the endothelial cells. This would create a potentially damaging microenvironment in which reactive oxygen products and lysosomal enzymes are not accessible to the circulating free radical scavengers and enzyme inhibitors. ANCA have been shown *in vitro* to augment the neutrophil chemotactic response to f-Met–Leu–Phe (Keogan *et al.*, 1992). In addition, it has been reported that ANCA can increase neutrophil adhesion to endothelial cells in culture, and this is enhanced by TNF stimulation of either cell (Ewert *et al.*, 1992*c*). The mechanism leading to increased neutrophil–endothelial adhesion may be mediated by up-regulation of specific endothelial cell surface adhesion molecules. Anti-PR3 antibodies have recently been reported to promote neutrophil adhesion through induction of E-selectin on endothelial cells. The binding of neutrophils was inhibited by a monoclonal antibody to E-selectin (Mayet & Meyer zum Büschenfelde, 1993).

ANCA-mediated injury might also be directed towards the endothelium by the localization there of MPO and PR3. It has been demonstrated that the anionic charge on endothelial cells *in vitro* can lead to the binding of the cationic proteins MPO and PR3 with the subsequent binding of ANCA (Varagunam *et al.*, 1992*a*; Savage *et al.*, 1993*a*). PR3 binds mainly to the extracellular matrix rather than to the endothelial cells themselves while MPO has been shown to bind both to the matrix and the cells (Ballieux *et al.*, 1994). Savage *et al.* were able to show that the binding of anti-MPO antibodies to MPO on HUVEC could result in complement-mediated cell damage (Savage *et al.*, 1993*a*). Recently Ballieux *et al.* reported that MPO and PR3 binding did not make endothelial cells susceptible to antibody-dependent cellular cytotoxicity (ADCC) (Ballieux *et al.*, 1994). However, it is not yet known whether the binding of ANCA to endothelial-bound MPO or PR3 can result in other sublethal but potentially harmful changes in endothelial cell function, as have been reported with AECA in scleroderma (see Chapter 7).

There is *in vivo* evidence from experimental studies and human renal biopsies in support of charge-mediated binding of granule enzymes. Johnson *et al.* (1987) infused MPO into rat renal arteries and were able to document its binding, presumably by charge, to the glomerular capillary wall and in the subepithelial space. Staining of renal biopsies from patients with Wegener's granulomatosis for MPO and PR3 has localized these enzymes on the glomerular endothelium and basement membrane (Brouwer *et al.*, 1994).

Mayet *et al.* (1993) recently reported that HUVEC intrinsically express PR3 in the cytoplasm and that this can be further induced and translocated to the plasma membrane by TNFα, interleukin (IL)-1α/β and interferon (IFN)γ. Such TNF-stimulated endothelial cells were shown to bind anti-PR3 antibodies. However, our own observations (unpublished data) using semi-quantitative polymerase chain reaction have failed to identify mRNA for PR3 in HUVEC and we have found no binding of cANCA-positive sera to TNFα-stimulated endothelial cells by ELISA. We did find low levels of expression of PR3 by cultured human renal tubular epithelial cells, and this may contribute to the interstitial inflammation seen in vasculitis. Histochemical staining for PR3 in the renal biopsies of patients with active Wegener's granulomatosis again failed to identify intracellular endothelial PR3 but did show PR3 in the tubular epithelium (Brouwer *et al.*, 1994).

Effects of ANCA on enzymic actions by PR3 and MPO. ANCA inhibit the proteolytic activity of PR3 towards elastin but also the binding of PR3 to its inhibitor, α1-antitrypsin (van de Wiel *et al.*, 1992). The overall effect of these properties of ANCA on PR3 is not known. PR3 is potentially very damaging and can result in the detachment and cytolysis of endothelial cells (Daha *et al.*, 1993).

MPO catalyses the conversion of H_2O_2 and halide ions to the highly toxic hypohalous acids. The MPO–H_2O_2–halide system may be important in neutrophil-mediated endothelial injury. When Johnson *et al.* (1987) infused H_2O_2 and iodide into a rat renal artery following MPO infusion, this resulted in significant glomerular injury, comprising endothelial cell swelling with occasional denudation, effacement of epithelial cell foot processes and proteinuria. The MPO–H_2O_2–halide system has also been incriminated in the rat model of human anti-MPO-associated necrotizing small vessel vasculitis and crescentic glomerulonephritis described earlier (Brouwer *et al.*, 1993).

Summary of the pathogenic effects of ANCA. Thus ANCA *in vitro* display a number of properties (summarized in Table 8.1) of potential pathogenic importance *in vivo*. They can activate neutrophils, promote their adhesion to the endothelium and induce neutrophil-mediated endothelial injury. Another potentially harmful effect on the endothelium mediated by the activation of neutrophils by ANCA is an increase in the permeability of endothelial monolayers, accentuated by pretreatment of endothelial cells by IL-1 (Beynon *et al.*, 1993).

The binding of MPO and PR3 by charge and the possibility of intrinsic expression of PR3 by endothelial cells provide additional means of localizing

Table 8.1. Summary of potential pathogenic properties of ANCA

ANCA–neutrophil interaction
- Bind to surface MPO/PR3 on activated neutrophils
- Neutrophil respiratory burst (reactive oxygen release)
- Neutrophil degranulation (enzyme release)
- Neutrophil chemotaxis

ANCA–enzyme interaction
- Inhibit PR3 to α1-antitrypsin complexation

ANCA–endothelial cell (EC) interaction
- Induce E-selectin on EC
- Bind to EC-bound MPO/PR3
- Complement-mediated EC injury after anti-MPO binding to EC-bound MPO
- Bind to ? endogenous PR3 in EC

ANCA–neutrophil–EC interaction
- Increase neutrophil adhesion to EC
- Neutrophil-mediated EC lysis
- Increase EC permeability

Abbrev: PR3, proteinase-3; MPO, myeloperoxidase

the injury to the endothelium. This may focus enzyme-mediated injury to the endothelium as well as ANCA-mediated damage (and possibly autoreactive T cells). It is important to note, however, that patients with active Wegener's granulomatosis and microscopic polyarteritis may be persistently ANCA-negative. This may be particularly so in microscopic polyarteritis (Lee *et al.*, 1990). In view of the pathogenic potential of ANCA, such ANCA-negative disease would be expected to differ in its pathogenesis and clinical outcome. However, in a retrospective analysis of ANCA-negative (n = 37) and ANCA-positive (n = 22) patients with microscopic polyarteritis we found no difference in clinical and laboratory parameters or in the outcome in terms of response to treatment, relapses or survival (unpublished data). It is possible that T cell mediated injury may predominate in these ANCA-negative patients.

Role of anti-endothelial cell antibodies (AECA)

The incidence of IgG and IgM AECA in Wegener's granulomatosis and microscopic polyarteritis has been variably reported by different centres ranging from 10–86% (Ferraro *et al.*, 1990; Frampton *et al.*, 1990; Savage *et al.*, 1991; Del Papa *et al.*, 1992; Varagunam *et al.*, 1992*b*). It is not clear whether AECA represent an important autoantibody system in systemic vasculitis. Some workers have suggested a correlation between AECA and disease activity, implying a pathogenic role of AECA (Ferraro *et al.*, 1990; Frampton *et al.*, 1990).

The AECA autoantigens on endothelial cells have not been elucidated but their expression is enhanced by various cytokines including TNF, IL-1 and IFNγ (Savage *et al.*, 1991). MHC Class I molecules and ANCA antigen determinants are not implicated. There is well-documented partial cross-reactivity of AECA with fibroblasts and peripheral mononuclear cells. AECA from patients with Wegener's granulomatosis immunoprecipitate five bands from 25–180 kD which are antigenic determinants on the endothelial cell surface (Del Papa *et al.*, 1994).

The results of cytotoxicity studies on HUVEC have been conflicting. Savage *et al.* (1991) demonstrated ADCC with peripheral blood mononuclear cells by a proportion of AECA-positive sera. No complement-mediated cytotoxicity was seen although this has been reported by others (Brasile *et al.*, 1988). It has been suggested that AECA may also induce functional changes on endothelial cells. Much of this has been observed in response to AECA from patients with systemic lupus erythematosus, with alterations in the coagulant properties of the endothelium (see Chapter 6). AECA from patients with scleroderma have been reported to upregulate endothelial cell adhesion molecule expression and neutrophil adhesion by inducing cytokine release from the endothelium in an autocrine manner (Carvalho *et al.*, 1994). It is not yet known whether this property is shared by AECA from patients with Wegener's granulomatosis or microscopic polyarteritis.

Role of T lymphocytes

Histological studies clearly show T lymphocytes in necrotizing small vessel vasculitis. Renal, lung and nasal biopsies contain $CD3^+$ cells, which are predominantly of the $CD4^+$ helper subset rather than the $CD8^+$ cytotoxic effector subset (Gephardt, Ahmad & Tubbs, 1983; Brouwer *et al.*, 1991*a*; Rasmussen & Petersen, 1993). Many of the $CD4^+$ cells are HLA DR-positive, indicative of activation. There are also increased numbers of $CD3^+$ cells in the bronchial lavage of patients with Wegener's granulomatosis (Rasmussen *et al.*, 1988; Barth *et al.*, 1991). Further, the presence of granulomatous lesions, which are seen particularly in Wegener's granulomatosis but which may also be found in microscopic polyarteritis, implies a delayed hypersensitivity type reaction mediated by T cells. In addition, a role for T cells in systemic vasculitis is suggested by the occurrence of ANCA-negative patients with microscopic polyarteritis and the response of some of these patients to monoclonal anti-T-cell treatment (Mathieson *et al.*, 1990). A role for T cells is consistent with the detection of immunoglobulin class switching of ANCA including IgG4, and some evidence of circulating activated T cells ($CD25^+$ and CD45RO) (Brouwer *et al.*, 1991*b*; Jayne, Weetman & Lockwood, 1991; Jannsen *et al.*, 1993).

There is, however, less evidence for peripheral T cell activation compared to lesional T cell activation. Stegeman *et al.* (1993) found no increase in soluble CD4 and CD8 levels in patients with active Wegener's granulomatosis. They did find a significant rise in soluble IL-2 receptor levels within the 2 months prior to clinical relapse. This occurred after increased levels of ANCA and may therefore reflect monocyte activation or even neutrophil activation, rather than T or B cell activation. They found no increase in the number of peripheral T cells that were HLA DR-positive compared to controls. Local rather than peripheral T cell involvement may therefore predominate in systemic vasculitis.

It is likely that ANCA production is through an antigen-specific T cell-mediated B cell response. As mentioned, the pattern of IgG ANCA subclasses seen would be consistent with T cell-dependent B cell immunoglobulin class switching. As with T cells it may be that the B cells are functionally active at the sites of vasculitic lesions rather than peripherally. This is supported by studies showing that peripheral B cells from patients with Wegener's granulomatosis have a diminished IgG production *in vitro* in response to both T cell-dependent (pokeweed mitogen) and T cell-independent (EB virus) stimuli (Rasmussen & Petersen, 1993). Thus ANCA production may occur through a local T cell-mediated B cell response. The ratio of cANCA to albumin measured in bronchial lavage fluid in patients with Wegener's granulomatosis suggested local ANCA production (Baltaro *et al.*, 1991). Certainly, the widely reported correlation of ANCA titres with disease activity would be consistent with ANCA being produced at the site of the vasculitic inflammatory focus.

The stimulus for the T cell and B cell response is not known. It may be antigen-specific, directed against the neutrophil antigens and truly autoreactive. Indeed, van der Woude, van Es & Daha (1990), and Rasmussen *et al.* (1988) have provided evidence for autoreactive T-lymphocytes directed at the neutrophil antigens. Using [^{3}H]thymidine incorporation, they have reported the proliferation of *ex-vivo* peripheral blood mononuclear cells, from cANCA positive patients, in response to neutrophil antigens including PR3. In common with most other autoimmune conditions, the reasons for the breakdown in self-tolerance to the neutrophil antigens are unknown.

Role of cell adhesion molecules and cytokines

Cell adhesion molecules (CAM) play a critical role in inflammation and in particular the interaction between the vascular endothelium and leukocytes (see Chapters 3 & 4; and Zimmerman *et al.*, 1992; Brady, 1994; Springer,

1994). Clearly, both the expression of CAM in inflammation and their role in leukocyte recruitment is complex and dependent on a number of factors constituting the local inflammatory milieu. In addition, the site of inflammation is likely to be of importance. It may be that the expression and regulation of CAM varies between venous and arterial endothelium and there may be also organ-specific differences. Such considerations may underlie the different patterns of organ involvement seen in vasculitis. For instance, Hauser, Johnson & Madri (1993) have reported no inducible VCAM-1 expression (an endothelial adhesion ligand for T-cell VLA-4) on human iliac artery compared to vein. Also, unlike in other vascular beds, there has been uncertainty as to whether human kidney glomerular endothelium can express E-selectin (an endothelial-specific adhesion ligand for neutrophils). Seron, Cameron & Haskard (1991) found no E-selectin in renal biopsies from patients with a variety of inflammatory kidney diseases. However, we have shown glomerular endothelial E-selectin expression in a diabetic patient with pyelonephritis (Pall *et al.*, 1993*a*) and Briscoe & Cotran (1993) demonstrated cytokine-inducible E-selectin on cultured kidney *in vitro*. Using glomerular kidney organ culture also, we found E-selectin could be induced in response to IL-1 and, interestingly, IFNγ but less so with TNF (unpublished data).

There is very little specific information available on the precise role of CAM in vasculitis. No studies have looked in detail at the correlation between CAM and the relative numbers of different leukocytes in vasculitic lesions. Renal biopsies from patients with Wegener's granulomatosis and microscopic polyarteritis show glomerular endothelial ICAM-1 expression, perhaps with more intense staining than that seen in the normal kidney (Lhotta *et al.*, 1991). In addition, there is glomerular endothelial VCAM-1 staining which is not seen in normal kidneys (Pall *et al.*, 1994*a*). We found a correlation between glomerular VCAM-1 staining and the severity of renal vasculitis (assessed by the proportion of glomeruli with segmental necrotizing glomerulonephritis) in the biopsies from patients with Wegener's granulomatosis or microscopic polyarteritis. This was not so in Henoch Schönlein nephritis, suggesting a specific role for VCAM-1 in Wegener's granulomatosis and microscopic polyarteritis. Cytokine stimulation of glomerular kidney culture in our studies failed to induce VCAM-1 expression implying that the *in vivo* expression seen in vasculitis is likely to be more complex than a direct consequence of cytokine stimulation.

As previously mentioned, ANCA and AECA have both been shown to stimulate the expression of E-selectin by cultured HUVEC (Mayet *et al.*, 1993; Carvalho *et al.*, 1994). However, we and others have failed to show any glomerular endothelial E-selectin expression in the biopsies of patients with renal vasculitis (Seron *et al.*, 1991; Pall *et al.*, 1994*a*). This does not necessarily imply that E-selectin is not important in vasculitic lesions, rather it may be that E-selectin has an important role in the early stages of inflammation, or its absence might reflect the extent of glomerular endothelial cell injury.

CAM may also exist in a soluble form and significant circulating levels have been found in a variety of diseases. They arise from proteolytic cleavage of the membrane-bound CAM. We have found significantly raised levels of soluble ICAM-1 and soluble E-selectin in patients with active Wegener's granulomatosis and microscopic polyarteritis, and these probably reflect endothelial activation and injury (Pall *et al.*, 1994*b*). There is no evidence to suggest that these soluble CAM have a pathogenic role in vasculitis, although they may provide a mechanism regulating leukocyte adhesion which has yet to be elucidated.

Like CAM, cytokines are likely to be important mediators of endothelial inflammation and injury in vasculitis, but again there are limited data on their specific involvement. Most of the studies have been aimed at identifying raised circulating levels of proinflammatory cytokines in active vasculitis. Different studies have variably reported increased levels of TNFα, IL-1β, IL-6, IFNγ and IL-8 in the circulation (Grau *et al.*, 1989; Deguchi, Shibata & Kishimoto, 1990; Kekow, Szymkowiak & Gross, 1992). The presence of soluble forms of the IL-2 receptor has been discussed previously in relation to potential markers of T cell activation.

Deguchi *et al.* (1990) reported increased TNFα gene expression by peripheral blood mononuclear cells from patients with Wegener's granulomatosis and microscopic polyarteritis, but found no correlation of raised levels of plasma TNFα with disease activity. Kekow *et al.* (1992) found a correlation between raised levels of IL-8 (a potent chemoattractant and activator of neutrophils) but not of TNFα or IL-6, and disease activity. In our own studies (unpublished data) of the plasma levels and peripheral blood mononuclear cell cytokine production from patients with ANCA-positive Wegener's granulomatosis and microscopic polyarteritis we found significantly raised plasma levels of IL-6, but not TNFα or IL-8. IL-6 in the supernatants of peripheral blood mononuclear cells from the same patients was not increased compared to controls, suggesting that the circulating IL-6 probably originates from activated endothelium (see Chapter 2).

Undoubtedly the local cytokine milieu that exists at the site of vasculitic lesions is important and this is almost certainly not reflected accurately by circulating levels or *in vitro* production by peripheral blood mononuclear cells. Data on local expression are lacking. Noronha *et al.* (1993) using *in situ* hybridization on kidney biopsies from patients with Wegener's granulomatosis, microscopic polyarteritis, or focal segmental, necrotizing glomerulonephritis reported the expression of TNF and IL-1 by glomerular and crescentic cells including infiltrating monocytes and macrophages as well as resident glomerular endothelial and mesangial cells.

Role of platelets and the clotting mechanism

Early vasculitic lesions are characterized by intravascular thrombosis with fibrin and platelet deposition in the vessel wall (Novak *et al.*, 1982; Weiss & Crissman, 1984; D'Agati *et al.*, 1986; Adu *et al.*, 1987; Antonovych *et al.*, 1989). Resting endothelium normally provides an anticoagulant, non-thrombogenic surface. IL-1 and TNFα activation of the endothelium stimulates the intrinsic and extrinsic coagulation pathways and also reduces its fibrinolytic ability (see Chapter 2; and Pober & Cotran, 1990). There is decreased synthesis of thrombomodulin, inhibiting the activation of protein C, increased tissue factor expression and increased synthesis of plasminogen activator inhibitor with consequent inhibition of tissue plasminogen activator. Furthermore, IL-1 and TNFα stimulate prostacyclin (PGI_2) and platelet-activating factor production resulting in the aggregation of platelets, their adhesion to injured endothelium (mediated by receptors for fibrinogen and von Willebrand factor (vWF) on the surface of the platelets), activation and degranulation. Apart from their role in clotting, platelets are known to release mediators of inflammation (Bracquet & Rola-Pleszczynski, 1987) although their precise role in vasculitis has not yet been analysed.

The significance of the procoagulant changes in vasculitic lesions may extend beyond the local endothelial damage in vasculitis. Our own observations in patients with Wegener's granulomatosis and microscopic polyarteritis suggest a prothrombotic tendency with a high incidence of systemic thromboembolic events (28%) (Pall *et al.*, 1994*c*). In patients with active diseases we have found significantly reduced partial thromboplastin time, increased numbers of circulating platelets, fibrinogen, vWF and plasminogen activator inhibitor (PAI-1) levels (Pall *et al.*, 1994*c*). Egbring, Seitz & Andrassy (1990), and Hergesell *et al.* (1993) similarly reported activated coagulation correlating with serological (ANCA) and clinical disease activity. They found increased thrombin–antithrombin, prothrombin fragments 1 and 2, D-dimers and plasma thrombomodulin in patients with active Wegener's granulomatosis and microscopic polyarteritis. Persistently increased plasmin, plasminogen inhibitor and reduced plasminogen activator have been reported in a patient with Wegener's granulomatosis following treatment with the fibrinolytic agent, Ancrod (Weiss & Crissman, 1984).

Potential role of other mediators of endothelial injury and inflammation in vasculitis

Future studies are likely to provide further details of the specific role played by the mediators discussed so far in the endothelial cell inflammation and injury of vasculitis. In addition, other mediators, including various cytokines and chemokines, not yet studied in vasculitis may prove to be important. One area yet to be explored is the possibility of a role for nitric oxide (NO) in vasculitis. There is now convincing evidence that NO has an important role in inflammation including experimental glomerulonephritis (Cattell, Cook & Moncada, 1990; Cook *et al.*, 1994). It is a highly reactive free radical, a potent vasodilator, inhibitor of platelet activation and has the capacity to attenuate neutrophil adhesion *in vitro* and *in vivo* which suggests a possible regulatory role in inflammation. A cytokine-inducible form of NO synthase has recently been identified in a number of cell types including endothelial cells (Radomski, Palmer & Moncada, 1990), human glomerular mesangial (Nicolson *et al.*, 1993) and epithelial cells (Wilkes *et al.*, 1994) as well as human neutrophils (Goode *et al.*, 1994) and macrophages (Hibbs *et al.*, 1990). Palmer *et al.* reported LPS and IFNγ mediated endothelial cell injury which was inhibited by an NO synthase inhibitor implying NO-mediated damage (Palmer *et al.*, 1992). The reaction of NO with superoxide anion produces peroxynitrite, a strong oxidant capable of endothelial cell injury. As in other aspects of vasculitis the endothelium may not only be a target of injury by NO but its ability to produce this molecule in response to cytokine stimulation potentially allows it to participate actively in the inflammatory process.

The endothelium as active participant

Clearly the endothelium is not just a passive target of injury but plays an active role in vasculitis. Localization and propagation of the leukocyte and autoantibody-mediated inflammation depends on the coordinated expression of CAM by the vascular endothelium and its production of cytokines, notably IL-1, IL-6, and IL-8 (see Chapter 2). Further, the ability of endothelial cells to bind ANCA autoantigens by charge may localize MPO (via MPO–H_2O_2–halide pathway) and PR3-mediated injury and as discussed may also lead to binding of ANCA and provide the possibility of transient deposition of immune complexes.

There is increasing evidence to support the view that endothelial cells can present antigen to, and activate T lymphocytes (reviewed in Chapter 11). Antigen presentation to $CD4^+$ T cells and to $CD8^+$ T cells requires binding of an antigenic peptide to MHC Class II and Class I molecules, respectively. TNF and IFNγ enhance MHC Class I while IFNγ induces MHC Class II molecule expression on the surface of endothelial cells (Pober & Cotran, 1990). Endothelial LFA-3 provides the secondary signals necessary to activate T cells and augment IL-2 production (Hughes, Savage & Pober, 1990). Savage *et al.* (1993*b*) have reported the proliferation of allogenic $CD4^+$ T cells by endothelial cells and their ability to process and present peptides to $CD4^+$ T cells. Cationic proteins, such as the ANCA autoantigens, are particularly well taken up by antigen-presenting cells. Therefore, endothelial cells may have the ability to present exogenous ANCA autoantigens (released from azurophil granules of neutrophils and monocytes) to $CD4^+$ T cells as well as any endogenous PR3 (recently described) to $CD8^+$ T cells, with subsequent T cell activation. The endothelium in vasculitis may be able to stimulate an antigen-specific T cell-mediated B cell response with the production of ANCA autoantibodies. Thus the endothelium may be important in the initiation and development of the autoimmune response in the ANCA-associated vasculitides.

The treatment of systemic vasculitis

Existing treatment of Wegener's granulomatosis and microscopic polyarteritis with combinations of corticosteroids and cytotoxic drugs is highly effective in inducing remission. Five-year patient survival is now around 80% (Fauci *et al.*, 1979; Balow, 1980; Fauci *et al.*, 1983; D'Amico & Sinico, 1979; Bacon *et al.*, 1992). However, long-term use of this therapy is potentially toxic, and there remains also a significant risk of relapse (Hoffman *et al.*, 1992; Gordon *et al.*, 1993). Monitoring disease activity is essential in initiating and assessing the response to treatment. In addition to clinical monitoring, most centres utilize serological markers which usually include acute phase proteins such as C-reactive protein (Hind *et al.*, 1983). The correlation of ANCA titres with disease activity has been discussed. Direct markers of endothelial injury and inflammation would be particularly useful. In this respect vWF has proved to be of some, albeit limited, value (Woolf *et al.*, 1987). Soluble CAM especially ICAM-1 and E-selectin are under investigation, as well as levels of circulating cytokines of endothelial origin such as IL-6 and coagulation factors.

Although effective, current therapy with combinations of cyclophosphamide, prednisolone and plasma exchange is non-specific and potentially highly toxic. Cyclophosphamide exerts effects on neutrophils as well as T and B lymphocytes. It also has been reported to reduce CAM expression and cytokine release from endothelial cells (Hengst & Kampf, 1984; Bacon, 1987). Plasma exchange, which is beneficial in severe renal vasculitis, is thought to be important through the removal of soluble mediators of inflammation (Hind *et al.*, 1983). Prednisolone has non-specific immunosuppressive effects but may, in addition, have more specific beneficial effects. It is hoped that increased understanding of the pathogenesis of systemic vasculitis will allow the targeting of therapy towards specific inflammatory mediators and mechanisms leading to endothelial cell injury in vasculitis, so that treatment will be more specific, less toxic and ultimately more effective.

Treatment, for instance, may be directed at neutrophils and their injurious reactive oxygen products. A monoclonal antibody to neutrophils (RP3) was found to reduce the severity of vasculitic lesions in the rat mercuric chloride model (Qasim *et al.*, 1993). In the same model there was some protective benefit from anti-oxidants (Mathieson *et al.*, 1993). In patients with active ANCA-associated systemic vasculitis Macconi *et al.* (1993) reported a decrease to normal levels in the release of superoxide anion from patient neutrophils following treatment with intravenous high dose methylprednisolone. This was reported to be mediated by increased production of the antioxidant manganese superoxide dismutase. Pentoxiphylline, a xanthine derivative, has a number of potentially useful anti-inflammatory and inhibitory effects on neutrophils which may prove helpful in vasculitis. It inhibits neutrophil activation, aggregation, superoxide anion and cytokine production as well as neutrophil-mediated endothelial cell injury *in vitro* (Bessler *et al.*, 1986; Zheng *et al.*, 1990). Neutrophil activation in experimental endotoxaemia in primates is attenuated by pentoxiphylline (van Leenen *et al.*, 1993). The use of pentoxiphylline in human vasculitis has yet to be fully examined.

Jayne *et al.* (1990) have suggested a beneficial effect of intravenous pooled normal human immunoglobulin (IVIG) in patients with ANCA-positive vasculitis. *In vitro* studies have shown that IVIG contains anti-idiotypic antibodies to ANCA and AECA, capable of inhibiting the binding of these autoantibodies to their autoantigens (Rossi *et al.*, 1991; Pall *et al.*, 1993*b*; Pall *et al.*, 1994*d*). *In vivo*, IVIG may also provide the immunoregulatory elements needed for the idiotype network and control of the autoimmune repertoire.

Mathieson *et al.* (1990) successfully used sequential monoclonal antibodies to T cells (Campath-H directed against CDw52 followed by monoclonal anti-CD4) in a patient with ANCA-negative dermal lymphocytic vasculitis. Of interest is that neither IVIG nor anti-CD4 were effective in ameliorating the histological lesions or reducing anti-MPO levels in the rat mercuric chloride model of vasculitis (Mathieson *et al.*, 1993).

Monoclonal antibodies to CAM have been used in human renal transplant rejection (Kirby, Lin & Browell, 1993) and reduced the inflammation and proteinuria in animal models of anti-glomerular basement membrane disease (Kawasaki *et al.*, 1993). In vasculitis, the use of specific anti-CAM therapy may result from further definition of the role of CAM.

Summary

Aetiology of the primary systemic vasculitides remains obscure. Recent years have seen significant advances in our understanding of inflammation and in particular the role of, and interactions between, the vascular endothelium, inflammatory mediators and immune effector cells. This has helped to elucidate further those specific processes relevant to vasculitis which result in endothelial cell damage. In Wegener's granulomatosis and microscopic polyarteritis the evidence favours an autoimmune inflammatory response, characterized by specific mediators in which the endothelium is both target and active participant. The focal nature of the lesions seen in systemic vasculitis as evident in the kidney is unlike that of other immune-mediated renal diseases and has yet to be explained. Similarly, in the absence of immune complex deposition, the mechanism of endothelial injury and the contribution to the injury by humoral and cell-mediated mechanisms need to be studied further. Other potential mechanisms of injury need to be explored. For instance, there may be a possible deficiency or delay in the phagocytosis of neutrophils by apoptosis, thus predisposing to neutrophil-mediated endothelial injury (discussed by Savill, 1993). Increased understanding of the pathogenesis of systemic vasculitis is likely to provide the basis for the use of more selective immunomodulatory therapies in the future.

Acknowledgement

We are grateful to Dr D. Adu, Renal Unit, Queen Elizabeth Hospital, Birmingham, for allowing us to report unpublished data.

References

Adu, D., Howie, A. J., Scott, D. G. I., Bacon, P. A., McGonigle, R. J. S. & Michael, J. (1987). Polyarteritis and the kidney. *Quarterly Journal of Medicine*, **62**, 221–37.

Adu, D., Luqmani, R. A. & Bacon, P. A. (1993). Polyarteritis, Wegener's granulomatosis and Churg–Strauss syndrome. In Maddison, P. J., Isenberg, D. A., Woo, P. & Blass, D. N., eds. *Oxford Textbook of Rheumatology*, vol. 2, 846–59, Oxford: Oxford Medical Publications.

Antonovych, T. T., Sabnis, S. G., Tuur, S. M., Sesterhenn, I. A. & Balow, J. E. (1989). Morphologic differences between polyarteritis and Wegener's granulomatosis using light, electron and immunohistochemical techniques. *Modern Pathology*, **2**, 349–59.

Bacon, P. A. (1987). Vasculitis–clinical aspects and therapy. *Acta Medica Scandinavica*, **715**, 157–63.

Bacon, P. A., Luqmani, R. A., Scott, D. G. I. & Adu, D. (1992). Immunopharmacology of vasculitic syndromes. In Rugstad, H. E., ed. *Immunopharmacology in Autoimmune Disease and Transplants*. pp. 273–89, New York: Plenum Publishing.

Ballieux, B. E. P. B., Zondervan, K. T., Kievit, P., Hagen, E. C., van Es, L. A., Van der Wonde, F. J. & Daha, M. R. (1994). Binding of proteinase 3 and myeloperoxidase to endothelial cells: ANCA-mediated endothelial damage through ADCC? *Clinical Experimental Immunology*, **97**, 52–60.

Balow, J. E. (1980). Wegener's granulomatosis: response of progressive glomerulonephritis to immunosuppressive therapy. In Schreiner, G., Winchester, J., Mattern, W. & Mendelson, B., eds. *Controversies in Nephrology*. pp. 243–7, Washington DC: Georgetown University Press.

Baltaro, R. J., Hoffman, G. S., Sechler, J. M. G., Suffredini, A. F., Shelhamer, J. H., Fauci, A. S. & Fleisher, T. A. (1991). Immunoglobulin G antineutrophil cytoplasmic antibodies are produced in the respiratory tract of patients with Wegener's granulomatosis. *American Review of Respiratory Disease*, **143**, 275–8.

Barrett, T. M., Thomason, P., Taylor, C. M., Pall, A. A. & Adu, D. (1993). Environmental trigger for anti-neutrophil cytoplasmic antibodies. *Lancet*, **342**, 369–70.

Barth, J., Petermann, W., Zemke, F., Kreipe, H. & Gross, W. L. (1991). Bronchoalveolar lavage in Wegener's granulomatosis. *Pneumologie*, **45**, 570–4.

Beynon, H. L. C., Haskard, D. O., Davies, K. A., Haroutanian, R. & Walport, M. J. (1993). Combinations of low concentrations of cytokines and acute agonists synergize in increasing the permeability of endothelial monolayers. *Clinical and Experimental Immunology*, **91**, 314–19.

Bessler, H., Gilgal, R., Djaldetli, M. & Zahari, I. (1986). Effect of pentoxifylline on the phagocytic activity, cAMP levels and superoxide anion production by monocytes and polymorphonuclear cells. *Journal of Leukaemia Biology*, **40**, 747.

Borrie, P. (1972). Cutaneous polyarteritis nodosa. *British Journal of Dermatology*, **87**, 87–95.

Brady, H. R. (1994). Leukocyte adhesion molecules and kidney diseases. *Kidney International*, **45**, 1285–300.

Braquet, P. & Rola-Pleszczynski, M. (1987). Platelet-activating factor and cellular immune response. *Immunology Today*, **8**, 345–52.

Brasile, L., Kremer, M., Clark, J. L. & Cerilli, J. (1988). Identification of an autoantibody to vascular endothelial cell-specific antigens in patients with systemic vasculitis. *American Journal of Medicine*, **87**, 74–80.

Braverman, I. M. & Yen, A. (1975). Demonstration of immune complexes in spontaneous and histamine-induced lesions and in normal skin of patients with leukocytoclastic angiitis. *Journal of Investigative Dermatology*, **64**, 105–12.

Briscoe, D. M. & Cotran, R. S. (1993). Role of leucocyte-endothelial cell adhesion molecules in renal inflammation: *in vitro* and *in vivo* studies. *Kidney International*, **44** (suppl 42), S27–34.

Brouwer, E., Cohen Tervaert, J. W., Horst, G., Huitema, M. G., Van der Geissen, M., Limburg, P. C. & Kallenburg, C. G. M. (1991*b*). Predominance of IgG1 and IgG4 subclasses of anti-neutrophil cytoplasmic autoantibodies (ANCA) in patients with Wegener's granulomatosis and clinically related disorders. *Clinical and Experimental Immunology*, **83**, 379–86.

Brouwer, E., Cohen Tervaert, J. W., Weening, J. J. & Kallenberg, C. G. M. (1991*a*). Immunohistopathology of renal biopsies in Wegener's granulomatosis (WG): clues to its pathogenesis? *Kidney International*, **39**, 1055–6.

Brouwer, E., Huitema, M. G., Klok, P. A., de Weerd, H., Cohen Tervaert, J. W., Weening, J. J. & Kallenburg, C. G. M. (1993) Antimyeloperoxidase-associated proliferative glomerulonephritis: an animal model. *Journal of Experimental Medicine*, **177**, 905–14.

Brouwer, E., Huitema, M. G., Mulder, A. H. L., Heeringa, P., Van Goo, H., Cohen Tervaert, J. W., Weening, J. J. & Kallenburg, C. G. M. (1994). Neutrophil activation *in vitro* and *in vivo* in Wegener's granulomatosis. *Kidney International*, **45**, 1120–31.

Calafat, J., Goldschmeding, R., Ringeling, P. L., Janssen, H. & van der Schoot, C. E. (1990). *In situ* localization by double-labeling immunoelectron microscopy of anti-neutrophil cytoplasmic autoantibodies in neutrophils and monocytes. *Blood*, **75**, 242–50.

Carrington, C. B. & Liebow, A. A. (1966). Limited forms of angiitis and granulomatosis of Wegener's type. *American Journal of Medicine*, **41**, 497–527.

Carvalho, D., Adamson, P., Savage, C. O. S. & Pearson, J. D. (1994). Antiendothelial cell autoantibodies (AECA) stimulate leukocyte adhesion by cytokine release from endothelium. *Nephrology Dial Transplant*, **9**, 889.

Cattell, V., Cook, T. & Moncada, S. (1990). Glomeruli synthesize nitrite in experimental nephrotoxic nephritis. *Kidney International*, **38**, 1056–60.

Charles, L. A., Caldas, M. L. R., Falk, R. J., Terrel, R. S. & Jennette, J. C. (1991). Antibodies against granule proteins activate neutrophils *in vitro*. *Journal of Leukaemia Biology*, **50**, 539–46.

Charles, L. A., Falk, R. J. & Jennette, J. C. (1992). Reactivity of antineutrophil cytoplasmic antibodies with mononuclear phagocytes. *Journal of Leukaemia Biology*, **51**, 65–8.

Cochrane, C. G. & Koffler, D. (1973) Immune complex disease in experimental animals and man. *Advances in Immunology*, **16**, 185–264.

Cohen Tervaert, J. W., Huitema, M. G., Hené, R. J., Sluiter, W. J., The, T. H., van der Hem, G. K. & Kallenburg, C. G. M. (1990). Prevention of relapses in Wegener's granulomatosis by treatment based on antineutrophil cytoplasmic titre. *Lancet*, **336**, 709–11.

Cohen Tervaert, J. W., van der Woude, F. J., Fauci, A. S., Ambrus, J. L., Velosa, J., Keane, W. F., Meizer, S., van der Giessen, M. (1989). Association between active Wegener's granulomatosis and anticytoplasmic antibodies. *Archives in Internal Medicine*, **149**, 2461–5.

Cook, H. T., Ebrahim, H., Jansen, A. S., Foster, G. R., Largen, P. & Cattell, V. (1994). Expression of the gene for inducible nitric oxide synthase in experimental glomerulonephritis in the rat. *Clinical and Experimental Immunology*, **97**, 315–20.

Csernok, E., Ernst, M., Schmitt, W., Bainton, D. F. & Gross, W. L. (1994). Activated neutrophils express proteinase 3 on their plasma membrane *in vitro* and *in vivo*. *Clinical and Experimental Immunology*, **95**, 244–50.

Csernok, E., Ludemann, J., Gross, W. L. & Bainton, D. F. (1990). Ultrastructural-localization of proteinase 3, the target antigen of anti-cytoplasmic antibodies circulating in Wegener's granulomatosis. *American Journal of Pathology*, **137**, 1113–20.

D'Agati, V., Chandler, P., Nash, M. E. & Mancilla-Jimenez, R. M. (1986). Idiopathic microscopic polyarteritis nodosa: ultrastructural observations on the renal vasculature and glomerular lesions. *American Journal of Kidney Disease*, **7**, 95–110.

Daha, M. R., Ballieux, B. E. P. B., Hagen, E. C., Hiemstra, P. I., van Es, L. A. & van der Woude, F. J. (1993). Detachment and cytolysis of endothelial cells by proteinase 3. *Clinical and Experimental Immunology*, **93** (Suppl 1), 26.

D'Amico, G. & Sinico, R. G. (1990). Treatment and monitoring of systemic vasculitis. *Nephrology Dial Treatment*, **1**, 53–7.

Davies, D. J., Moran, J. E., Niall, J. F. & Ryan, G. B. (1982). Segmental necrotizing glomerulonephritis with antineutrophil antibody: possible arbovirus aetiology? *British Medical Journal*, **285**, 606.

Deguchi, Y., Shibata, N. & Kishimoto, S. (1990). Enhanced expression of the tumour necrosis factor/cachectin gene in peripheral blood mononuclear cells from patients with systemic vasculitis. *Clinical and Experimental Immunology*, **81**, 311–14.

Del Papa, N., Conforti, G., Gambini, D, La Rosa, L., Tincani, A., D'Cruz, D., Khamashta, M., Hughes, G. R. V., Balestrieri, G. & Meroni, P. L. (1994). Characterisation of endothelial surface proteins recognized by anti-endothelial antibodies in primary and secondary autoimmune vasculitis. *Clinical Immunological Immunopathology*, **70**, 211–16.

Del Papa, N., Meroni, P. L., Barcellini, W., Sinico, A., Radice, A., Tincani, A., D'Cruz, D., Nicoletti, F., Borghi, M. O., Khamashta, M. A., Hughes, G. R. V. & Balestrieri, G. (1992). Antibodies to endothelial cells in primary vasculitides mediate in vitro endothelial cytotoxicity in the presence of normal peripheral blood mononuclear cells. *Clinical Immunological Immunopathology*, **63**, 267–74.

DeRemee, R. A., McDonald, T. J. & Weiland, L. H. (1985). Wegener's granulomatosis: observations on treatment with antimicrobial agents. *Mayo Clinical Proceedings*, **60**, 27–32.

Donald, K. J., Edwards, R. L. & McEvoy, J. D. S. (1976). An ultrastructural study of the pathogenesis of tissue injury in limited Wegener's granulomatosis. *Pathology*, **8**, 161–9.

Egbring, R., Seitz, R. & Andrassy, K. (1990). Activation of blood coagulation and endothelial dysfunction in patients with Wegener's granulomatosis and related diseases. *APMIS*, **98**, Suppl 19, 42–3.

Egner, W. & Chapel, H. M. (1990). Titration of antibodies against neutrophil cytoplasmic antigens is useful in monitoring disease activity in systemic vasculitis. *Clinical and Experimental Immunology*, **82**, 244–9.

Elkon, K. B., Sutherland, D. C., Rees, A. J., Hughes, G. R. V. & Batchelor, J. R. (1983). HLA frequencies in systemic vasculitis. Increase in HLA-DR2 in Wegener's granulomatosis. *Arthritis and Rheumatology*, **26**, 102–5.

Esnault, V. L. M., Mathieson, P. W., Thiru, S., Oliveira, D. B. G. & Lockwood, C. M. (1992). Autoantibodies to myeloperoxidase in Brown Norway rats treated with mercuric chloride. *Laboratory Investigation*, **67**, 114–20.

Ewert, B., Becker, M., Falk, R. J. & Jennette, J. C. (1992*c*). Anti-myeloperoxidase antibodies stimulate neutrophils to adhere to human umbilical vein endothelium. *Kidney International*, **41**, 375–83.

Ewert, B. H., Jennette, J. C. & Falk, R. J. (1992*b*). Anti-myeloperoxidase antibodies stimulate neutrophils to damage human endothelial cells. *Kidney International*, **41**, 375–83.

Ewert, B. H., Terrell, R. S., Wright, C., Jennette, J. C. & Falk, R. J. (1992*a*). Anti-myeloperoxidase antibodies (αMPO) activate neutrophils using a phospholipase D-containing signal transduction pathway. *Journal of the American Society of Nephrology*, **3**, 585.

Falk, R. J. & Jennette, J. C. (1988). Anti-neutrophil cytoplasmic autoantibodies with specificity for myeloperoxidase in patients with systemic vasculitis and idiopathic necrotising and crescentic glomerulonephritis. *New England Journal of Medicine*, **318**, 1651–7.

Falk, R. J., Terrell, R. S., Charles, L. A. & Jennette, J. C. (1990). Anti-neutrophil cytoplasmic autoantibodies induce neutrophils to degranulate and produce oxygen radicals *in vitro*. *Proceedings of the National Academy of Sciences, USA*, **87**, 4115–19.

Fauci, A. S., Haynes, B. F., Katz, P. & Wolff, S. M. (1983). Wegener's granulomatosis: prospective clinical and therapeutic experience with 85 patients for 21 years. Clinical Review. *Annals Internal Medicine*, **98**, 76–85.

Fauci, A. S., Katz, P., Haynes, B. F. & Wolff, S. M. (1979). Cyclophosphamide therapy of severe systemic vasculitis. *New England Journal of Medicine*, **301**, 235–8.

Ferraro, G., Meroni, P. L., Tincani, A., Sinico, A., Barcellini, W., Radice, A., Gregorini, G., Froldi, M., Borghi, M. O. & Balestrieri, G. (1990). Anti-endothelial cell antibodies in patients with Wegener's granulomatosis and micropolyarteritis. *Clinical and Experimental Immunology*, **79**, 47–53.

Frampton, G., Jayne, D. R. W., Perry, G. J., Lockwood, C. M. & Cameron, J. S. (1990). Autoantibodies to endothelial cells and neutrophil cytoplasmic antigens in systemic vasculitis. *Clinical and Experimental Immunology*, **82**, 227–32.

Gallicchio, M. C. & Savige, J. A. (1991). Detection of anti-myeloperoxidase and anti-elastase antibodies in vasculitides and infection. *Clinical and Experimental Immunology*, **84**, 232–7.

Gaskin, G., Ryan, J. J., Rees, A. J. & Pusey, C. D. (1991*a*). ANCA specificity in microscopic polyarteritis, Churg-Strauss syndrome, and polyarteritis nodosa. *American Journal of Kidney Disease*, **18**, 207–8.

Gaskin, G., Savage, C. O. S., Ryan, J. J., Jones, S., Rees, A. J., Lockwood, C. M. & Pusey, C. D. (1991*b*). Anti-neutrophil cytoplasmic antibodies and disease activity during follow-up of 70 patients with systemic vasculitis. *Nephrology Dial Transplant*, **6**, 689–94.

Gephardt, G., Ahmad, M. & Tubbs, R. (1983). Pulmonary vasculitis (Wegener's granulomatosis). Immunohistochemical studies of T and B cell markers. *American Journal of Medicine*, **74**, 700–3.

Goldschmeding, R., van der Schoot, C. E., ten Bokkel Huinink, D., Hack, C. E., van den Ende, M. E., Kallenberg, C. G. M. & von dem Borne, A. E. G. K. (1989). Wegener's granulomatosis autoantibodies identify a novel diisopropylfluorphosphate-binding protein in the lysosomes of normal human neutrophils. *Journal of Clinical Investigation*, **84**, 1577–87.

Goode, H. F., Webster, N. R., Howdle, P. D. & Walker, B. E. (1994). Nitric oxide production by human peripheral blood polymorphonuclear leukocytes. *Clinical Sciences*, **86**, 411–15.

Gordon, M., Luqmani, R. A., Adu, D., Greaves, I., Richards, N., Michael, J., Emery, P., Howie, A. J. & Bacon, P. A. (1993). Relapses in Patients with a Systemic Vasculitis. *Quarterly Journal Medicine*, **86**, 779–89.

Gower, R. G., Sams, W. M., Thorne, E. G., Kohler, P. F. & Claman, H. N. (1977). Leukocytoclastic vasculitis: sequential appearance of immunoreactions and cellular changes in serial biopsies. *Investigative Dermatology*, **69**, 477–84.

Grau, G. E., Roux-Lombard, P., Gysler, C., Lambert, C., Dayer, J. M. & Guillevin, L. (1989). Serum cytokine changes in systemic vasculitis. *Immunology*, **68**, 196–8.

Hauser, I. A., Johnson, D. R. & Madri, J. A. (1993). Differential induction of VCAM-1 on human iliac venous and arterial endothelial cells and its role in adhesion. *Journal of Immunology*, **151**, 5172–85.

Hay, E. M., Beaman, M., Ralston, A. J., Ackrill, P., Bernstein, R. M. & Holt, P. J. L. (1991). Wegener's granulomatosis occurring in siblings. *British Journal of Rheumatology*, **30**, 144–5.

Hengst, J. C. D. & Kempf, R. A. (1984). Immunomodulation by cyclophosphamide. In Mitchell, M. S., Fahey, J. L., eds. Immune suppression and modulation. *Clinics in Immunology and Allergy*. vol. 4, pp. 199–216. Saunders, W. B.

Hergesell, O., Andrassy, K., Nawroth, P. & Gabat, S. (1993). Endothelial dysfunction and activation of haemostasis (anticardiolipin antibodies, thrombin-antithrombin complexes (TAT), prothrombin fragments (F1+2), D-Dimers) as markers of disease activity in patients with systemic necrotizing vasculitis. *Thrombosis and Haemostasis*, **69**, 953.

Hibbs, J. B., Taintor, R. R., Vavrin, Z., Granger, D. L., Drapier, J. C., Amber, I. J. & Lancaster, J. R. (1990). Synthesis of nitric oxide from a terminal guanidine nitrogen atom of L-arginine: a molecular mechanism regulating cellular proliferation that targets intracellular iron. In Moncada, S. & Higgs, E. A., eds. *Nitric oxide from L-arginine. A Bioregulatory System*. pp. 189–223. Amsterdam: Elsevier.

Hind, C. R. K., Lockwood, C. M., Peters, D. K., Paraskevakou, H., Evans, D. J. & Rees, A. J. (1983). Prognosis after immunosuppression of patients with crescentic nephritis requiring dialysis. *Lancet*, **i**, 263–5.

Hind, C. R. K., Savage, C. O. S., Winearls, C. G. & Pepys, M. B. (1984). Objective monitoring of disease activity in polyarteritis by measurement of serum C reactive protein concentrations. *British Medical Journal*, **288**, 1027–30.

Hoffman, G. S., Kerr, G. S., Leavitt, R. Y *et al.* (1992). Wegener's granulomatosis: An analysis of 158 patients. *Annals of International Medicine*, **116**, 488–98.

Hughes, C. C. W., Savage, C. O. S. & Pober, J. S. (1990). The endothelial cell as a regulator of T-cell function. *Immunology Review*, **117**, 85–102.

Janssen, B. A., Schlesinger, B., Matthews, N., Salmon, M., Bacon, P. A. & Emery, P. (1993). Evidence for involvement of circulating T cells in vasculitis. *Clinical and Experimental Immunology*, **93**, 23.

Jayne, D. R. W., Davies, M. J., Fox, C. J. V., Black, C. M. & Lockwood, C. M. (1990). Treatment of systemic vasculitis with pooled intravenous immunoglobulin. *Lancet*, **337**, 1137–9.

Jayne, D. R. W., Jones, S. J., Severn, A., Shaunak, S., Murphy, J. & Lockwood, C. M. (1989). Severe pulmonary hemorrhage and systemic vasculitis in association with circulating anti-neutrophil cytoplasm antibodies of IgM class only. *Clinical Nephrology*, **32**, 101–6.

Jayne, D. R. W., Weetman, A. P. & Lockwood, C. M. (1991). IgG subclass distribution of autoantibodies to neutrophil cytoplasmic antigens in systemic vasculitis. *Clinical and Experimental Immunology*, **84**, 476–81.

Jenne, D. E., Tschopp, J., Ludemann, J., Utecht, B. & Gross, W. L. (1990). Wegener's autoantigen decoded. *Nature*, **346**, 520.

Jennette, J. C., Falk, R. J., Andrassy, K., Bacon, P. A., Churg, J., Gross, W. L., Hagen, E. C., Hoffman, G. S., Hunder, G. G., Kallenberg, C. G. M., McCluskey, R. T., Sinico, R. A., Rees, A. J., van Es, L. A., Waldnerr, R. & Wiik, A. (1994). Nomenclature of systemic vasculitides: the proposal of an international consensus conference. *Arthritis and Rheumatology*, **37**, 187–92.

Jennette, J. C., Hoidal, J. H. & Falk, R. J. (1990). Specificity of anti-neutrophil cytoplasmic autoantibodies for proteinase 3. *Blood*, **78**, 2263–4.

Jennette, J. C., Wilkman, A. S. & Falk, R. J. (1989). Anti-neutrophil cytoplasmic autoantibody-associated glomerulonephritis and vasculitis. *American Journal of Pathology*, **135**, 921–30.

Johnson, R. J., Couser, W. G., Chi, E. Y., Adler, S. & Klebanoff, S. J. (1987). New mechanism for glomerular injury. Myeloperoxidase-hydrogen peroxidase-halide system. *Journal of Clinical Investigations*, **79**, 1379–87.

Katz, P., Alling, D. W., Haynes, B. F. & Fauci, A. S. (1979). Association of Wegener's granulomatosis with HLA-B8. *Clinical Immunology and Immunopathology*, **14**, 268–70.

Kawasaki, K., Yaoita, E., Yamamoto, T., Tamatani, T., Miyasaka, M. & Kihara, I. (1993). Antibodies against intercellular adhesion molecule-1 and lymphocyte function-associated antigen-1 prevent glomerular injury in rat experimental crescentic glomerular nephritis. *Journal of Immunology*, **150**, 1074–83.

Kekow, J., Szymkowiak, C. & Gross, W. L. (1992). Involvement of cytokines in granuloma formation within primary systemic vasculitis. In Romagni, S., ed. *Cytokines: Basic Principles and Clinical Applications*. pp. 341–8, New York: Raven Press.

Keogan, M. T., Esnault, V. L. M., Green, A. J., Lockwood, C. M. & Brown, D. L. (1992). Activation of normal neutrophils by anti-neutrophil cytoplasm antibodies. *Clinical and Experimental Immunology*, **90**, 228–34.

Kirby, J. A., Lin, Y. & Browell, D. A. (1993). Renal allograft rejection: examination of adhesion blockade by antilymphocyte antibody drugs. *Nephrology Dial Treatment*, **8**, 544–50.

Koderisch, J., Andrassy, K., Rasmussen, N., Hartmann, M. & Tilgen, W. (1990). 'False-positive' anti-neutrophil cytoplasmic antibodies in HIV infection. *Lancet*, **ii**, 1227–8.

Lai, K. N. & Lockwood, C. M. (1991). The effect of anti-neutrophil cytoplasm autoantibodies on the signal transduction in human neutrophils. *Clinical and Experimental Immunology*, **85**, 396–401.

Lee, S. S., Adu, D. & Thompson, R. A. (1990). Anti-myeloperoxidase antibodies in systemic vasculitis. *Clinical and Experimental Immunology*, **79**, 41–6.

Lhotta, K., Neumayer, H. P., Joannidis, M., Geissler, D. & Konig, P. (1991). Renal expression of intercellular adhesion molecule-1 in different forms of glomerulonephritis. *Clinical Science*, **81**, 477–81.

Macconi, D., Zanoli, A. F., Orisio, S., Longaretti, L., Magrini, L., Rota, S., Radice, A., Pozzi, C. & Remuzzi, G. (1993). Methylprednisolone normalizes superoxide anion production by polymorphs from patients with ANCA-positive vasculitides. *Kidney International*, **44**, 215–20.

Mark, E. J., Matsubara, O., Tan-liu, N. S. & Fienberg, R. (1988). The pulmonary biopsy in the early diagnosis of Wegener's (pathergic) granulomatosis. *Human Pathology*, **19**, 1065–71.

Mathieson, P. W., Cobbold, S. P., Hale, G., Clark, M. R., Oliveira, D. B. G., Lockwood, C. M. & Waldmann, H. (1990). Monoclonal-antibody therapy in systemic vasculitis. *New England Journal of Medicine*, **323**, 250–4.

Mathieson, P. W., Qasim, F. J., Esnault, V. L. M. & Oliveira, D. B. G. (1993). Animal models of systemic vasculitis. *Journal of Autoimmunity*, **6**, 251–64.

Mayet, W. J. & Meyer zum Büschenfelde, K. H. (1993). Antibodies to proteinase 3 increase adhesion of neutrophils to human endothelial cells. *Clinical and Experimental Immunology*, **94**, 440–6.

Mayet, W. J., Csernok, E., Szymkowiak, C., Gross, W. L. & Meyer zum Büschenfelde, K. H. (1993). Human endothelial cells express proteinase 3, the target antigen of anticytoplasmic antibodies in Wegener's granulomatosis. *Blood*, **82**, 1221–9.

Mulder, A. H. L., Horst, G., Limburg, P. C. & Kallenberg, C. G. M. (1993). Activation of neutrophils by anti-neutrophils cytoplasmic antibodies (ANCA) is FcR dependent. *Clinical and Experimental Immunology*, **93**, 16.

Nicolson, A. G., Haites, N. E., McKay, N. G., Wilson, H. M., MacLeod, A. M. & Benjamin, N. (1993). Induction of nitric oxide synthase in human mesangial cells. *Biochemica et Biophysica Research Communications*, **193**, 1269–74.

Niles, J. L., McCluskey, R. T., Ahmad, M. F. & Arnaout, M. A. (1989). Wegener's granulomatosis autoantigen is a novel neutrophil serine proteinase. *Blood*, **74**, 1888–93.

Noronha, I. L., Krüger, C., Andrassy, K., Ritz, E. & Waldherr, R. (1993). In situ production of TNFα, IL-1β and IL-2R in ANCA-positive glomerulonephritis. *Kidney International*, **43**, 682–92.

Novak, R. F., Christiansen, R. G. & Sorensen, E. T. (1982). The acute vasculitis of Wegener's granulomatosis in renal biopsies. *American Journal of Clinical Pathology*, **78**, 367–71.

Orbo, A. & Bostad, L. (1989). Vasculitis of the breast. *APMIS*, **97**, 1003–6.

Pall, A. A., Adu, D., Drayson, M. Taylor, C. M., Richardson, N. T. & Michael, J. (1994*b*). Circulating soluble adhesion molecules in systemic vasculitis. *Nephrology Dialysis Transplant*, **9**, 770–4.

Pall, A. A., Adu, D., Richards, N. T. & Michael, J. (1993*b*). Pooled human immunoglobulin (PHIG) inhibits the binding of antiendothelial cell antibodies to endothelial cells. *Nephrology Dialysis Transplant*, **8**, 1428–9.

Pall, A. A., Adu, D., Wilde, J. T., Roper, J., George, J., Richards, N. T. & Michael, D. (1994*c*). Prothrombotic tendency in systemic vasculitis. *Nephrology Dialysis Transplant*, **9**, 941.

Pall, A. A., Garner, C. M., Richards, G. M., Howie, A. J., Adu, D., Taylor, C. M., Richards, N. T. & Michael. J. (1993*a*). Expression of E-selectin in the human kidney. *Nephrology Dialysis Transplant*, **8**, 1429–30.

Pall, A. A., Howie, A. J., Adu, D., Richards, G. M., Inward, C. D., Milford, D. V., Richards, N. T., Michael, J. & Taylor, C. M. (1994*a*). Glomerular VCAM-1 expression in renal vasculitis. *Nephrology Dialysis Transplant*, **9**, 897.

Pall, A. A., Varagunam, M., Adu, D., Smith, N., Richards, N. T., Taylor, C. M. & Michael, J. (1994*d*). Anti-idiotypic activity against anti-myeloperoxidase antibodies in pooled human immunoglobulin. *Clinical Experimental Immunology*, **95**, 257–62.

Palmer, R. M. J., Bridge, L., Foxwell, N. A. & Moncada, S. (1992). The role of nitric oxide in endothelial cell damage and its inhibition by glucocorticoids. *British Journal of Pharmacology*, **105**, 11–12.

Pettersson, E. & Heigl, Z. (1992). Antineutrophil cytoplasmic antibody (cANCA and pANCA) titers in relation to disease activity in patients with necrotizing vasculitis: a longitudinal study. *Clinical Nephrology*, **37**, 219–28.

Pinching, A. J., Rees, A. J., Pussell, B. A., Lockwood, C. M., Mitchison, R. S. & Peters, D. K. (1984). Relapses in Wegener's granulomatosis: the role of infection. *British Medical Journal*, **281**, 836–8.

Pober, J. S. & Cotran, R. S. (1990). Cytokines and endothelial cell biology. *Physiology Review*, **70**, 427–51.

Pudifin, D. J., Duursma, J., Gathiram, V. & Jackson, T. F. H. G. (1994). Invasive amoebiasis is associated with the development of anti-neutrophil cytoplasmic antibody. *Clinical and Experimental Immunology*, **97**, 48–51.

Qasim, F. J., Thiru, S., Sgotto, B., Sendo, F. & Oliveira, D. B. G. (1993). The effects of antibodies against neutrophils on experimental vasculitis. *Clinical and Experimental Immunology*, **93** (Suppl.), 22.

Radomski, M. W., Palmer, R. M. J. & Moncada, S. (1990). Glucocorticoids inhibit the expression of an inducible, but not the constituitive, nitric oxide synthase in vascular endothelial cells. *Proceedings of the National Academy of Sciences, USA*, **87**, 10043–7.

Rasmussen, N., Petersen, J., Ralfkiaer, E., Avnstrom, S. & Wiik, A. (1988). Spontaneous and induced immunoglobulin synthesis and anti-neutrophil cytoplasm antibodies in Wegener's granulomatosis: relation to leukocyte subpopulations in blood and active lesions. *Rheumatology International*, **8**, 153–8.

Rasmussen, N. & Petersen, J. (1993). Cellular immune response and pathogenesis in c-ANCA positive vasculitides. *Journal of Autoimmunity*, **6**, 227–36.

Reinisch, C. L. & Moyer, C. F. (1991). Animal models of vasculitis. In Churg, A. & Churg, J., eds. *Systemic Vasculitides*. pp. 31–40, New York Tokyo: Igaku-Shoin.

Ronco, P., Verroust, P., Mignon, F., Korailsky, O., Vanhille, Ph., Meyrier, A., Mery, O. Ph. & Morel Maroger, L. (1993). Immunopathological studies of polyarteritis nodosa and Wegener's granulomatosis: a report of 43 patients with 51 renal biopsies. *Quarterly Journal of Medicine*, **52**, 212–23.

Rossi, F., Jayne, D. R. W., Lockwood, C. M. & Kazatchkine, M. D. (1991). Anti-idiotypes against anti-neutrophil cytoplasmic antigen autoantibodies in normal human polyspecific IgG for therapeutic use and in the remission serum of patients with systemic vasculitis. *Clinical and Experimental Immunology*, **83**, 298–303.

Savage, C. O. S., Brooks, C., Picard, J., Harcourt, G. & Willcox, N. (1993*b*). Processing and presentation of peptides by vascular endothelial cells to CD4+ T cell lives. *Clinical and Experimental Immunology*, **93**, 19.

Savage, C. O. S., Gaskin, G., Pusey, C. D. & Pearson, J. D. (1993*a*). Anti-neutrophil cytoplasm antibodies can recognize vascular endothelial cell-bound anti-neutrophil cytoplasm antibody-associated autoantigens. *Experimental Nephrology*, **1**, 190–5.

Savage, C. O. S., Pottinger, B., Gaskin, G., Lockwood, C. M., Pusey, C. D. & Pearson, J. (1991). Vascular damage in Wegener's granulomatosis and microscopic polyarteritis: presence of anti-endothelial cell antibodies and their relation to anti-neutrophil cytoplasm antibodies. *Clinical and Experimental Immunology*, **85**, 14–19.

Savage, C. O. S., Pottinger, B. E., Gaskin, G., Pusey, C. D. & Pearson, J. D. (1992). Autoantibodies developing to myeloperoxidase and proteinase 3 in systemic vasculitis stimulate neutrophil cytotoxicity towards cultured endothelial cells. *American Journal of Pathology*, **141**, 335–42.

Savage, C. O. S., Winearls, C. G., Evans, D. J., Rees, A. J. & Lockwood, C. M. (1985). Microscopic polyarteritis: presentation, pathology and prognosis. *Quarterly Journal of Medicine*, **56**, 467–83.

Savage, C. O. S., Winearls, C. G., Jones, S., Marshall, P. D. & Lockwood, C. M. (1987). Prospective study of radioimmunoassay for antibodies against neutrophil cytoplasm in diagnosis of systemic vasculitis. *Lancet*, **i**, 1389–93.

Savige, J. A., Gallicchio, M. C., Stockman, A., Cummingham, T. J. & Rowley, M. J. (1991). Anti-neutrophil cytoplasm antibodies in rheumatoid arthritis. *Clinical and Experimental Immunology*, **86**, 92–8.

Savill, J. (1993). The fate of the neutrophil in vasculitis. *Clinical and Experimental Immunology*, **93**, 2–5.

Saxon, A., Shanahan, F. & Landers, C. (1990). A distinct subset of antineutrophil cytoplasmic antibodies is associated with inflammatory bowel disease. *Journal of Allergy Clinical Immunology*, **86**, 202–10.

Scott, D. G. I. (1993). Classification of vasculitis. In Maddison, P. J., Isenberg, D. A., Woo, P. & Glass, D. N., eds. *Oxford Textbook of Rheumatology*, vol. 2, pp. 842–6. Oxford Medical Publications.

Segelmark, M., Baslund, B. & Wieslander, J. (1994). Some patients with anti-myeloperoxidase autoantibodies have a C-ANCA pattern. *Clinical and Experimental Immunology*, **96**, 458–65.

Seron, D., Cameron, J. S. & Haskard, D. O. (1991). Expression of VCAM-1 in the normal and diseased kidney. *Nephrology Dialysis Transplant*, **6**, 917–20.

Spencer, S. J. W., Burns, A., Gaskin, G., Pusey, C. D. & Rees, A. J. (1992). HLA class II specificities and the development and duration of small vessel vasculitis. *Kidney International*, **41**, 1059–63.

Springer, T. A. (1994). Traffic signals for lymphocyte recirculation and leukocyte emigration: the multistep paradigm. *Cell*, **76**, 301–11.

Stegeman, C. A., Cohen Tervaert, J. W., Huitema, M. G. & Kallenberg, C. G. M. (1993). Serum markers of T cell activation in relapses of Wegener's granulomatosis. *Clinical and Experimental Immunology*, **91**, 415–20.

Stegeman, C. A., Cohen Tervaert, J. W., Sluiter, W. J., Manson, W. L., de Jong, P. E. & Kallenberg, C. G. M. (1994). Association of chronic nasal carriage of staphylococcus aureus and higher relapse rates in Wegener's granulomatosis. *Annals of Internal Medicine*, **120**, 12–17.

van de Wiel, B. A., Dolman, K. M., van der Meer-Gerritsen, C. H., Hack, C. E., von dem Borne, A. E. G. K. & Goldschmeding, R. (1992). Interference of Wegener's granulomatosis autoantibodies with neutrophil proteinase 3 activity. *Clinical and Experimental Immunology*, **90**, 409–14.

van der Woude, F. J., Rasmussen, N., Lobatto, S., Wiik, A., Permin, H., van Es, L. A., van der Geissen, M., van der Hem, G. K. & The. T. H. (1985). Autoantibodies against neutrophils and monocytes: tool for diagnosis and marker of disease activity in Wegener's granulomatosis. *Lancet*, **i**, 425–9.

van der Woude, F. J., van Es, L. A. & Daha, M. R. I. (1990). The role of the c-ANCA antigen in the pathogenesis of Wegener's granulomatosis. A hypothesis based on both humoral and cellular mechanisms. *Netherlands Journal of Medicine*, **36**, 169–71.

van Leenen, D., van der Poll, T., Levi, M., ten Cate, H., van Deventer, S. J. H., Hock, C. F., Aarden, L. A. & ten Cate, J. W. (1993). Pentoxifylline attenuates neutrophil activation in experimental endotoxinemia in chimpanzees. *Journal of Immunology*, **151**, 2318–25.

Varagunam, M., Adu, D., Taylor, C. M., Michael, J., Neuberger, J. & Richards, N. (1992*a*). Endothelium myeloperoxidase-antimyeloperoxidase interaction in vasculitis. *Nephrology Dialysis Transplant*, **7**, 1077–81.

Varagunam, M., Nwosu, Z., Adu, D., Garner, C., Taylor, C. M., Michael, J. & Thompson, R. A. (1992*b*). Little evidence for anti-endothelial cell antibodies in microscopic polyarteritis and Wegener's granulomatosis. *Nephrology Dialysis Transplant*, **8**, 113–17.

Warfield, A. T., Lees, S., Phillips, S. & Pall, A. A. (1994). Isolated testicular vasculitis mimicking a testicular neoplasm. *Journal of Clinical Pathology*. In press.

Weiss, M. A. & Crissman, J. D. (1984). Renal biopsy findings in Wegener's granulomatosis: segmental necrotizing glomerulonephritis with glomerular thrombosis. *Human Pathology*, **15**, 943–56.

Wilkes, M., Pall, A. A., Garner, C., Wellington, M., Richards, N. T., Adu, D. & Hutton, P. (1994). Induction of nitric oxide synthase by TNF in human glomerular epithelial cells. *Nephrology Dialysis Transplant*, **9**, 932.

Woolf, A. D., Wakerley, G., Wallington, T. B., Scott, D. G. I. & Dieppe, P. A. (1987). Factor VIII related antigen in the assessment of vasculitis. *Annals of Rheumatic Diseases*, **46**, 441–7.

Yang, J. J., Tuttle, R., Jennette, J. C. & Falk, R. J. (1993). Glomerulonephritis in rats immunized with myeloperoxidase (MPO). *Clinical and Experimental Immunology*, **93** (Suppl.) 22.

Zimmerman, G. A. Prescott, S. M. & McIntyre, T. M. (1992). Endothelial cell interactions with granulocytes: tethering and signalling molecules. *Immunology Today*, **13**, 93–100.

Zheng, H., Crowley, J. J., Chan, J. C., Hoffman, H., Hatherill, J. R., Ishizaka, A. & Raffin, J. A. (1990). Attenuation of tumor necrosis factor-induced endothelial cell cytotoxicity and chemiluminescence. *American Review of Respiratory Diseases*, **142**, 1073.

–9–
Endothelial involvement in childhood Kawasaki disease

M. J. DILLON

Vasculitis is a feature of many different diseases and syndromes of childhood (Hicks, 1988). In some, it is the predominant manifestation of the condition; in others, it may be one aspect of a multisystem disease. Of the various vasculitic syndromes seen in children, Kawasaki disease (mucocutaneous lymph node syndrome) is comparatively common and is of some importance since, unlike many vasculitides, there is good evidence pointing to an infective initiating agent.

In this chapter the clinical and laboratory features of Kawasaki disease are described with current views on management and prognosis. In addition, the evidence supporting endothelial involvement is outlined, providing further support for the general importance of endothelial cell pathology in the variety of immunologically mediated diseases described in other chapters of this volume.

Kawasaki disease–clinical and therapeutic aspects

This childhood systemic vasculitis was first described in Japan in 1967 (Kawasaki, 1967). Since then over 80 000 cases have been reported from that country alone (Yanagawa & Nakamura, 1986), although it is of worldwide distribution, affecting predominantly infants and young children under five years of age (Tizard *et al.*, 1991*a*). There is an ethnic bias towards Oriental or Afro-Caribbean children, a male preponderance, some seasonality, and occasional epidemics (Hicks & Melish, 1986; Rowley, Gonzalez-Crussi & Shulman, 1988).

Clinical features

The principal manifestations are outlined in Table 9.1, based on the diagnostic guidelines prepared by the Japan Kawasaki Disease Research Committee (1984). At least five of the six items in Table 9.1 should be

Table 9.1. *Principal symptoms of Kawasaki disease*

- Fever persisting for five days or more
- Changes in the peripheral extremities (reddening of palms and soles, indurative oedema in initial stage, and membranous desquamation of the finger tips in the convalescent phase)
- Polymorphous exanthema
- Bilateral conjunctival injection
- Changes of lips and oral cavity (reddening of lips, strawberry tongue, diffuse injection of oral and pharyngeal mucosa)
- Acute non-purulent cervical lymphadenopathy

Table 2. *Other significant symptoms and findings in Kawasaki disease*

- *Cardiovascular system*: heart murmurs, gallop rhythm, ECG changes, cardiomegaly, two-dimensional echo findings of pericardial effusion, coronary artery aneurysms, aneurysms of peripheral arteries, angina pectoris and myocardial infarction
- *Gastrointestinal tract*: diarrhoea, vomiting, abdominal pain, hydrops of the gallbladder, ileus and jaundice
- *Blood*: leukocytosis, thrombocytosis, increased erythrocyte sedimentation rate, increased C-reactive protein, hypoalbuminaemia and anaemia
- *Urine*: proteinuria, increased leukocytes in sediment
- *Skin*: transverse furrows of finger nails
- *Respiratory tract*: cough and rhinorrhoea
- *Joints*: pain and swelling
- *Neurological system*: pleocytosis in cerebrospinal fluid, convulsions and facial palsy

present for the diagnosis to be established. Patients with four items can be diagnosed as having Kawasaki disease if coronary artery aneurysms are also present on two-dimensional echocardiography or coronary angiography. However, there may be a need to review the diagnostic criteria in the future in view of the increasing number of cases of incomplete Kawasaki disease that are being recognized (Rowley *et al.*, 1987). Other significant symptoms or findings seen in Kawasaki disease are listed in Table 9.2.

Incidence

In Japanese populations, the incidence is 150 per 100 000 children less than five years of age per year (Yanagawa & Nakamura, 1986). Elsewhere the incidence is substantially less: 10.3 (USA), and in several European countries, including the UK approximately 3.0 per 100 000 children less than five years of age (Shulman, 1987; Kawasaki, 1988; Hall & Newton, 1992).

Cardiovascular complications

Cardiovascular complications are variable but may be up to 35% if transient coronary artery dilation, pericardial effusion, ECG abnormalities, pericarditis, myocardial infarction, ventricular aneurysm, mitral incompetence and cardiac failure are included (Kato *et al.*, 1975; Suzuki *et al.*, 1985; Tizard *et al.*, 1991*b*; Rowley *et al.*, 1988). The incidence of coronary artery aneurysms ranges from 20–30% depending on which series is being considered. Mortality is of the order of 1–2% although this is decreasing since the introduction of immunoglobulin therapy.

Laboratory investigations

Investigations reveal a polymorphonuclear leukocytosis, thrombocythaemia, circulating immune complexes (Levin *et al.*, 1985) and both antineutrophil cytoplasmic antibodies (ANCA) (Savage *et al.*, 1989; Tizard & Dillon, 1990) and anti-endothelial cell antibodies (AECA) (Leung *et al.*, 1986; Tizard *et al.*, 1991*a*; Kaneko *et al.*, 1993*a*) which may have diagnostic as well as aetiopathological roles. The ANCA findings on immunofluorescence are very characteristic, with a diffuse cytoplasmic staining that is distinct from the granular cytoplasmic pattern seen in Wegener's granulomatosis or the perinuclear pattern in renal-associated disease (Kaneko *et al.*, 1993*b*). These findings will be further discussed in the section dealing with pathogenetic mechanisms.

Treatment

Aspirin and high-dose intravenous gamma-globulin either as four or five daily doses of 400 mg/kg/day (Newburger *et al.*, 1986), or one dose of 2 g/kg (Newburger *et al.*, 1991), are currently recommended. Dipyridamole has also been used in addition to aspirin by some groups. In the presence of very large coronary artery aneurysms, especially if there is myocardial ischaemia, intravenous prostacyclin (Tizard *et al.*, 1991*b*) or plasma exchange or exchange transfusions (Tizard & Dillon, 1991) may also have a place. Intra-arterial or intravenous urokinase has been used when a coronary artery becomes occluded with thrombus (Terai *et al.*, 1985). Coronary revascularization surgery may be indicated for critical stenotic lesions in the convalescent phase of the illness (Suzuki *et al.*, 1985). Steroids remain controversial and are not advocated, but some argue that they might have a role if used in conjunction with aspirin therapy. In support of this is the observation that steroid treatment has been of value in children at the Hospital for Sick Children with aggressive disease who appear resistant to gamma-globulin and aspirin therapy.

Prognosis

The general outlook for children with Kawasaki disease is good, although there is an acute mortality rate of 1–2% due to myocardial infarction. This may be reduced by alertness of clinicians to the diagnosis, and the early use of gamma-globulin and antiplatelet therapy. After the acute phase there is morbidity and occasionally mortality due to coronary artery stenotic lesions in later life (Tatara *et al.*, 1989) with ischaemic myocardial sequelae. Interestingly it has been postulated that adult atheromatous coronary heart disease may have its origins in childhood and be due to previous covert or overt Kawasaki disease (Brecker, Gray & Obedershaw, 1988).

Aetiology of Kawasaki disease

Most workers agree that Kawasaki disease has an infective basis, although the nature of the organism and the mechanism involved remains in doubt. A number of organisms have been considered including *Streptococcus sanguis*, *Propionibacterium acnes*, EB virus, human herpes virus-6, *Chlamydia*, *Rickettsia*, and retroviruses, but none has been clearly implicated (Shulman, 1987; Kawasaki, 1988). A retroviral role was considered because of the profound immunoregulatory disturbance in the acute phase of the illness, suggesting the involvement of a lymphotropic agent (Shulman & Rowley, 1986; Burns *et al.*, 1986). In spite of much effort to confirm this, the consensus is that retroviruses are not involved (Melish *et al.*, 1989). At present, there is interest in the possible role of a toxin-producing organism in view of the finding of selective expansion of T cells expressing T cell receptor variable regions $V\beta2$ and $V\beta8$ in Kawasaki disease patients (Abe *et al.*, 1992). These observations might be caused by new clones of toxic shock syndrome toxin-producing *Staphylococcus aureus* since a substantial proportion of Kawasaki disease patients have been shown to be infected with such bacteria (Leung *et al.*, 1993). A much smaller percentage of patients appear to be infected with Streptococci producing pyrogenic exotoxin and this may be the aetiological agent in some children affected by Kawasaki disease (Leung *et al.*, 1993).

Pathology

Although the coronary arteries appear to be markedly affected in Kawasaki disease, it is important to note that any small or medium-sized blood vessel can be involved (Hirose & Hamashima, 1978).

On reviewing autopsy cases of Kawasaki disease, post-mortem pathology varies according to the duration of the illness (Fujiwara & Hamashima, 1978; Hirose & Hamashima, 1978; Leung, 1988). If death occurs less than 10 days after the onset of fever the post-mortem pathology is characterized by acute inflammation involving the endothelial surface of arterioles, venules and capillaries, as well as the intima of small and medium-sized arteries, especially the coronaries, with, in addition, a perivasculitis. The latter is associated with acute inflammation of the vasa vasorum without inflammatory changes in the media (Fujiwara & Hamashima, 1978).

Microscopically the acute vascular lesion in Kawasaki disease is associated with evidence of endothelial activation and endothelial cell damage (Hirose & Hamashima, 1978). This consists of endothelial swelling, increased endothelial replication, the adhesion of leukocytes to the endothelial walls and endothelial necrosis, with or without immunoglobulin deposition (Leung, 1988, 1991). The lesion is also associated with infiltration of both neutrophils and mononuclear cells. The mononuclear cells consist of activated $CD4^+$ cells and monocyte macrophages. Class II major histocompatibility complex (MHC) antigens have been demonstrated on coronary artery endothelium in Kawasaki disease patients, but not in normal controls (Terai *et al.*, 1990). The presence of Class II MHC antigens on endothelial cells, as well as the observation of leukocyte adhesion to endothelial cells in the vascular lesion of Kawasaki disease, suggests that cytokine-induced endothelial antigens (see Chapter 2) play a role in the pathogenesis of the disease (Leung, 1991; Cotran & Pober, 1988).

If death occurs 12–35 days after onset of fever, the characteristic finding is marked infiltration of inflammatory cells into the media of the coronary and other medium-sized arteries. There is medial destruction in the blood vessel wall with aneurysm formation and thrombosis, presumably as a result of tissue destruction that follows local release of inflammatory mediators (Leung, 1988). Subsequently, the acute inflammatory process regresses and granulation of the coronary arteries is noted and in patients dying 40 days to 4 years after onset, there is scar formation and organization of thrombi.

Thus there is a major involvement of the endothelium in the early phase of the disease process, and with healing of severe arterial disease intimal findings are reported that are very similar to those seen in early atherosclerosis (Sasaguri & Kato, 1982).

One interesting aspect of Kawasaki disease is that vascular lesions, although affecting other vessels, appear to localize markedly to the coronary arteries (Fujiwara *et al.*, 1980). This is difficult to explain, although it is known that spontaneous endothelial injury is non-randomly distributed over the aortic surface in the rat, with foci of increased cell death and replication (Hansson *et al.*, 1985). Haemodynamic factors, however, such as turbulence and regions of low and/or high shear may promote the development of endothelial injury (Fry, 1968; Nerem & Cornhill, 1980; Davies *et al.*, 1986). It is also obvious from epidemiological studies that certain risk factors are more important in some regions of the vasculature than in others; for example, hypercholesterolaemia is an important risk factor for coronary atherosclerosis but less important for leg artery atherosclerosis where smoking is a major factor (Hopkins & Williams, 1981). None of these observations explains the predilection of the coronaries for vasculitic damage in Kawasaki disease, but they emphasize that the endothelium is not an homogeneous cell layer throughout the vasculature, but is subject to variations in structure, metabolism and response to injury as part of regional specialization (Hansson, 1987).

Pathogenetic mechanisms

The major pathological feature is a vasculitis affecting small and medium-sized blood vessels, not only in the coronary circulation but in many other organs of the body. The vasculitis, with endothelial cell necrosis, leukocytic infiltration into the media and adventitia of arteries and venules, and medial disruption, often coexists with dilatation of the blood vessel and intraluminal thrombosis (Fujiwara & Hamashima, 1978). A number of cellular and humoral immunological abnormalities have been documented during the acute phase of Kawasaki disease. These include deficient CD8-positive suppressor/cytotoxic T-cells, increased CD4-positive activated helper T-cells bearing HLA-DR surface antigens, and grossly increased numbers of B-cells spontaneously secreting IgG and IgM (Leung, Chu & Wood, 1983). High levels of the plasma cytokines interleukin-1 (IL-1) and tumour necrosis factor (TNF) and spontaneous secretion of cytokines have also been documented (Furukawa *et al.*, 1988; Maury, Salo & Pelkonen, 1988), which are likely to contribute to the activation of endothelial cells noted above (Leung, 1991). Immune complexes have also been detected in the circulation two to four weeks after onset of the disease in several studies (Levin *et al.*, 1985; Kohsaka *et al.*, 1988) and have been shown to induce platelet activation and release of vasoactive mediators (Levin *et al.*, 1985). Furthermore, there appeared to be an association between the presence of immune complexes and the characteristic thrombocytosis occurring in the second and third weeks of the illness.

Anti-endothelial cell antibodies and endothelial injury

The presence of vasculitis in Kawasaki disease has focused the attentions of several workers on the mechanisms of vascular injury in the condition. Leung *et al.* (1986, 1989) demonstrated complement-dependent endothelial cell toxicity of Kawasaki serum for cultured endothelial cells treated with tumour necrosis factor, interleukin 1 and gamma interferon. Since Kawasaki disease is associated with marked T cell and macrophage activation (Leung, 1991) it was argued that immune activation present in the disease results in the elaboration of cytokines that activate endothelium and induce new surface antigens and that the ensuing antibody response resulted in vascular injury.

On the other hand, the binding of anti-endothelial cell antibodies (AECA) detected by ELISA (Tizard *et al.*, 1991*a*; Kaneko *et al.*, 1993*a*) did not depend on prior cytokine stimulation of target endothelium. It has also been shown that cytotoxicity can occur without pre-stimulation of endothelial cells with cytokine, although it was enhanced by such pretreatment (Kaneko *et al.*, 1993*a*). These data suggest that cytokine stimulation may be necessary to promote maximal cytotoxic effects of AECA but may not be necessary for their formation.

Further work in Kawasaki disease has involved, as mentioned above, an interest in the effects of cytokine stimulation of endothelium. Increased secretion of interleukin 1 (Maury *et al.*, 1988), tumour necrosis factor (Furakawa *et al.*, 1988) and gamma interferon (Rowley *et al.*, 1988) has been shown by several groups. Extending this work Leung *et al.* (1989) demonstrated that endothelial activation antigens were expressed *de novo* (for example, E-selectin) or showed increased expression (for example ICAM-1) in skin biopsies of children in the acute stages of the disease. Although E-selectin and ICAM-1 do not appear to be the target antigens of AECA, they do serve as markers for cytokine-inducible endothelial cell activation. Interestingly, following treatment with gamma globulin, which is known to decrease the incidence of coronary artery aneurysms in the disease, the endothelial cell activation disappears in the majority of cases. The mechanism of action of gamma globulin is not known, but Leung postulated that gamma globulin could inhibit cytokine-mediated endothelial cell activation either by neutralising the effects of the cytokines or by inhibiting the endothelial cell response, thus making the endothelium less susceptible to damage by AECA (Leung *et al.*, 1989).

As yet the antigens against which the AECA are directed have not been identified. A probability that has been considered is that AECA may be directed against epitopes on as yet unidentified infective agents that cross-react with antigenic sites on endothelial cells, thus causing endothelial injury and clinical vasculitis. Although this might be relevant, so many other factors play a part in the vasculitic process that such a simple explanation is unlikely to apply. However, until the antigens to which AECA are directed are identified, this issue will have to remain in abeyance.

Antineutrophil cytoplasmic antibodies and neutrophil-induced injury

In addition to the potential role of AECA and cytokines in inducing endothelial injury there is, in Kawasaki disease, evidence to support a contribution from neutrophils as well. IgG and IgM antineutrophil cytoplasmic antibodies are elevated in acute Kawasaki disease (Savage *et al.*, 1989; Tizard & Dillon, 1990; Tizard *et al.*, 1991*b*; Dillon & Tizard, 1991; Kaneko *et al.*, 1993*b*) and this is a finding that links this important childhood arteritis to systemic necrotizing vasculitis in adults. (See Chapter 8). These antibodies have been detected by solid phase RIA (Savage *et al.*, 1989), by ELISA (Tizard *et al.*, 1991*b*; Kaneko *et al.*, 1993*b*) and by indirect immunofluorescence (Savage *et al.*, 1989; Kaneko *et al.*, 1993*b*). The indirect immunofluorescence appearances are unusual in that there is a diffuse cytoplasmic staining, distinct from the granular pattern seen in Wegener's granulomatosis and the perinuclear staining seen in renal associated disease thought to be due to antibodies directed against proteinase 3 and myeloperoxidase, respectively (Jennette & Falk, 1990). Studies on the antigenic specificities of these antibodies have provided varying results. Kaneko *et al.* (1993*b*) showed that a proportion of patients had antibodies to the α fraction of neutrophil primary granules but not to myeloperoxidase. This left, in their study, a number of patients who had positive ANCA for acid extracts of neutrophils in whom the precise epitope to which the antibodies were raised was unknown. More recently, Gilbert *et al.* (1993) showed that a substantial proportion of acute Kawasaki disease patients sera contained antibodies directed against cathepsin G. The question, however, arises as to whether the specificity is in anyway meaningful in terms of the pathophysiology of the disease or its diagnosis or whether variable findings might occur in individual patients reflecting non-specific B cell activation.

There is, however, evidence that in vasculitides ANCA can induce neutrophil activation, and contribute as a result to endothelial injury (Savage *et al.*, 1992; Ewart *et al.*, 1992). What is more, an unidentified endothelial cell ligand, which does not appear to be 1CAM-1, appears to be able to stimulate adherent TNF-primed neutrophils via MAC-1 (CD11b/CD18) and trigger the release of reactive oxygen species, suggesting that endothelial cells may also have the ability to contribute to neutrophil activation (Von Asmuth *et al.*, 1991; Savage, 1993). Savage *et al.* (1993) have also been able to show that endothelial bound myeloperoxidase and proteinase 3 can be recognized by ANCA, and there are reports that proteinase 3 is expressed under the influence of cytokines by endothelial cells and can bind anti-proteinase 3 ANCA though others have failed to confirm these findings (see Chapter 8; Mayet & Meyer zum Buschenfelde, 1993; Mayet *et al.*, 1993). These observations point to important relationships between ANCA, neutrophils and endothelial cells that may have implications in terms of the vasculitic process, which are discussed in more detail in Chapter 8.

Data of this sort have not been generated in Kawasaki disease, but clearly there is the potential for these various pathophysiological processes to be operative in patients with this condition and they may well play a major part in causing the endothelial injury that occurs.

Conclusions

The pathogenesis of the vascular injury in Kawasaki disease, as in other vasculitides, is complex and involves a range of mechanisms as outlined in this chapter and in other chapters of this book. The increasing recognition that endothelial and other vascular wall component injury is dependent on both effector and target cell involvement with cytokines playing a major role as mediators will hopefully lead to a clearer understanding of the nature of this condition and hence lead to more rational therapeutic approaches. Kawasaki disease might be a suitable model for study in this respect because of its very circumscribed nature and the possibility that, in view of its potentially infective aetiology, some clarification might emerge as to the type of infective agent involved in precipitating the vasculitic process, and hence the mechanisms of injury, that could be applied to other systemic vasculitides whose aetiology is generally unknown.

References

Abe, J., Kotzin B. L., Jujo, K., Melish, M. E., Glode, M. P., Kohsaka, T. & Leung, D. Y. M. (1992). Selective expansion of T cells expressing T-cell receptor variable regions Vβ2 and Vβ8 in Kawasaki disease. *Proceedings of the National Academy of Sciences USA*, **89**, 4066–70.

Brecker, S. J. D., Gray, H. H. & Obedershaw, P. J. (1988). Coronary artery aneurysms and myocardial infarction: adult sequelae of Kawasaki disease. *British Heart Journal*, **59**, 509–12.

Burns, J. C., Geha, R. S., Schneeberger, E. E., Newburger, J. W., Rosen, F. S., Glezen, L. S., Huang, A. S., Natale, J. & Leung, D. Y. M. (1986). Polymerase activity in lymphocyte culture supernatants from patients with Kawasaki disease. *Nature*, **323**, 814–16.

Cotran, R. S. & Pober, J. S. (1988). Endothelial activation: its role in inflammatory and immune reactions. In Simionescu, N. & Simionescu, M. eds. *Endothelial Cell Biology*, pp. 335–47. New York: Plenum.

Davies, P. F., Remuzzi, A., Gordon, E. J., Dewey, C. F. Jr. & Gimbrone, M. A. Jr. (1986). Turbulent fluid shear stress induces vascular endothelial cell turnover *in vitro*. *Proceedings of the National Academy of Sciences USA*, **83**, 2114–17.

Dillon, M. J. & Tizard, E. J. (1991) Anti-neutrophil cytoplasmic antibodies and anti-endothelial cell antibodies. *Pediatric Nephrology*, **5**, 256–9.

Ewert, B. H., Jennette, J. C. & Falk, R. J. (1992). Anti-myeloperoxidase antibodies stimulate neutrophils to damage human endothelial cells. *Kidney International*, **41**, 375–83.

Fry, D. L. (1968). Acute vascular endothelial changes associated with increased blood velocity gradients. *Circulation Research*, **22**, 165–97.

Fujiwara, H., Fujiwara, T., Kao, T.-C. *et al.* (1980). Pathology of Kawasaki disease in the healed state. Relationships between typical and atypical cases of Kawasaki disease. *Acta Pathology Japan*, **36**, 857–67.

Fujiwara, H. & Hamashima, Y. (1978). Pathology of the heart in Kawasaki disease. *Pediatrics*, **61**, 100–7.

Furukawa, S., Matsubara, T., Jujoh, K., Yone, K., Sugawara, T., Sasai, K., Kato, H. & Yabuta, K. (1988). Peripheral blood monocyte/macrophages and serum tumour necrosis factor in Kawasaki disease. *Clinical Immunology and Immunopathology*, **42**, 247–51.

Gilbert, R. D., Shah, V., Reader J. & Dillon, M. J. (1993). Cathepsin G specific IgM anti neutrophil cytoplasmic antibodies (ANCA) and anti endothelial cell antibodies (AECA) in acute Kawasaki disease. *Clinical and Experimental Immunology*, **93**(Suppl 1), 30.

Hall, S. & Newton, L. (1992). Kawasaki disease. In *British Paediatric Surveillance Unit Seventh Annual Report*, pp. 8–9.

Hansson, G. (1987). Pathogenetic mechanisms of arteritis in Kawasaki disease—a critical analysis. In Shulmam, S. T. ed. *Kawasaki Disease*, pp. 383–394. New York: Alan R. Liss Inc.

Hansson, G. K., Chao, S., Schwartz, S. M. & Reidy, M. A. (1985). Aortic endothelial cell death and replication in normal and lipopolysaccharide-treated rats. *American Journal of Pathology*, **121**, 123–7.

Hicks, R. V., ed. (1988). *Vasculopathies of Childhood*. Littleton: PSG Publishing.

Hicks, R. V. & Melish, M. E. (1986). Kawasaki syndrome. *Pediatric Clinics of North America*, **33**, 1151–75.

Hirose, S. & Hamashima, Y. (1978). Morphological observations on the vasculitis in the mucocutaneous lymph node syndrome. *European Journal of Pediatrics*, **129**, 17–27.

Hopkins, P. N. & Williams, R. R. (1981). A survey of 246 suggested coronary risk factors. *Atherosclerosis*, **40**, 1–52.

Japan Kawasaki Disease Research Committee (1984). *Diagnostic Guidelines of Kawasaki Disease*, 4th revised edn. Tokyo, Japan: Red Cross Medical Center.

Jennette, J. C. & Falk, R. J. (1990). Antineutrophil cytoplasmic autoantibodies and associated diseases: a review. *American Journal of Kidney Disease*, **15**, 517–29.

Kaneko, K., Savage, C. O. S., Pottinger, B. E. *et al.* (1993*a*). Cytotoxic autoantibodies to endothelial cells in Kawasaki disease. In Takahashi, M. & Taubert, K. eds. *Proceedings of 4th International Symposium on Kawasaki Disease*, pp. 185–91. American Heart Association.

Kaneko, K., Shah, V., Gaskin, G. *et al.* (1993*b*). Kawasaki disease has distinct anti-neutrophil cytoplasmic antibodies. In Takahashi, M. & Taubert, K. eds. *Proceedings of 4th International Symposium on Kawasaki Disease*, pp. 192–7. American Heart Association.

Kato, H., Koike, S., Yamamoto, M. *et al.* (1975). Coronary aneurysms in infants and young children with acute febrile mucocutaneous lymph node syndrome. *Journal of Pediatrics*, **86**, 892–8.

Kawasaki, T. (1967). Acute febrile mucocutaneous syndrome with lymphoid involvement with specific desquamation of the fingers and toes in children. *Japanese Journal of Allergy*, **16**, 178–222.

Kawasaki, T. ed. (1988). *Proceedings of the Third International Kawasaki Symposium*. Tokyo: Japan Heart Foundation.

Kohsaka, T., Abe, J., Nakayama, M. *et al.* (1988). The significance of IgM-immune complex and complement breakdown products in Kawasaki syndrome. In Kawasaki, T. ed. *Proceedings of the 3rd International Kawasaki Disease Symposium*, pp. 138–40. Toyko: Japan Heart Foundation.

Leung, D. Y. M. (1988). Cytokine production and vascular endothelial cell activation in Kawasaki disease. In Kawasaki, T. ed. *Proceedings of the 3rd International Kawasaki Disease Symposium*, pp. 113–6. Tokyo: Japan Heart Foundation.

Leung, D. Y. M. (1991). Immunologic aspects of Kawasaki disease: implications for pathogenesis and therapy. *Clinical Cardiology*, **14**(Suppl 11), 11–15.

Leung, D. Y. M., Chu, E. T. & Wood, N. (1983). Immunoregulatory T cell abnormalities in mucocutaneous lymph node syndrome. *Journal of Immunology*, **130**, 2002–4.

Leung, D. Y. M., Collins, T., Lapierre, L. A., Geha, R. S. & Pober, J. S. (1986). Immunoglobulin M antibodies present in the acute phase of Kawasaki syndrome lyse cultured vascular endothelial cells stimulated by gamma interferon. *Journal of Clinical Investigation*, **77**, 1428–35.

Leung, D. Y. M., Cotran, R. S. & Kurt-Jones, E. (1989). Endothelial cell activation and high interleukin 1 secretion in the pathogenesis of acute Kawasaki disease. *Lancet*, **ii**, 1298–302.

Leung, D. Y. M., Meissner, H. C., Fulton, D. R., Murray, D. L., Kotzin, B. L. & Schlievert, P. M. (1993). Toxic shock syndrome toxin-secreting *Staphylococcus aureus* in Kawasaki syndrome. *Lancet*, **342**, 1385–8.

Levin, M., Holland, P. C., Nokes, T. J., Novelli, V., Mola, M., Levinsky, R. J., Dillon, M J., Barratt, T. M. & Marshall, W. C. (1985). Platelet immune complex interaction in pathogenesis of Kawasaki disease and childhood polyarteritis. *British Medical Journal*, **290**, 1456–60.

Maury, C. P. J., Salo, E. & Pelkonen, P. (1988). Circulating interleukin-1β in patients with Kawasaki disease. *New England Journal of Medicine*, **319**, 1670–1.

Mayet, W. J., Hermann, E. H., Csernok, E. *et al.* (1993). *In vitro* interactions of C-ANCA (antibodies to proteinase 3) with human endothelial cells. In Gross, W. K. ed. *ANCA-Associated Vasculitides*, pp. 109–13. New York: Plenum Press.

Melish, M. E., Marchette, N. J., Kaplan, J. C., Kihara, S., Ching, D. & Ho, D. D. (1989). Absence of significant RNA-dependent DNA polymerase in lymphocytes from patients with Kawasaki syndrome. *Nature*, **337**, 288–90.

Nerem, R. M. & Cornhill, J. F. (1980). Hemodynamics and atherosclerosis. *Atherosclerosis*, **36**, 55–65.

Newburger, J. W., Takahashi, M., Beiser, A. S., Burns, J. C., Bastian, J., Chung, K. J., Colan, S. D., Duffy, C. E., Fulton, D. R., Glode, M. P., Mason, W. H., Meissner, H. C., Rowley, A. H., Shulman, S. T., Reddy, V., Sundel, R. P., Wiggins, J. W., Colton, T., Melish, M. E. & Rosen, F. S. (1991). A single intravenous infusion of gammaglobulin as compared with four infusions in the treatment of acute Kawasaki syndrome. *New England Journal of Medicine*, **324**, 1633–9.

Newburger, J. W., Takahashi, M., Burns, J. C., Beiser, A. S., Chung, K. J., Duffy, C. E., Glode, M. P., Mason, W. H., Reddy, V., Sanders, S. P., Shulman, S. T., Wiggins, J. W., Hicks, R. V., Fulton, D. R., Lewis, A. B., Leung, D. Y. M., Colton, T., Rosen, F. S. & Melish, M. E. (1986). The treatment of Kawasaki syndrome with intravenous gamma globulin. *New England Journal of Medicine*, **315**, 341–7.

Rowley, A. H., Gonzales-Crussi, F., Gidding, S. S., Duffy, C. F. & Shulman, S. T. (1987). Incomplete Kawasaki disease with coronary artery involvement. *Journal of Pediatrics*, **110**, 409–13.

Rowley, A. H., Gonzalez-Crussi, F. & Shulman, S. T. (1988). Kawasaki syndrome. *Review of Infectious Diseases*, **10**, 1–15.

Rowley, A. H., Shulman, S. T., Preble, O. T., Poiesz, B. J., Ehrlich, G. D. & Sullivan, J. R. (1988). Serum interferon concentrations and retroviral serology in Kawasaki syndrome. *Pediatric Infectious Disease Journal*, **7**, 663–6.

Sasaguri, Y. & Kato, H. (1982). Regression of aneurysms in Kawasaki disease: a pathological study. *Journal of Paediatrics*, **100**, 225–31.

Savage, C. O. S. (1993). The endothelial cell: active participant or innocent bystander in primary vasculitis? *Clinical and Experimental Immunology*, **93**(Suppl 1), 6–7.

Savage, C. O. S., Gaskin, G., Pusey, C. D. & Pearson, J. D. (1993). Anti-neutrophil cytoplasm antibodies (ANCA) can recognize vascular endothelial cell-bound ANCA-associated autoantigens. *Experimental Nephrology*, **1**, 190–5.

Savage, C. O. S., Pottinger, B. E., Gaskin, G., Pusey, C. D. & Pearson, J. D. (1992). Autoantibodies developing to myeloperoxidase and proteinase 3 in systemic vasculitis stimulate neutrophil cytotoxicity towards cultural endothelial cells. *American Journal of Pathology*, **141**, 335–42.

Savage, C. O. S., Tizard, E. J., Jayne, D., Lockwood, C. M. & Dillon, M. J. (1989). Antineutrophil cytoplasm antibodies in Kawasaki disease. *Archives of Disease in Childhood*, **64**, 360–3.

Shulman, S. T. ed. (1987). Kawasaki disease: Proceedings of the Second International Kawasaki Disease Symposium. *Progress in Clinical Biological Research*, vol. 250. New York: Alan R. Liss.

Shulman, S. T. & Rowley, A. H. (1986). Does Kawasaki disease have a retroviral aetiology? *Lancet*, **ii**, 545–6.

Suzuki, A., Kamiya, T., Ono, Y., Takahashi, N., Naito, Y. & Kou, Y. (1985). Indication of aortocoronary by-pass for coronary arterial obstruction due to Kawasaki disease. *Heart and Vessels*, **1**, 94–100.

Suzuki, A., Tizard, E. J., Gooch, V., Dillon, M. J. & Haworth, S. G. (1990). Kawasaki disease: echocardiographic features in 91 cases presenting in the United Kingdom. *Archives of Disease in Childhood*, **65**, 1142–6.

Tatara, K., Kusakawa, S., Itoh, K., Kazuma, N., Lee, K., Hashimoto, K., Shimohora, T., Kondoh, C. & Hiroe, M. (1989). Long term prognosis of Kawasaki disease in patients with coronary artery obstruction. *Heart Vessels*, **5**, 47–51.

Terai, M., Kohno, Y., Namba, M., Umemiya, T., Niwa, K, Nakajima, H. & Mikata, A. (1990). Class II major histocompatibility antigen expression in coronary arterial endothelium in a patient with Kawasaki disease. *Human Pathology*, **21**, 231–4.

Terai, M., Ogata, M., Sugimoto, K., Nagai, K., Toba, T., Tamai, K., Aotsuka, H., Niwa, K. & Nakajima, H. (1985). Coronary arterial thrombi in Kawasaki disease. *Journal of Pediatrics*, **106**, 76–8.

Tizard, E. J., Baguley, E., Hughes, G. R. V. & Dillon, M. J. (1991*a*). Anti-endothelial cell antibodies detected by a cellular based ELISA in Kawasaki disease. *Archives of Disease in Childhood*, **66**, 189–92.

Tizard, E. J. & Dillon, M. J. (1990). Laboratory investigation in the diagnosis and management of childhood vasculitis. *Prospective in Pediatrics*, **20**, 35–9.

Tizard, E. J. & Dillon, M. J. (1991). Plasmapheresis in childhood. *Care of the Critically Ill*, **7**, 51–5.

Tizard, E. J., Suzuki, A., Levin, M. & Dillon, M. J. (1991*b*). Clinical aspects of 100 patients with Kawasaki disease. *Archives of Disease in Childhood*, **66**, 185–8.

Von Asmuth, E. J. U., Van der Linden, C. J., Leeuwenberg, J. F. M. & Buurman, W. A. (1991). Involvement of the CD 11b/CD18 integrin, but not the endothelial cell adhesion molecules ELAM-1 and ICAM-1 in tumour necrosis factor induced neutrophil toxicity. *Journal of Immunology*, **147**, 3869–75.

Yanagawa, H. & Nakamura, Y. (1986). Nationwide epidemic of Kawasaki disease in Japan during winter of 1985–1986. *Lancet*, **ii**, 1138–40.

-10-

The role of the endothelium in thrombotic thrombocytopaenic purpura and haemolytic uraemic syndrome

CARLA ZOJA and GIUSEPPE REMUZZI

Introduction

Thrombotic thrombocytopaenic purpura (TTP) is an uncommon and severe multi-system disease characterized by intravascular platelet aggregation, thrombocytopaenia, central nervous system (and other organ) ischaemia and microangiopathic haemolytic anaemia that mainly occurs in adults (Bukowski, 1982). TTP shows many similarities to haemolytic uraemic syndrome (HUS), a disorder of thrombocytopaenia, microangiopathic haemolytic anaemia and acute renal failure that mainly affects young children (Kaplan & Remuzzi, 1991).

Although many attempts have been made to differentiate TTP and HUS, none of the proposed criteria clearly separates the two syndromes (Remuzzi, 1987*a*). A clinical distinction based on multi-organ involvement in TTP and renal involvement in HUS is not always apparent (Nalbandian, Henry & Bick, 1979). Even the most widely used criteria, the presence of neurological symptoms in TTP and of renal failure in HUS, fails to distinguish TTP from HUS since neurological involvement has been observed in HUS (Gianantonio, 1964; Sheth, Swick & Haworth, 1986) and many patients classified as having TTP also have renal failure (Amorosi & Ultmann, 1966; Dunea *et al.*, 1966; Eknoyan & Riggs, 1986). The fundamental pathological lesion, thrombotic microangiopathy, is identical in TTP and HUS, and identical aetiological agents and pathogenetic mechanisms have been proposed for both syndromes. Most of the available morphological evidence indicates that endothelial injury is probably the inciting event to the development of microangiopathic lesions.

Factors known to cause TTP and HUS (bacterial endotoxins, antibodies and immune complexes, immunosuppressive agents) can all induce vascular endothelial damage (Remuzzi, 1987*b*). This is true also for verocytotoxin produced by *E. coli*, whose association with HUS and subsequently also with TTP has been consistently documented in the last ten years (Karmali *et al.*, 1983, 1985; Kavi & Wise, 1989; Morrison, Tyrrel & Jewell, 1986; Windler *et al.*, 1989). The initial injury to endothelium is followed by a number of biochemical abnormalities that contribute to the development of the lesions. Thus abnormalities in haemostatic mediators of endothelial cell origin, including prostacyclin (PGI_2), von Willebrand factor (vWf) and tissue plasminogen activator (TPA) have been described in patients with TTP and HUS. Loss of functional and/or morphological integrity of endothelial cells, as occurs in TTP/HUS, may also result in a defect in nitric oxide production or be associated with enhanced endothelin release. The possible role of nitric oxide or endothelin in the pathogenesis of TTP/HUS still needs to be appropriately addressed.

Histological evidence of endothelial injury in TTP and HUS

Microvascular thrombosis is the typical lesion of TTP and HUS (Remuzzi, Ruggenenti & Bertani, 1993) (Fig. 10.1). Widespread platelet thrombi and fibrin occluding capillaries, arterioles and arteries of various organs, including kidney, pancreas, adrenals, spleen, heart and brain is the most striking microscopic feature of TTP (Amorosi & Ultmann, 1966; Berkowitz, Dalldorf & Blatt, 1979). In the kidney, thrombosis affects arterioles and less frequently interlobular arteries. Frequently, arterioles show pale material in the subendothelial space and a proliferation of endothelial and myointimal cells. When the proliferative process is severe, the arterioles near the glomeruli may assume the appearance and size of glomeruli and are called glomeruloid structures (Goodman *et al.*, 1978; Umlas & Kaiser, 1970). Aneurysmal dilatation of the vessel wall of arterioles can be also observed. Glomerular changes in TTP have not been described in the same detail in the literature as they have for HUS. Glomerular capillaries may be thickened with double contours. Due to the arteriolar involvement in the microangiopathic process, glomeruli undergo ischaemic changes with retraction of the tufts and thickening and wrinkling of capillary loops. At the ultrastructural level those vessels with thrombosis or with intramural lesions contain endothelial cells that are swollen and show signs of activation, such as multiple cytoplasmic projections, an increased number of mitochondria, lipid granules and expansion of the Golgi apparatus. Glomerular endothelium is swollen and the subendothelial space is enlarged because of the deposition of non-homogeneous material. According to Habib *et al.* (1969) the glomerular lesions of TTP are identical to those of HUS.

In young children under 2 years of age who are affected by HUS, the typical lesion is a thickening of the glomerular capillary wall with double

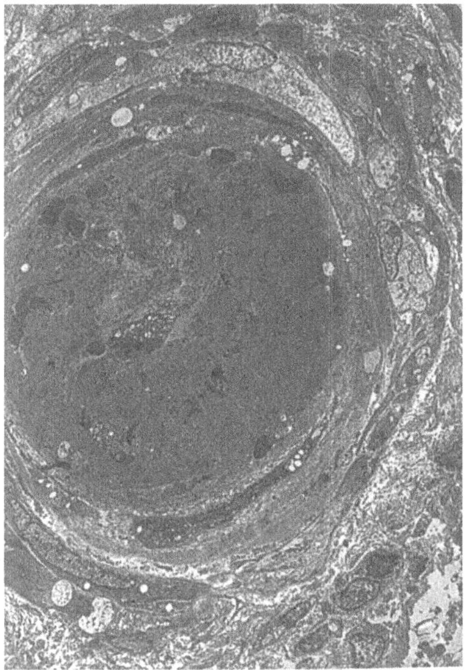

Fig. 10.1. Electron micrograph of a renal arteriole in HUS. The lumen is occluded by a thrombus formed by electron dense material that includes red blood cells and cellular debris (magnification ×550).

contours associated with a pronounced swelling of endothelial cells, marked reduction or occlusion of the glomerular capillary lumina, and occasional fragmentation of erythrocytes and intraluminal thrombi (Levy, Gagnadoux & Habib, 1980). At electron microscopy, glomerular endothelial cells are swollen with an electron-lucent cytoplasm. A marked widening of the subendothelial space resulting from detachment of endothelium from the glomerular basement membrane is observed, which may lead to complete obliteration of the lumen. The subendothelial space is filled with fluffy glomerular material containing fibrin or cellular debris (Fig. 10.2). Glomerular capillary lumina may become occluded by thrombi consisting of fibrin and platelets. In older children and adults, the microangiopathic process mainly involves arteries and arterioles, and the prognosis is poorer than in young children (Levy *et al.*, 1980; Kanfer *et al.*, 1980). The main findings are oedema and proliferation of the intima, necrosis of the arterial wall (Fig. 10.3); some vessels are thrombosed. In some cases, a 'glomeruloid' structure of the small arteries is detected which is probably the result of endothelial and myointimal proliferation of small arteries adjacent to glomeruli (Pirani, 1983). Extrarenal lesions have been found at autopsy in 35 of 62 HUS cases,

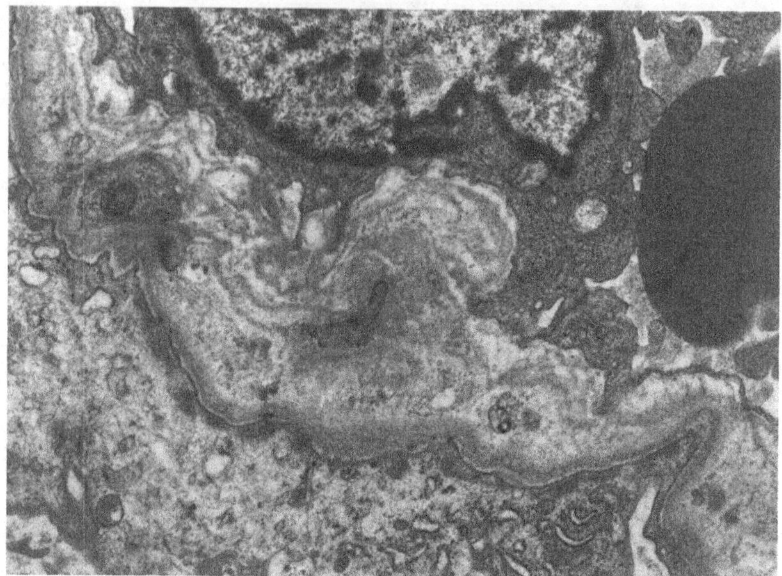

Fig. 10.2. Electron micrograph of a segment of glomerular capillary in a patient with HUS. The endothelium is detached from glomerular basement membrane. The subendothelium is occupied by electron-lucent fluffy material. Beneath the endothelium a thin layer of new formed glomerular basement membrane is observed. Foot processes are extensively fused (magnification ×4000).

studied by Gianantonio (1984); these included microthrombotic lesions in the colon, heart, brain and pancreas. Intracranial haemorrhages were also described (Gianantonio, 1984).

Triggering agents of TTP and HUS may cause endothelial injury

Various agents capable of causing TTP and HUS are toxic to vascular endothelium under various experimental conditions (Remuzzi, 1987*b*). They include bacterial endotoxin and verocytotoxin, viruses, antibodies, immune complexes and drugs. Cases of HUS associated with endotoxin-producing bacteria (*Shigella* and *Salmonella* species) have been consistently reported (Koster *et al.*, 1978; Baker *et al.*, 1974). Endotoxin is a well-known trigger of endothelial damage as documented by *in vitro* studies showing that lipopolysaccharide derived from *E. coli*, *Salmonella minnesota* or *Salmonella typhosa* could directly injure cultured bovine endothelial cells, inducing cell detachment and lysis (Harlan *et al.*, 1983). In rabbits, two

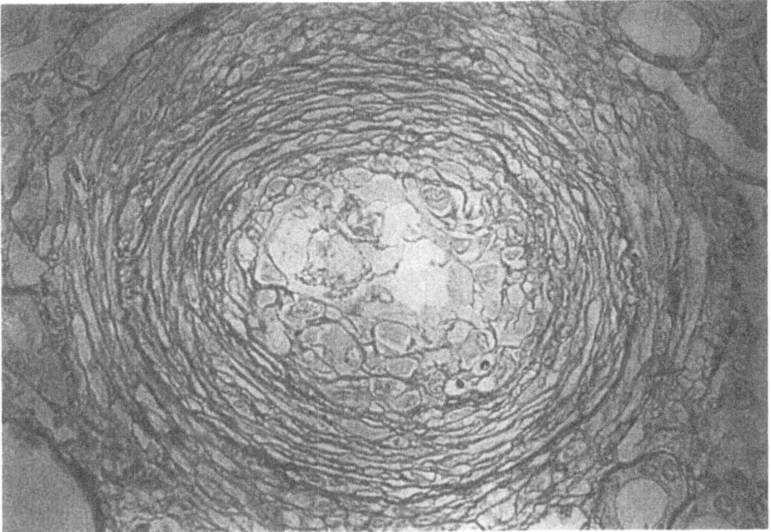

Fig. 10.3. Interlobular artery of a patient with HUS showing a marked myointimal proliferation and marked swelling of endothelium (PAS; magnification ×175).

intravenous injections of endotoxin from gram-negative bacteria, spaced 18–24 hours apart, produced a generalized Schwartzmann reaction with disseminated intravascular coagulation and bilateral cortical necrosis of the kidneys (Thomas & Good, 1952). In other studies, a five hour continuous infusion of endotoxin in rabbits induced a syndrome that closely resembled human HUS (Bertani *et al.*, 1989). Sequential histological examination of kidneys revealed focal irregularities of endothelial fenestrae and endothelial swelling that developed a few minutes after the start of the infusion, followed by leukocyte and platelet accumulation within glomerular capillaries. After 1 hour a marked glomerular polymorphonuclear cell infiltration was detected; after 5 hours fibrin-like material, as free strands in the lumina or as large clumps along the luminal surface of the endothelial layer, was observed (Fig. 10.4). Damage was completely reversible: 48 hours after the end of the infusion only mild endothelial changes and occasional polymorphs, but no fibrin deposits, were found in the glomeruli. This rabbit model therefore shows close similarities with the so-called glomerular type of HUS occurring in young children (Levy *et al.*, 1980) in which the favourable outcome of HUS indicates a spontaneous resolution of the microangiopathic process and active removal of fibrin.

Karmali *et al.* (1983) first noted an association between HUS and enteric infections with verocytotoxin-producing *E. coli* (VTEC). Human VTEC

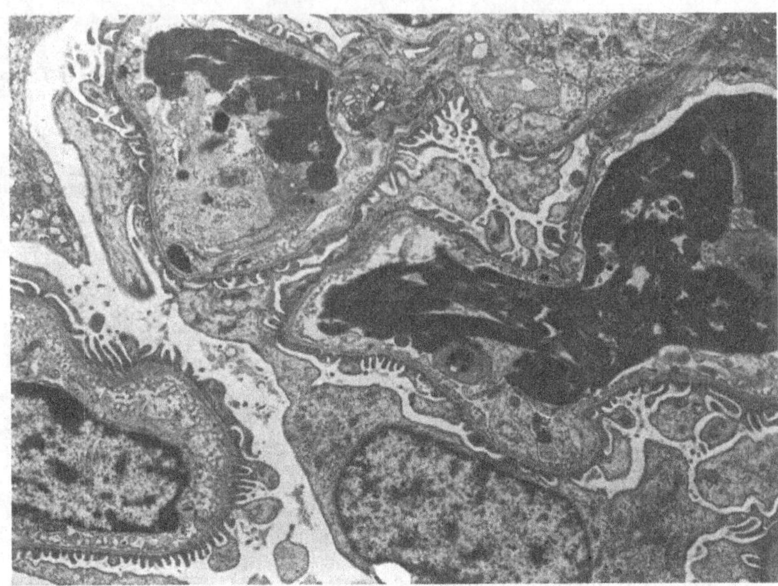

Fig. 10.4. Electron micrograph of a glomerular capillary loop in a rabbit infused with endotoxin for 5 hours. Fibrin deposits are present in the glomerular capillary lumen (magnification ×1800).

strains produce two distinct bacteriophage-mediated protein exotoxins, VT-1 and VT-2, that are closely related to Shiga toxin (O'Brien & Holmes, 1987). The VTEC consists of a biologically active subunit A and a number of B subunits that allow binding of the toxin to glycolipids, mainly ceramide derivatives, containing a terminal disaccharide, galactose-(α1-4)-galactose (Lindberg *et al.*, 1987; Lingwood *et al.*, 1987). Binding is followed by internalization of the A subunit, which inhibits protein synthesis by inactivating 60S ribosomal subunits and leads to cell death (O'Brien & Holmes, 1987). VTEC and Shiga toxin are directly cytotoxic to human umbilical vein endothelial cells (HUVEC) in culture (Obrig *et al.*, 1987; Kavi *et al.*, 1987). The cytopathic effect of VTEC on vascular endothelium is accompanied by release of vWF by HUVEC (Kavi *et al.*, 1987) and by reduced synthesis of PGI_2 in rat aortic tissue (Karch *et al.*, 1988). Endothelial damage by VT-1 or Shiga toxin *in vitro* is potentiated by additional exposure to inflammatory mediators such as tumour necrosis factor-α (TNF-α) or interleukin-1 (IL-1) (Van de Kar *et al.*, 1991; Tesh *et al.*, 1991; Louise & Obrig, 1991). A recent study reported that preincubation of HUVEC with TNF-α resulted in a 10- to 100-fold increase of specific binding sites for VT-1 (Van de Kar *et al.*, 1992). Similar effects were elicted by IL-1 although to a lesser extent. Glycolipid extracts of TNF-α treated cells demonstrated an increase of the verotocytotoxin receptor, globotriaosylceramide, suggesting that preincubation of HUVEC with TNF-α leads to an increase in globotriaosylceramide synthesis in these cells. It is likely that the reduction of protein synthesis and the increased cytotoxicity caused by VT-1 is primarily the consequence of enhanced VT-1 binding to endothelial cells.

In vivo studies by Richardson *et al.* (1987) showed that in rabbits verotoxin induced a reproducible illness characterized by neurologic and enteric dysfunction, with endothelial swelling and luminal occlusion of small arteries and arterioles. Whether or not the kidney was involved in the disease process was not reported in this study. More recently, we have shown that rabbits challenged with VT-1 purified from *E. coli* 0157:H7 developed anorexia, lethargia and limb paralysis but renal function was normal (Zoja *et al.*, 1992). Microvascular damage was confined to brain, cerebellum, lungs and colon, and no kidney lesions were documented. This can be explained by the presence in the rabbit of verotoxin receptors in all of the foregoing organs, except the kidney. It follows that organ localization of the microangiopathic process in various animal species infected with VTEC follows the distribution of verocytotoxin receptors in different organs. Thus the susceptibility of rabbits to neurological and enteric disease associated with verotoxin challenge may be explained by the receptor distribution that prevails in the central nervous system and gastrointestinal tract (Zoja *et al.*, 1992). Rabbits do not develop renal dysfunction since verotoxin receptors are not expressed in their kidneys. On the other hand, piglets, which have both brain and kidney receptors for verotoxin, develop both neurologic abnormalities (Tzipori, Chow & Powell, 1988) and renal dysfunction (Gyles & Vilcock, 1987) when infected with Shiga-like toxin. If a preliminary finding that human glomerular endothelial cells express high affinity receptors for verotoxin (Boyd & Lingwood, 1989) is confirmed by further studies, this could be relevant to the glomerular localization of lesions in children with classic HUS and diarrhoea prodromes.

In a review Amorosi & Ultmann (1966) reported that a prodromal illness resembling viral infection occurs in about 40% of TTP patients. An association between TTP/HUS and viruses such as Coxsackie A (Glasgow & Balduzzi, 1965), Coxsackie B (Berberich, Cuene & Chard, 1974), other unspecified viruses (Wasserstein *et al.*, 1981) and with influenza vaccination (Brown *et al.*, 1973*b*) has been recognized in a number of patients. Viruses can induce endothelial damage. This has been very well documented in *in vitro* studies showing the cytopathic effect of an avian haemangioma retrovirus and its envelope glycoprotein on cultured human and bovine endothelial cells (Resnick-Roguel *et al.*, 1990). Of interest, endothelial cell perturbation was associated with a reduced release of PGI_2 and an increased expression of tissue factor.

Antibodies and immune complexes can also induce endothelial injury and trigger massive sequestration of platelets and polymorphonuclear leukocytes in the microvasculature, as occurs in acute graft rejection in humans (see Chapter 11). Leung *et al.* (1988) reported the presence of complement-fixing IgG and IgM antibodies cytotoxic to cultured HUVEC in the sera from 13 of 14 children with acute HUS and in sera from three to five adult patients with TTP, suggesting an autoimmune pathogenesis for these disorders. Immune complexes also induce platelet and inflammatory cell activation with fibrin deposits within the glomerular capillaries, promoting extensive endothelial damage. An interesting study by Forsyth *et al.* (1989), in children with the diarrhoea-associated form of HUS which is accompanied by neutrophil leukocytosis, showed increased adherence of the patients' neutrophils to endothelial cells in culture compared to control neutrophils. Patients' neutrophils induced endothelial injury which was abrogated in four of ten subjects when the hyperadhesive neutrophils were incubated with a CD18 antibody directed against the common β-chain of the leukocyte integrin molecules which mediate neutrophil adhesion to endothelium. It was suggested that the HUS neutrophils can release proteases which attack the surface of the endothelium. This has been supported by finding increased concentrations of neutrophil elastase in plasma from children with the diarrhoea-associated form of HUS compared with uninfected children with chronic renal failure.

An association between HUS- and TTP-like lesions and certain drugs including oral contraceptives (Brown *et al.*, 1973*a*; Schoolwerth *et al.*, 1976) and immunosuppressive agents such as cyclosporin (Cy A) (Bonser *et al.*, 1984; Van Buren *et al.*, 1985) and mitomycin (Proia, Harden & Silberman, 1984; Lesesne *et al.*, 1989) has been extensively reported. Some evidence indicates that Cy A and more frequently mitomycin can cause endothelial damage. In cultured bovine aortic endothelial cells Cy A caused cell detachment and lysis (Zoja *et al.*, 1986). Moreover, exposure of cultured rat microvascular endothelial cells to Cy A resulted in inhibition of cell replication (Lau, Wong & Hwang, 1989). It was suggested that, through its direct inhibition of endothelial cell replication, Cy A could potentiate glomerular endothelial injury *in vivo* by impairing the regenerative response of endothelium to injury. *In vivo* studies in rats showed that Cy A induced glomerular endothelial injury with swelling of endothelium, focal loss of fenestrae, doubling of glomerular basement membrane and mononuclear cell infiltration and platelet accumulation (Bertani *et al.*, 1987). Perfusion of the rat renal artery with mitomycin also induced the ultrastructural changes of HUS with an initial lesion to vascular endothelium followed by platelet deposition and obliteration of capillary lumina (Cattell, 1985).

Abnormalities of endothelial cell function associated with TTP and HUS

Defective PGI_2 bio-availability

PGI_2 is the major arachidonic acid metabolite generated by vascular endothelial cells and plays a major role in the regulation of platelet/vessel wall interactions. It possesses potent platelet anti-aggregatory as well as vasodilatory properties (Moncada, 1980). In 1978 it was first reported that vein biopsy specimens from patients with HUS had a reduced ability to produce PGI_2 (Remuzzi *et al.*, 1978). It was also noted that plasma obtained before, but not after plasma exchange, failed to stimulate the *ex vivo* production of PGI_2 by rat aortic rings, as measured by bioassay. Based on these observations, a deficiency of a plasma factor(s) that stimulates vascular PGI_2 synthesis was suggested to play a role in the pathogenetic sequence of thrombotic microangiopathy (Remuzzi *et al.*, 1978). This factor is present in normal plasma and stimulates PGI_2 production by cultured endothelial cells (MacIntyre, Pearson & Gordon, 1978). It has been partially purified and characterized in plasma from healthy humans and is a stable highly polar substance with a molecular weight of 300 to 400 D that protects the vascular PGI_2-forming system from inactivation during persistent endothelial damage, probably by acting as a reducing co-factor for cyclo-oxygenase (Deckmyn *et al.*, 1985). The hypothesis of a defective capacity of plasma to stimulate PGI_2 activity in TTP and HUS gained further support from several studies (Siegler, 1993; Remuzzi, Zoja & Rossi, 1987; Remuzzi *et al.*, 1979; Machin *et al.*, 1980; Wiles *et al.*, 1981; Jorgensen & Pedersen, 1981; Stuart, Spitzer & Coppe, 1983; Levin *et al.*, 1983; Walters *et al.*, 1985; Turi *et al.*, 1986; Siegler *et al.*, 1986; Alam, Abdal & Wahed, 1991; Schlegel, Maclouf & Loirat, 1987).

As shown in Table 10.1, defective PGI_2 activity appears to be a feature of the adult and the atypical childhood forms of the disease. The classic (previously termed typical or epidemic) form occurring mainly in infants under 2 years of age with a prodrome of bloody diarrhoea, is predominantly characterized by glomerular thrombotic microangiopathy, has a good prognosis and is not associated with consistent abnormalities in PGI_2 function. Forms other than the classic disease (previously termed sporadic) occur in older children, have an insidious onset with predominantly arterial renal microangiopathy, severe hypertension and a poor prognosis (Drummond, 1985). Children with the atypical form may lack the plasma factor needed for PGI_2 generation. However, whether this missing factor contributes to the development of the thrombotic microangiopathy or is merely a consequence or a marker of it is not yet firmly established. As outlined by Siegler *et al.*

Table 10.1. *Prostacyclin stimulating activity in TTP and HUS plasma or serum*

Syndrome	Pts Age/Sex	System	Activity	Reference
HUS	54/F 56/F	Rat aorta	Decreased	Remuzzi *et al.*, 1979
TTP	27/F	Rat aorta	Absent	Machin *et al.*, 1980
HUS	19/F	Rat aorta	Decreased	Wiles *et al.*, 1981
TTP	39/M	Rabbit aorta	Decreased	Jorgensen & Pedersen, 1981
HUS	4 mo/M (recurrent)	Human umbilical artery rings	Decreased	Stuart *et al.*, 1983
HUS	13 children with sporadic and epidemic form	Rat aorta	Decreased in sporadic form	Levin *et al.*, 1983
HUS	37 children with typical and atypical form	Rat aorta	Decreased in 100% of atypical and 12% of typical cases	Walters *et al.*, 1985
HUS	10 children	Human umbilical artery rings	Absent in 9 decreased in 1	Turi *et al.*, 1986
HUS	22 children	Cultured human endothelial cells	Decreased	Siegler *et al.*, 1986
HUS	19 children	Rat aorta	Increased	Schlegel *et al.*, 1987
HUS	11 children	Rabbit aorta	Decreased	Alam *et al.*, 1991

(1986) not all the methods used to evaluate PGI_2 stimulating activity of plasma from HUS patients measure the PGI_2 produced by the endothelial cells actually involved in the microangiopathic process. Therefore, although plasma or serum samples from patients with TTP and HUS often have a decreased ability to support or modulate PGI_2 by endothelial cells, the relationship of this finding to the pathogenesis of the disease remains difficult to establish. In this context, the data of some studies that are at variance with the majority and which have shown normal or increased PGI_2 activity in patient serum or plasma, can be reconciled if one recognizes that while PGI_2 stimulating activity diminishes as the thrombotic microangiopathy proceeds and the 'stimulating factor' is used, consumption relative to production is probably quite variable from patient to patient (Siegler, 1993). Moreover, although one might expect increased PGI_2 biosynthesis, at least initially following endothelial injury, the response of the endothelial cells to perturbation in TTP/HUS probably represents the net effect of various factors that either promote or inhibit its biosynthesis. Factors which may be important in promoting PGI_2 biosynthesis in TTP/HUS include direct endothelial cell injury, endotoxins, cytokines and thrombin, while factors inhibiting its biosynthesis may include platelet derived beta-thromboglobulin, lipid peroxidation products and verotoxin or Shiga-like toxin. It has been reported recently that Shiga-like toxin inhibits endothelial cell PGI_2 production by blocking the *de novo* synthesis of cyclo-oxygenase (Huang *et al.*, 1989).

Recently, Noris *et al.* (1992) studied the urinary excretion of PGI_2 metabolites, taken as a marker of the actual biosynthesis, in six children with HUS during the acute phase of the disease and again when remission was achieved. Urinary excretion of the PGI_2 hydrolysis product, 6-keto-PGF1α, was significantly reduced in children with acute HUS as compared with controls indicating a defective renal synthesis of PGI_2. At remission urinary 6-keto-PGF1α level increased to values higher than those of controls. By contrast, the urinary excretion of the major PGI_2 β-oxidation product, 2,3,-dinor-6-keto-PGF1α, was comparable to controls indicating normal systemic PGI_2 biosynthesis. It was concluded that renal, but not systemic, PGI_2 biosynthesis is reduced in the context of systemic platelet activation in the acute phase of HUS. Moreover it was speculated that renal localization of the defect might explain the predominant renal involvement in childhood HUS.

Other mechanisms implicated in the defective PGI_2 bioavailability in TTP and HUS include; a) an inhibition of PGI_2 synthesis at the site of microvascular injury because of an excess of oxygen-free radicals (Deckmyn *et al.*, 1985) or enhanced lipid peroxidation (Ham *et al.*, 1979); b) defective PGI_2 serum binding (Wu *et al.*, 1985); or c) an accelerated PGI_2 degradation (Chen *et al.*, 1981).

vWF abnormalities

Vascular damage is associated with vWF abnormalities (Zucker, Broeckman & Kaplan, 1979; Ruggeri *et al.*, 1982) so that unusually large multimers of vWF (supranormal multimers) with platelet activating properties are released in circulating plasma following endothelial injury. Moake *et al.* (1982) described unusually large vWF multimers in plasma samples from four patients with chronic relapsing forms of TTP, which were detected during clinical remission but not during relapses. They suggested that these patients were unable to process the multimers secreted by endothelial cells and that large multimers could persist in the circulation, predisposing the patients to microvascular thrombosis and relapses. During relapses the multimers would be 'consumed' in the microcirculation because of their interaction with activated platelets and would no longer be detected in circulating blood (Moake *et al.*, 1982). It has been shown that the unusually large vWF multimers produced by human endothelial cells are exceptionally effective in supporting shear-stress induced platelet aggregation (Moake *et al.*, 1986). Shear stress induces alterations in GPIb-IX or GPIIb-IIIa (the platelet vWF receptors) and may potentiate the attachment of unusually large vWF multimers to GPIIb-IIIa (Moake *et al.*, 1986; Peterson *et al.*, 1987). *In vivo* it is likely that unusually large vWF multimers, along with the largest normal plasma vWF forms, may be induced to attach to platelet GPIb-IX and GPIIb-IIIa receptors by the elevated fluid shear stresses in glomerular capillaries and arterioles that are narrowed by swollen endothelial cells, thus contributing to the development of thrombosis.

The multimeric structure of vWF has also been studied in HUS and a variety of abnormalities have been described (Moake *et al.*, 1984; Rose *et al.*, 1984). Moake *et al.* (1984) found a relative decrease in the levels of the largest multimers in acute HUS, which then returned to normal when the platelet count normalized. It was suggested that the largest vWF multimer forms could have been deposited selectively onto the exposed subendothelial surfaces of damaged renal vessels, thereby increasing platelet-subendothelial attachments. Alternatively, selective interactions between the largest plasma vWF forms and platelets could have occurred during the acute HUS episode, so that these largest plasma vWF multimers were then relatively diminished in peripheral venous samples. At variance with patients with chronic relapsing TTP, there was no evidence that HUS patients had a defect in the conversion of unusually large vWF multimers derived from endothelial cells to the vWF forms normally present in the circulation. In order to interpret this heterogeneous pattern of abnormalities in vWF multimeric structure in HUS and TTP it should be taken into account that artifacts due to *in vitro* proteolysis may have influenced the data, since most studies did not use protease inhibitors during sampling.

Mannucci *et al.* (1989) by collecting samples from eight patients with acute HUS and TTP into an anticoagulant cocktail of protease inhibitors, demonstrated plasma-enhanced proteolytic fragmentation of vWF in all. This was expressed by a relative decrease in the intact 225 kD subunit of vWF and a relative increase in the 176 kD fragment. However, instead of the loss of larger forms of normal multimers described by Moake *et al.* (1984), the plasma of all but one of the patients contained a set of larger than normal (supranormal) multimers. Hence, although proteolytic fragmentation of vWF was enhanced during acute HUS/TTP, this was not associated with the loss of larger multimers. It has been suggested (Mannucci *et al.*, 1989) that, during the acute phase of the disease, supranormal multimers leak from endothelial cells perhaps damaged by cytolytic antiendothelial antibodies.

Recently Ruggenenti *et al.* (1993) reported a case of a patient with chronic relapsing TTP who had 21 relapsing episodes over three years, and demonstrated that infusion rather than removal of plasma induced remission of the disease. Unusually large vWF multimers were found during both acute and remission phases. This could be taken as an evidence that the mechanism(s) responsible for the abnormal release of vWF in the circulation still operates between relapses. It is likely that unusually large vWF multimers circulating during remission act as a predisposing factor to microvascular thrombosis. Proteolytic enzymes such as plasmin, calcium-dependent cysteine protease, and elastase may account for the loss of larger multimers in the acute phases of the disease. Moore, Murphy & Kelton (1990) reported that vWF proteolyzed by calpain (calcium-dependent cysteine protease) binds to activated platelets and induces platelet aggregation. A report from Berkowitz *et al.* (1988) also described 170 kD and 150 kD fragments after treating vWF with calpain. Of relevance, normal plasma prevented calpain-induced abnormal fragmentation of vWF. Normal plasma contains potent inhibitors of calpain such as high molecular weight kininogen (Schmaier *et al.*, 1986), an alpha-cysteine proteinase inhibitor (Schmaier *et al.*, 1986) and $\alpha 2$-macroglobulin (Waxman, 1981). This suggests that an abnormal calpain-like protease activity in TTP plasma induces abnormal fragmentation of unusually large vWF (Murphy, Moore & Kelton, 1987). Such fragments differ from the normal circulating ones and because of their high affinity to platelet receptors, may cause platelet adhesion and aggregation in the microcirculation. It is possible that infusion of normal plasma normalizes protease inhibitory activity in the circulation of patients with recurrent TTP.

Fibrinolytic activity abnormalities

In addition to PGI_2 and vWF, other substances of endothelial origin are involved in the antithrombotic properties of normal endothelium and may be produced abnormally in TTP/HUS. Bergstein, Kuederli & Bang (1982) described the presence of a circulating inhibitor of glomerular fibrinolysis in HUS plasma and suggested that the inhibitor may be crucial for the persistence of glomerular fibrin deposition. This inhibitor is now recognized as type 1 plasminogen-activator inhibitor (PAI-1) (Bergstein & Bang, 1989) and is released in its active form chiefly from endothelial cells. More recently a close correlation between the clinical course of HUS and duration of elevated PAI-1 activity has been described (Bergstein, Riley & Bang, 1992). Of interest, when the inhibitor was removed from the circulation by peritoneal dialysis renal function improved. It is likely that increased PAI-1 activity interferes with tissue plasminogen activator and urokinase mediated intraglomerular fibrinolysis, thus favouring microvascular thrombosis.

Nitric oxide and endothelin

Abnormal production of the recently described endothelium-dependent vasoactive mediators, nitric oxide and endothelin (Vane, Anggard & Botting, 1990) may be implicated in the pathogenesis of TTP/HUS. Thus loss of functional and/or morphological integrity of endothelial cells, as occurs in TTP/HUS, could result in a defect in nitric oxide production that would favour vasoconstriction, platelet aggregation and adhesiveness and, ultimately, vaso-occlusion. That this can occur is suggested by data from experimental animals showing that Cy A which, as described above, causes endothelial damage and an acute arteriolopathy resembling HUS, induced a diminished endothelium-dependent relaxation of renal resistance arteries, reflecting impaired generation of nitric oxide (Dieterich *et al.*, 1990). A possible role for the vasoconstrictor peptide endothelin in the pathogenesis of TTP/HUS is suggested by the observation that one of the main aetiological factors for TTP/HUS, bacterial endotoxin, induced an increased production of endothelin by endothelial cells in culture (Sugiura, Inagami & Kon, 1989). Moreover, endotoxin-treated animals had higher plasma endothelin levels than controls (Sugiura, Inagami & Kon, 1989). It is likely that the enhanced endothelin production during endothelial cell damage causes vasoconstriction and a local reduction in blood flow, thereby potentiating thrombus formation in TTP/HUS. Finally, an increased urinary excretion of endothelin has been found in children with HUS (Siegler *et al.*, 1991).

Acknowledgement

We thank Tullio Bertani for his help with the present work and Antoinette Faccio for preparing the manuscript.

References

Alam, A. N., Abdal, N. M. & Wahed, M. A. (1991). Prostacyclin concentrations in haemolytic–uraemic syndrome after acute shigellosis in children. *Archives of Disease in Childhood*, **66**, 1231–5.

Amorosi, E. L. & Ultmann, J. E. (1966). Thrombotic thrombocytopenic purpura: report of 16 cases and review of the literature. *Medicine*, **45**, 139–59.

Baker, N. M., Mills, A. E., Rachman, I. & Thomas, J. E. P. (1974). Haemolytic–uraemic syndrome in typhoid fever. *British Medical Journal*, **2**, 84–7.

Berberich, F. R., Cuene, S. A. & Chard, R. L. (1974). Thrombotic thrombocytopenic purpura. Three cases with platelet and fibrinogen survival studies. *Journal of Pediatrics*, **84**, 503–9.

Bergstein, J. M., Kuederli, Y. & Bang, N. U. (1982). Plasma inhibitor glomerular fibrinolysis in the hemolytic–uremic syndrome. *American Journal of Medicine*, **73**, 322–7.

Bergstein, J. M. & Bang, N. U. (1989). Plasminogen activator inhibitor-1 (PAI-1) is the circulating inhibitor of fibrinolysis (PAI-HUS) in the hemolytic uremic syndrome (HUS). *Kidney International*, **37**, 254.

Bergstein, J. M., Riley, M. & Bang, N. U. (1992). Role of plasminogen-activator inhibitor type 1 in the pathogenesis and outcome of the hemolytic–uremic syndrome. *New England Journal of Medicine*, **327**, 755–9.

Berkowitz, L. R., Dalldorf, F. G. & Blatt, P. M. (1979). Thrombotic thrombocytopenic purpura: a pathology review. *Journal of the American Medical Association*, **241**, 1709–20.

Berkowitz, S. D., Nozaki, H., Titani, K., Murachi, T., Plow, E. F., Zimmerman, T. S. & Scott, D. (1988). Evidence that calpains and elastase do not produce the von Willebrand factor fragments present in normal plasma and IIA von Willebrand disease. *Blood*, **72**, 721–7.

Bertani, T., Perico, N., Abbate, M., Battaglia, C. & Remuzzi, G. (1987). Renal injury induced by long-term administration of cyclosporin A to rats. *American Journal of Pathology*, **127**, 569–79.

Bertani, T., Abbate, M., Zoja, C., Corna, D. & Remuzzi, G. (1989). Sequence of glomerular changes in experimental endotoxemia: a possible model of hemolytic uremic syndrome. *Nephron*, **53**, 330–7.

Bonser, R. S., Adu, D., Franklin, I. & McMaster, P. (1984). Cyclosporin-induced haemolitic–uraemic syndrome in liver allograft recipient. *Lancet*, **ii**, 1337.

Boyd, B. & Lingwood, C. (1989). Verotoxin receptor glycolipid in human renal tissue. *Nephron*, **51**, 207–10.

Brown, C. B., Clarkson, A. R., Robson, J. S., Cameron, J. S., Thomson, P. & Ogg, C. S. (1973*a*). Haemolytic–uraemic syndrome in women taking oral contraceptives. *Lancet*, **i**, 1479–1481.

Brown, R. C., Blecher, T. E., French, E. A. & Toghill, P. J. (1973*b*). Thrombotic thrombocytopenic purpura after influenza vaccination. *British Medical Journal*, **2**, 303.

Bukowski, R. M. (1982). Thrombotic thrombocytopenic purpura: a review. In T. H. Spaet, ed. *Progress in Hemostasis and Thrombosis*, pp. 287. New York: Grune & Stratton.

Cattell, V. (1985). Mitomycin-induced hemolytic uremic kidney. An experimental model in the rat. *American Journal of Pathology*, **121**, 88–95.

Chen, Y. C., McLeod, B., Hall, E. R. & Wu, K. K. (1981). Accelerated prostacyclin degradation in thrombotic thrombocytopenic purpura. *Lancet*, **ii**, 267–9.

Deckmyn, H., Zoja, C., Arnout, J., Todisco, A., Bulcke, F. V., D'Hond, T. L., Henrickx, N., Gresele, P. & Vermylen, J. (1985). Partial isolation and function of the prostacyclin regulating plasma factor. *Clinical Science*, **69**, 383–93.

Dieterich, D., Jameson, M., Dai Fu-Xiang, A., Skopek, J. & Dieterich, A. (1990). Cyclosporine treatment impairs endothelial function in resistance arteries in rats. *Journal of the American Society of Nephrology*, **1**, 609. (Abstract).

Drummond, K. N. (1985). Hemolytic–uremic syndrome then and now. *New England Journal of Medicine*, **312**, 116–18.

Dunea, G., Muerke, R. C., Nakamoto, S. & Schwartz, F. D. (1966). Thrombotic thrombocytopenic purpura with acute anuric renal failure. *American Journal of Medicine*, **41**, 1000–6.

Eknoyan, G. & Riggs, S. A. (1986). Renal involvement in patients with thrombotic thrombocytopenic purpura. *American Journal of Nephrology*, **6**, 117–31.

Forsyth, K. D., Simpson, A. C., Fitzpatrick, M. M., Barratt, T. M. & Levinsky, R. J. (1989). Neutrophil-mediated endothelial injury in haemolytic–uraemic syndrome. *Lancet*, **ii**, 411–14.

Gianantonio, C. A. (1964). The hemolytic–uremic syndrome. *Journal of Pediatrics*, **64**, 478–91.

Gianantonio, C. A. (1984). Extrarenal manifestations of the hemolytic–uremic syndrome. In *Acute Renal Disorders and Renal Emergencies*, Strauss, J. ed. pp. 43. Boston: Martinus Nijhoff.

Glasgow, L. A. & Balduzzi, P. (1965). Isolation of coxsackie virus group A, type 4 from a patient with hemolytic–uremic syndrome. *New England Journal of Medicine*, **273**, 754–6.

Goodman, A., Ramos, R., Petrelli, M., Hirsch, S. A., Bukowski, R. & Harris, J. W. (1978). Gingival biopsy in thrombotic thrombocytopenic purpura. *Annals of Internal Medicine*, **89**, 501–4.

Gyles, C. L. & Vilcock, B. (1987). Response of conventional pigs to infection with verotoxigenic *E. coli* 0157:H7. *International Symposium on Verocytotoxin-Producing* E. coli, Toronto, AMV-17. (Abstract).

Habib, R., Cortecuisse, V., Leclerc, F., Mathieu, H. & Royer, P. (1969). Etude anatomopathologique de 35 observations de syndrome hemolytique et uremique de l'enfant. *Archives Françaises de Pediatrie*, **26**, 391–416.

Ham, E. A., Egan, R. W., Soderman, D. D., Gale, P. H. & Kuehl, F. A. (1979). Peroxidase-dependent deactivation of prostacyclin synthetase. *Journal of Biological Chemistry*, **254**, 2191–4.

Harlan, J. M., Harker, L. A., Reidy, M. A., Gajdusek, C. M., Schwartz, S. M. & Striker, G. E. (1983). Lipopolysaccharide-mediated bovine endothelial cell injury *in vitro*. *Laboratory Investigation*, **48**, 269–74.

Huang, P. S., Sanduja, R., Cleary, T. & Wu, K. K. (1989). Influence of Shiga-like toxins on endothelial cell arachidonate metabolism. *Blood*, **74**, 39a.

Jorgensen, K. A. & Pedersen, R. S. (1981). Familial deficiency of prostacyclin production stimulating factor in the hemolytic–uremic syndrome of childhood. *Thrombosis Research*, **21**, 311–15.

Kanfer, A., Morel-Maroger, L., Solez, K. *et al.* (1980). The value of renal biopsy in hemolytic–uremic syndrome in adults. In Remuzzi, G., Mecca, G. & De Gaetano, G. eds. *Hemostasis, Prostaglandins and Renal Disease*, pp. 399. New York: Raven Press.

Kaplan, B. S. & Remuzzi, G. (1991). The haemolytic uraemic syndrome. In Remuzzi, G. & Rossi, E. C. eds. *Haemostasis and the Kidney*, pp. 201. London: Butterworths.

Karch, H., Bitzan, M., Pietsch, R. *et al.* (1988). Purified verotoxins of *Escherichia coli* 0157:H7 decrease prostacyclin synthesis by endothelial cells. *Microbial Pathogenesis*, **5**, 215–21.

Karmali, M. A., Steele, B. T., Petric, M. & Lim, C. (1983). Sporadic cases of hemolytic–uraemic syndrome associated with faecal verotoxin and cytotoxin producing *Escherichia coli* in stools. *Lancet*, **i**, 619–20.

Karmali, M. A., Petric, M., Lim, C., Fleming, P. C., Arbus, G. S. & Lior, H. (1985). The association between idiopathic hemolytic–uremic syndrome and infection by verotoxin-producing *Escherichia coli*. *Journal of Infectious Diseases*, **151**, 775–82.

Kavi, J., Chant, I., Maris, M. & Rose, P. E. (1987). Cytopathic effect of verotoxin on endothelial cells. *Lancet*, **ii**, 1035.

Kavi, J. & Wise, R. (1989). Causes of the haemolytic–uraemic syndrome. It might be verocytotoxin produced by *Escherichia coli*. *British Medical Journal*, **298**, 65–6.

Koster, F., Levin, J., Walker, L., Tung, K. S. K., Gilman, R. M., Rahaman, M. M., Najid, M. A., Islam, S. & Williams, R. C. Jr. (1978). Hemolytic–uremic syndrome after shigellosis: relation to endotoxemia and circulating immune complexes. *New England Journal of Medicine*, **298**, 927–33.

Lau, D. C. W., Wong, K. L. & Hwang, W. S. (1989). Cyclosporine toxicity on cultured rat microvascular endothelial cells. *Kidney International*, **35**, 604–13.

Lesesne, J. B., Rothschild, N., Erickson, B., Korec, S., Sisk, R., Keller, J., Arbus, M., Woolley, P. V., Chiazze, L., Schein, P. S. & Neefe, J. R. (1989). Cancer-associated hemolytic–uremic syndrome: analysis of 85 cases from a national registry. *Journal of Clinical Oncology*, **7**, 781–9.

Leung, Y. D., Moake, J. L., Havens, P. L., Kim, M. L. & Pober, J. (1988). Lytic anti-endothelial cell antibodies in haemolytic–uraemic syndrome. *Lancet*, **ii**, 183–6.

Levin, M., Elkon, K. B., Nokes, T. J. C., Buckle, A. M., Dillon, M. J., Hardisty, R. M. & Barratt, T. M. (1983). Inhibitor of prostacyclin production in sporadic haemolytic–uraemic syndrome. *Archives of Disease in Childhood*, **58**, 703–8.

Levy, M., Gagnadoux, M. F. & Habib, R. (1980). Pathology of hemolitic–uremic syndrome in children. In Remuzzi, G., Mecca, G. & de Gaetano, G. eds. *Hemostasis, Prostaglandins and Renal Disease*, pp. 383–397. New York: Raven Press.

Lindberg, A. A., Brown, J. E., Stronberg, N., Westling-Ryd, M., Schultz, J. E. & Karlsson, K.-A. (1987). Identification of the carbohydrate receptor for Shiga toxin produced by *Shigella dysenteriae* type 1. *Journal of Biological Chemistry*, **262**, 1779–85.

Lingwood, C. A., Law, H., Richardson, S. *et al.* (1987). Glycolipid binding of purified and recombinant *Escherichia coli* produced verotoxin *in vitro*. *Journal of Biological Chemistry*, **262**, 8834–9.

Louise, C. B. & Obrig, T. G. (1991). Shiga toxin associated hemolytic uremic syndrome: combined cytotoxic effects of Shiga toxin, interleukin-1β, and tumor necrosis factor alpha on human vascular endothelial cells *in vitro*. *Infection and Immunity*, **59**, 4173–9.

Machin, S. J., Defreyn, G., Chamone, D. A. F. *et al.* (1980). Plasma 6-keto-PGF1α levels after plasma exchange in thrombotic thrombocytopenic purpura. *Lancet*, **i**, 661.

MacIntyre, D. E., Pearson, J. D. & Gordon, J. L. (1978). Localisation and stimulation of prostacyclin production in vascular cells. *Nature*, **271**, 549–51.

Mannucci, P. M., Lombardi, R., Lattuada, A., Ruggenenti, P., Viganò, G. L., Barbui, T. & Remuzzi, G. (1989). Enhanced proteolysis of plasma von Willebrand factor in thrombotic thrombocytopenic purpura and the hemolytic–uremic syndrome. *Blood*, **74**, 978–83.

Moake, J. L., Rudy, C. K., Troll, I. H., Weinstein, M. J., Colannino, N. M., Azocar, J., Seder, R. H., Hong, S. L. & Deykin, D. (1982). Unusually large plasma factor VIII: von Willebrand factor multimers in chronic relapsing thrombotic thrombocytopenic purpura. *New England Journal of Medicine*, **307**, 1432–5.

Moake, J. L., Byrnes, J. J., Troll, J. H., Rudy, C. K., Weinstein, M. J., Colannino, N. M. & Hong, S. L. (1984). Abnormal VIII: von Willebrand factor patterns in the plasma of patients with the hemolytic–uremic syndrome. *Blood*, **64**, 592–8.

Moake, J. L., Turner, N. A., Stathopoulos, N. A., Nolasco, L. H. & Hellums, J. D. (1986). Involvement of large plasma von Willebrand factor (vWF) multimers and unusually large vWF forms derived from endothelial cells in shear stress-induced platelet aggregation. *Journal of Clinical Investigation*, **78**, 1456–61.

Moncada, S. (1980). Prostacyclin and thromboxane A2 in the regulation of platelet–vascular interactions. In Remuzzi, G., Mecca, G. & De Gaetano, G. eds. *Hemostasis, Prostaglandins and Renal Disease*, pp. 175. New York: Raven Press.

Moore, J. C., Murphy, W. G. & Kelton, J. G. (1990). Calpain proteolysis of von Willebrand factor enhances its binding to platelet membrane glycoprotein IIb/IIIa: an explanation for platelet aggregation in thrombotic thrombocytopenic purpura. *British Journal of Haematology*, **74**, 457–64.

Morrison, D. M., Tyrrel, D. L. & Jewell, L. D. (1986). Colonic biopsy in verotoxin-induced hemorrhagic colitis. *American Journal of Clinical Pathology*, **86**, 108–12.

Murphy, W. G., Moore, J. C. & Kelton, J. C. (1987). Calcium-dependent cysteine protease activity in the sera of patients with thrombotic thrombocytopenic purpura. *Blood*, **70**, 1683–7.

Nalbandian, R. M., Henry, R. L. & Bick, R. L. (1979). Thrombotic thrombocytopenic purpura an extended editorial. *Seminars in Thrombosis and Hemostasis*, **5**, 216–40.

Noris, M., Benigni, A., Siegler, R., Gaspari, F., Casiraghi, F., Mancini, M. & Remuzzi, G. (1992). Renal prostacyclin biosynthesis is reduced in children with hemolytic–uremic syndrome in the context of systemic platelet activation. *American Journal of Kidney Disease*, **20**, 144–9.

O'Brien, A. D. & Holmes, R. K. (1987). Shiga and Shiga-like toxins. *Microbiological Review*, **51**, 206–20.

Obrig, T. G., Del Vecchio, P. J., Karmali, M. A., Petric, M., Moran, T. P. & Judge, T. K. (1987). Pathogenesis of haemolytic–uraemic syndrome. *Lancet*, **ii**, 687.

Peterson, D. M., Stathopoulos, N. A., Giorgio, T. D., Hellums, J. D. & Moake, J. L. (1987). Shear-induced platelet aggregation requires von Willebrand factor and platelet membrane glycoproteins Ib and IIb/IIIa. *Blood*, **69**, 625–8.

Pirani, C. L. (1983). Coagulation and renal disease. In Bertani, T. & Remuzzi, G. eds. *Glomerular Injury 300 Years After Morgagni*, pp. 119. Milano: Wichtig.

Proia, A. D., Harden, E. A. & Silberman, H. R. (1984). Mitomycin-induced hemolytic–uremic syndrome. *Archives of Pathology and Laboratory Medicine*, **108**, 959.

Remuzzi, G., Misiani, R., Marchesi, D., Livio, M., Mecca, G., de Gaetano, G. & Donati, M. B. (1978). Haemolytic–uraemic syndrome: deficiency of plasma factor(s) regulating prostacyclin activity? *Lancet*, **ii**, 871–2.

Remuzzi, G., Misiani, R., Marchesi, D., Livio, M., Mecca, G., de Gaetano, G. & Donati, M. B. (1979). Treatment of the haemolytic–uraemic syndrome with plasma. *Clinical Nephrology*, **12**, 279–84.

Remuzzi, G. (1987*a*). HUS and TTP: variable expression of a single entity. *Kidney International*, **32**, 292–308.

Remuzzi, G. (1987*b*). Thrombotic thrombocytopenic purpura and allied disorders. In Verstraete, M., Vermylen, J., Lijnen, H. R., & Arnout, J. eds. *Thrombosis and Haemostasis*, pp. 673. Leuven: Leuven University Press.

Remuzzi, G., Zoja, C. & Rossi, E. C. (1987). Prostacyclin in thrombotic microangiopathy. *Seminars in Hematology*, **2**, 110–18.

Remuzzi, G., Ruggenenti, P. & Bertani, T. (1994). Thrombotic microangiopathies. In Tischer, T. T. & Brenner, B. M. eds. *Renal Pathology*, pp. 1154. Philadelphia: J. B. Lippincott Co.

Resnick-Roguel, N., Eldor, A., Burstein, H., Hy-Am, E., Vlodavsky, I., Panet, A., Blajchman, M. A. & Kotler, M. (1990). Envelope glycoprotein of avian hemangioma retrovirus induces a thrombogenic surface on human and bovine endothelial cells. *Journal of Virology*, **64**(8), 4029–32.

Richardson, S. E., Jagadha, V., Smith, C. R., Becker, L. E., Petric, M. & Karmali, M. A. (1987). Pathological effects of injected H.30 verotoxin (VT) in rabbits (abstract). *Annual Meeting of the American Society for Microbiology, Atlanta, 1-6 March*, 42. (Abstract).

Rose, P. E., Enayat, S. M., Sunderland, R., Short, P. E., Williams, C. E. & Hill, F. G. H. (1984). Abnormalities of factor VIII related protein multimers in the haemolytic–uraemic syndrome. *Archives of Disease in Childhood*, **59**, 1135–40.

Ruggenenti, P., Galbusera, M., Plata Cornejo, R., Bellavita, P. & Remuzzi, G. (1993). Thrombotic thrombocytopenic purpura: evidence that infusion rather than removal of plasma induces remission of the disease. *American Journal of Kidney Disease*, **21**, 3,314–18.

Ruggeri, Z. M., Mannucci, P. M., Lombardi, R., Federici, A. M. & Zimmerman, T. S. (1982). Multimeric composition of factor VIII/von Willebrand factor following administration of DDAVP: implications for pathophysiology and therapy of von Willebrand's disease subtypes. *Blood*, **59**, 1272–8.

Schlegel, N., Maclouf, J. & Loirat, C. (1987). Absence of plasma prostacyclin stimulating activity deficiency in hemolytic–uremic syndrome. *Journal of Pediatrics*, **111**, 71–8.

Schmaier, A. H., Bradford, H., Silver, L. D., Farber, A., Scott, C. F., Schutsky, D. & Colman, R. W. (1986). High molecular weight kininogen is an inhibitor of platelet calpain. *Journal of Clinical Investigation*, **77**, 1565–73.

Schoolwerth, A. C., Sandler, R. S., Klahr, S. & Kissane, J. M. (1976). Nephrosclerosis postpartum and in women taking oral contraceptives. *Archives of Internal Medicine*, **136**, 178–85.

Sheth, K. J., Swick, H. M. & Haworth, N. (1986). Neurological involvement in hemolytic–uremic syndrome. *Annals of Neurology*, **19**, 90–3.

Siegler, R. L., Smith, J. B., Lynch, M. B. & Mohammad, S. F. (1986). *In vitro* prostacyclin production in the hemolytic–uremic syndrome. *Western Journal of Medicine*, **144**, 165–8.

Siegler, R. L., Edwin, S. S., Christofferson, R. D. & Mitchell, M. D. (1991). Endothelin in the urine of children with the hemolytic–uremic syndrome. *Pediatrics*, **88**, 1063–9.

Siegler, R. L. (1993). Prostacyclin in the hemolytic–uremic syndrome. *Journal of Nephrology*, **6**, 64–71.

Stuart, M. J., Spitzer, R. E. & Coppe, D. (1983). Abnormal platelet and vascular prostaglandin synthesis in an infant with hemolytic–uremic syndrome. *Pediatrics*, **71**, 120–4.

Sugiura, M., Inagami, T. & Kon, V. (1989). Endotoxin stimulates endothelin-release *in vivo* and *in vitro* as determined by radioimmunoassay. *Biochemical and Biophysical Research Communications*, **161**, 1220–7.

Tesh, V. L., Samuel, J. E., Perera, L. P., Sharefkin, J. B. & O'Brien, A. D. (1991). Evaluation of the role of Shiga and Shiga-like toxins in mediating direct damage to human vascular endothelial cells. *Journal of Infectious Diseases*, **164**, 344–52.

Thomas, L. & Good, R. A. (1952). Studies on the generalized Swartzman reaction. I. General observations concerning the phenomenon. *Journal of Experimental Medicine*, **96**, 605.

Turi, S., Beattie, T. J., Belch, J. J. & Murphy, A. V. (1986). Disturbances of prostacyclin metabolism in children with hemolytic–uremic syndrome in first degree relatives. *Clinical Nephrology*, **25**, 193–8.

Tzipori, S., Chow, C. W. & Powell, H. R. (1988). Cerebral infection with *Escherichia coli* 0157:H7 in humans and gnotobiotic piglets. *Journal of Clinical Pathology*, **41**, 1099–103.

Umlas, J. & Kaiser, J. (1970). Thrombohemolytic thrombocytopenic purpura (TTP): a disease or a syndrome? *American Journal of Medicine*, **49**, 723–8.

Van Buren, D., Van Buren, C. T., Flechner, S. M., Maddox, A. M., Verani, R. & Kahan, B. D. (1985). *De novo* hemolytic–uremic syndrome in renal transplant recipients immunosuppressed with cyclosporin. *Surgery*, **98**, 54–62.

Van de Kar, N. C. A. J., Van Hinsberg, V. W. M., Karmali, M. A. & Monnens, L. A. H. (1991). Endothelial damage by verocytotoxin depends on the additional exposure to inflammatory mediators. *Thrombosis and Haemostasis*, **65**, 1123.

Van de Kar, N. C. A. J., Monnens, L. A. H., Karmali, M. A. & Van Hinsbergh, V. W. M.

(1992). Tumor necrosis factor and interleukin-1 induce expression of the verocytotoxin receptor globotriaosylceramide on human endothelial cells: implications for the pathogenesis of the hemolytic–uremic syndrome. *Blood*, **80**, 2755–64.

Vane, J. R., Anggard, E. E. & Botting, R. M. (1990). Regulatory functions of the vascular endothelium. *New England Journal of Medicine*, **325**, 27–36.

Walters, S., Smith C., Levin, M. *et al.* (1985). Platelet activation in the haemolytic–uraemic syndrome (HUS). In *57th Annual Meeting of the British Pediatric Association*, York: April 16–20.

Wasserstein, A., Hill, G., Goldfarb, S. & Goldberg, M. (1981). Recurrent thrombotic thrombocytopenic purpura after viral infection. Clinical and histologic simulation of chronic glomerulonephritis. *Archives of Internal Medicine*, **141**, 685–7.

Waxman, L. (1981). Calcium-activated proteases in mammalian tissues. *Methods in Enzymology*, **80**, 664–80.

Wiles, P. G., Solomon, L. R., Lawler, W., Mallick, N. P. & Johnson, M. (1981). Inherited plasma factor deficiency in haemolytic–uraemic syndrome. *Lancet*, **i**, 1105–6.

Windler, F., Weh, H. J., Hossfeld, D. K., Franz, H. R., Karch, H., Heesemann, J. & Laufs, R. (1989). Verotoxin in thrombotic thrombocytopenic purpura (letter). *European Journal of Haematology*, **42**, 103.

Wu, K. K., Hall, E. R., Rossi, E. C. & Papp, A. C. (1985). Serum prostacyclin binding defects in thrombotic thrombocytopenic purpura. *Journal of Clinical Investigation*, **75**, 168–74.

Zoja, C., Furci, L., Ghilardi, F., Zilio, P., Benigni, A. & Remuzzi, G. (1986). Cyclosporin-induced endothelial cell injury. *Laboratory Investigation*, **55**, 455–62.

Zoja, C., Corna, D., Farina, C., Sacchi, G., Lingwood, C., Doyle, M. P., Padhye, V. V., Abbate, M. & Remuzzi, G. (1992). Verotoxin glycolipid receptors determine the localization of microangiopathic process in rabbits given Verotoxin-1. *Journal of Laboratory and Clinical Medicine*, **120**, 229–38.

Zucker, M. B., Broeckman, M. J. & Kaplan, K. L. (1979). Factor VIII-related antigen in human blood platelets: localization and release by thrombin and collagen. *Journal of Laboratory and Clinical Medicine*, **94**, 675–82.

–11–
The immunological role of the endothelium in organ transplantation

JOHN R. BRADLEY

Vascular endothelial cells form the interface between the tissues and the circulation and are therefore uniquely positioned to participate in inflammatory reactions at sites of antigenic stimulation. In the setting of transplantation the first foreign surface to be encountered by circulating host leukocytes is the endothelial lining of the donor organ. Donor endothelial cells have the capacity to both express antigens which may be recognized as foreign, including major histocompatibility complex molecules, and to present such antigens to host lymphocytes. In addition, endothelial cells are capable of undergoing a number of functional changes, collectively termed 'activation' (Pober, 1988; see Chapter 2), which enable them to promote inflammatory reactions. These include the modulation of vascular tone and permeability, the synthesis and expression of surface glycoproteins and soluble factors which promote the local accumulation, activation and subsequent extravasation into the tissues of leukocytes, and alterations in surface molecules which promote intravascular coagulation. Endothelial cells may thus both initiate allogenic immune responses and become active participants in the development of immune inflammatory reactions.

Endothelial cells as initiators of immune inflammation

The initiation of an immune response to foreign antigen generally requires activation of CD4 helper T cells. Activated helper T cells are necessary for the growth and differentiation of B cells into antibody producing plasma cells in the case of humoral immunity, or activation of macrophages and cytolytic T lymphocytes in the effector phase of cell-mediated immune responses. CD4 lymphocytes recognize antigen in association with a polymorphic determinant of a class II MHC molecule on the surface of a specific antigen-presenting cell, whereas CD8 lymphocytes recognize peptides bound to class I MHC molecules. The quantitative surface expression of class I and II MHC molecules are thus important determinants of the capacity of a cell to interact with CD8 and CD4 lymphocytes, respectively. Whereas most cells express class I MHC molecules and are able to present antigen to cytolytic CD8 cells, constitutive expression of class II MHC molecules is limited principally to bone marrow derived cells such as B lymphocytes and dendritic cells. Therefore it was initially felt that the ability to present foreign antigen to CD4 helper T lymphocytes, and thus initiate an immune response, was restricted to these bone marrow derived class II bearing cells which were regarded as 'professional antigen presenting cells'.

Endothelial cell MHC molecule expression

Cultured human endothelial cells constitutively express class I but not class II MHC molecules. However, although unstimulated endothelial cells do not express class II MHC molecules they are able to participate in the development of an immune response by causing proliferation of allogenic peripheral blood lymphocytes (Hirschberg *et al.*, 1975). This apparent dilemma was resolved by demonstrating that cultured endothelial cells could be induced to express class II MHC molecules by allogenic peripheral blood lymphocytes, and that the induction could be attributed to the production of interferon-γ (Pober *et al.*, 1983*a*,*b*). Interferon-γ induces new transcription of mRNA for class II MHC molecules in cultured endothelial cells. Maximal steady-state mRNA levels are achieved after about two days of exposure to interferon-γ and surface expression of class II MHC molecules becomes maximal after four to six days. The α and β chains of all three Class II loci (HLA-DR, DP and DQ) and the associated invariant chain are coordinately regulated (Collins *et al.*, 1984). Interferon-γ also increases expression of class I MHC molecules by increasing transcription, although this action is shared by interferon-α and β, tumour necrosis factor and lymphotoxin.

Induction of class II molecules by interferon-γ is not unique to endothelial cells. Many cell types including epithelial cells, smooth muscle cells and fibroblasts can be induced to express class II MHC molecules by interferon-γ. However, induction of class II MHC molecules on the cell surface does not necessarily equate with the ability to present antigen. The functional activation of T cells requires additional signals, or costimulator activities, which may be provided as surface membrane bound or secreted products of accessory cells.

Costimulator activities of endothelial cells

Several studies have shown that endothelial cells are able to act as antigen presenting cells *in vitro* (a proposition which is supported by *in vivo* studies of the distribution of class II MHC molecule expression during immune inflammatory reactions), and that this capacity may not be shared by other cell types which can be induced to express class II MHC molecules (Hirschberg, Bergh & Thorsby, 1980; Wagner, Vetto & Burger, 1984; Savage *et al.*, 1993).

Although the majority of CD4 cells are helper cells, a population of CD4 cytolytic cells which recognize class II MHC antigens has been defined. Cloned cytolytic CD4 T cell lines specific for an HLA-DR can recognize and kill endothelial cells (and fibroblasts) which have been induced to express class II MHC molecules by interferon-γ (Pober *et al.*, 1983*c*). Such killing is restricted to interferon-γ treated cells and can be blocked by monoclonal antibodies against HLA-DR, suggesting that it is a function of the class II MHC molecule expression. However, although T cells can recognize class II MHC molecules on both endothelial cells and fibroblasts, endothelial cells are distinguished by their ability to activate and stimulate proliferation of resting T cells. These results suggest that endothelial cells are able to provide additional signals which enable them to present foreign antigen to and activate helper T lymphocytes. Although these additional signals are as yet incompletely defined, several costimulatory activities which may be provided by endothelial cells have been characterized.

The first cytokine that was shown to have costimulator activity was IL-1. IL-1 is produced as two distinct gene products, IL-1α and IL-1β, both of which have the capacity to act as costimulators for T cell activation *in vitro* (March *et al.*, 1985). Endothelial cells can be induced to produce IL-1 by endotoxin, tumour necrosis factor, lymphotoxin or IL-1 itself (Kurt-Jones, Fiers & Pober, 1987). The predominant gene product synthesized by endothelium is IL-1α, which is expressed on the endothelial cell surface in a membrane associated form. As such, it may be optimally positioned to act as a costimulator for T cells bound to MHC molecules on the endothelial cell surface. However, IL-1 synthesis alone cannot account for all of the costimulatory activity provided by endothelial cells. Other cytokines with known costimulator activities include IL-6 and 7 and tumour necrosis factor. Endothelial cells are known to synthesize IL-6 (Jirik *et al.*, 1989), but the majority of costimulatory activity is probably provided by contact-dependent signalling via surface receptors.

CD4 T lymphocytes that are activated by MHC associated antigen and receive adequate costimulation synthesize interleukin 2. IL-2 is the principal autocrine and paracrine growth progression factor for T cells, serving to move T cells from G_1 to S phase of the cell cycle. The quantity of IL-2 produced by antigen activated T cells may thus provide a measure of the level of costimulatory activity, and is in turn an important determinant of the magnitude of an immune response.

T cells can be activated by lectins such as phytohaemagglutinin (PHA) which bind to surface glycoproteins including the T cell receptor, stimulating T cell IL-2 secretion and proliferation. IL-2 production by PHA activated CD4 T cells can be markedly increased by the presence of cultured endothelial cells (Guinan *et al.*, 1989; Hughes, Savage & Pober, 1990). This capacity to augment IL-2 synthesis is not shared by fibroblasts or smooth muscle cells, suggesting that endothelial cells have unique costimulator functions which endow them with specialized antigen presenting capacity (Hughes *et al.*, 1990). The signal leading to increased T cell IL-2 production is unlikely to be provided by endothelial cell secretion of cytokines. Neither IL-1, IL-6 nor media conditioned by endothelial cells under various conditions can replace endothelial cells in the augmentation of IL-2 synthesis by PHA activated CD4 cells. Furthermore, costimulation can be provided by paraformaldehyde-fixed endothelial cells, and the use of culture systems in which cells can be separated by porous membranes has shown that such augmentation of IL-2 synthesis is dependent upon contact between endothelial cells and T cells.

Antibody blocking studies have shown that costimulation is, at least in part, mediated by interaction between CD2, a glycoprotein expressed on the surface of over 90% of mature T cells, and endothelial cell leukocyte function associated antigen-3 (LFA-3) (Savage *et al*, 1991). Other ligands which have been implicated in endothelial cell costimulator activity include the adhesion molecules ICAM-1 or VCAM-1 (the ligands for T cell LFA-1 and VLA-4, respectively) (Damle & Aruffo, 1991). Thus endothelial cells may both act as antigen presenting cells, and play an important role in the activation of T cells as they migrate through the vessel wall.

Endothelial cell MHC molecule expression *in vivo*

Further evidence that endothelial cells may have a specialized role as antigen presenting cells comes from *in vivo* studies. Human venular endothelial cells basally express low levels of class II MHC molecules *in situ*. The significance of this is, however, uncertain as basal expression of class II MHC molecules in the dog is reduced by cyclosporin suggesting that it may not be constitutive but may depend on circulating cytokines (Groenewegen, Buurman & Van der Linden, 1985). In human skin organ culture, endothelial cells respond to interferon-γ by increasing class II MHC molecule expression, whereas other cell types such as keratinocytes, fibroblasts and smooth muscle cells do not (Messadi, Pober & Murphy, 1988). Furthermore interferon-γ readily increases endothelial cell class II MHC molecule expression in baboon skin (Munro, Pober & Cotran, 1989).

Increased endothelial cell class II MHC molecule expression can also be observed *in vivo* in experimental immune inflammatory reactions (Sobel *et al.*, 1984; Pober, 1988), but perhaps most notably during allograft rejection. It is not limited to venular endothelial cells, but has been observed in allograft coronary arteries following heart transplantation (Salomon *et al.*, 1991) and also in the arteritic lesions of immune mediated vasculitides such as Kawasaki disease (Terai *et al.*, 1990).

Thus the ability of endothelial cells to transcribe and express class II MHC molecules which can be functionally recognized by T cells, and the finding of increased vascular class II MHC molecule expression in the setting of immune mediated inflammation provide support for the role of endothelial cells in the development of immune responses. In this respect, endothelial cells differ from other cells such as fibroblasts which can express class II MHC molecules but cannot present antigen in a way that can activate resting T cells.

Endothelial cells as participants in the allograft immune response

Vascular endothelial cells in organ transplants may present foreign antigens, together with the necessary costimulator activities, to host lymphocytes, thereby initiating an immune response against the graft. In turn foreign endothelial cells may become a target for either cellular or antibody mediated immune reactions, in addition to contributing to allograft destruction by participating in the development of an inflammatory response. Thus endothelial cells may take part in all aspects of allograft rejection. It should be emphasized, however, that the evidence that endothelial cells are participants in immune inflammation is based largely on *in vitro* studies. Evidence that endothelial cells participate in immune responses *in vivo* is, however, accumulating in various clinical settings, particularly in the field of transplantation.

Endothelial cells as targets for injury

As kidneys were the first organ to be commonly transplanted much of the evidence that vascular endothelium is an active participant in rejection comes from histological studies of renal tissue. Early studies of renal transplantation emphasized the importance of vascular endothelium as a target for immune mediated injury (Busch *et al.*, 1971; Williams *et al.*, 1967, 1973). In hyperacute rejection, which is mediated by pre-existing antibodies to donor antigens, endothelial immunoglobulin and complement deposition in association with severe microvascular destruction can be demonstrated within minutes of transplantation (Rowlands, Hill & Zmijewski, 1976;

Forbes & Guttman, 1982). Perhaps the clearest role for antibodies in the development of endothelial cell injury during graft rejection is in xenotransplantation. In this setting it is generally accepted that rejection is initiated by complement activation mediated by pre-existing antibodies against the donor endothelium. This in turn sets in motion a series of events resulting in loss of endothelial cell functional integrity (Dalmasso, 1992).

The pathogenesis of acute rejection, in which both humoral and cell mediated immunity may play a role, is more complex. As in hyperacute rejection, endothelial cell antibody and complement deposition with loss of structural and functional vascular integrity occurs in humoral rejection, whereas mononuclear cell margination and migration into the tissues accompanied by variable combinations of endothelial cell hyperplasia, lysis and necrosis are the predominant features of cellular rejection.

Prevention of hyperacute rejection and the successful treatment of acute rejection episodes has led to the recognition of a different pattern of vascular pathology in chronic rejection. Arterial and arteriolar narrowing as a result of intimal hyperplasia progressing to frank proliferation and thickening are the most significant lesions both histologically and functionally. With time, glomerular and interstitial fibrosis, presumably as a consequence of chronic ischaemia, result in a gradual deterioration in renal function.

Similar patterns of rejection are recognized in cardiac transplantation (Bieber *et al.*, 1970), although with improved immunosuppressive regimes for acute rejection, obliteration of coronary arteries and arterioles, comparable to that seen in chronic rejecting kidney grafts, has emerged as the major cause of graft failure (Billingham, 1987). The term transplant-associated arteriosclerosis has been used to describe these changes, which generally differ from those of atherosclerosis in several respects (Salomon *et al.*, 1991). The lesions tend to be concentric rather than focal, often affecting the entire vessel, and neither necrosis nor lipid deposition are prominent features. Cellularity is increased due to a combination of smooth muscle proliferation in the arterial intima and variable numbers of inflammatory cells. The inflammatory cell infiltrate, which is composed predominantly of macrophages and lymphocytes, tends to be localized below the endothelium which itself is usually intact, suggesting that, whilst endothelial cells may be involved in the development of the lesions, they are not the principal target of injury. Similar arteriosclerotic lesions have been observed in the pulmonary vasculature of long-term heart–lung transplants (Yousem, Burke & Billingham, 1985).

Endothelial cells in cell-mediated rejection

The immune response in allograft rejection is directed against foreign antigens within the graft. The most important (although by no means the only) antigens are foreign MHC molecules. In this respect, the participation of MHC molecules in the generation of an immune response differs from their usual physiological function of presenting foreign antigens to autologous T cells. Indeed, it is unclear how T cells, which are usually restricted to the recognition of foreign peptides presented by self MHC molecules, recognize foreign MHC molecules (Lechler *et al.*, 1990). It is possible that alloreactive T cells recognize endogenous peptides presented by foreign MHC molecules or that the alloresponse is directed against the MHC molecules themselves, which are perceived as self MHC molecules associated with foreign peptides. Whatever mechanism is involved the frequency of alloreactive T cells that recognize foreign MHC molecules is remarkably high in all individuals, and the ability of MHC incompatible tissues to invoke strong primary immune responses is readily demonstrated by the mixed leukocyte reaction (Bach, Bach & Sondel, 1976).

When lymphocytes from one individual (the responder) are cultured with stimulating mononuclear leukocytes from a second individual, the responder lymphocytes proliferate. The major source of stimulation is provided by MHC antigens, and genetic differences in HLA-DR are recognized as the most important determinant of the magnitude of proliferation. The mixed leukocyte reaction provides an *in vitro* model for transplant rejection, and as such is a useful predictor of graft outcome. Cultured venous and arterial endothelial cells (but not smooth muscle cells or fibroblasts) can also stimulate allogenic lymphocytes to proliferate in mixed culture, and the expanded population of lymphocytes recovered from such a culture contains cytotoxic cells directed against antigens on the endothelium itself (Hirschberg *et al.*, 1975; Groenewegen & Buurman, 1984). Venous endothelial cells may differ from arterial endothelial cells in the generation of such cell mediated cytotoxicity. Lymphocytes stimulated with venous endothelial cells are capable of lysing both venous and arterial cells, whereas lymphocytes stimulated with arterial cells only develop cytotoxicity against arterial cells, suggesting that antigenic expression may differ between the cell types (Groenewegen *et al.*, 1984).

In vivo class I MHC antigens are constitutively expressed on arterial and venous endothelial cells in the tissues of all species studied. Class II MHC antigens can be detected by immunofluorescence and immunoperoxidase staining on the capillary endothelium of most human organs (Koyama *et al.*, 1979; Natali *et al.*, 1981*a*). In contrast, basal expression of class II MHC molecules by large vessels is less consistent. Constitutive expression by both arterial and venous endothelium has been described, although there appear to be variations between tissues (Hart *et al.*, 1981; Hayry, von Willebrand & Andersson, 1980; Taylor, Rose & Yacoub, 1989), and differences in the level of staining may occur even between vessels within the same tissue (Darr *et al.*, 1984).

Expression of class II MHC molecules by endothelial cells also varies between species. Unlike primate and canine venous and venular endothelial cells, mouse, rabbit, guinea pig and rat endothelial cells generally do not express class II MHC molecules (Natali *et al.*, 1981*b*).

Venular endothelial cells of most species can however be induced to express class II MHC molecules in the presence of inflammatory immune reactions. Indeed, evidence that endothelial cell class II MHC expression may be an important mediator of allograft rejection comes from observations concerning responses to organ transplants in different species.

Immune-mediated up-regulation of class II MHC molecules was first described in mouse skin allografts in which Ia antigens were found to be present on allograft vascular endothelial cells (de Waal *et al.*, 1983). The level of expression was found to depend on the immunological status of the recipient, increasing during rejection episodes but being reduced by immunosuppressive agents or T cell deficiency.

Rodent endothelial cells are constitutively negative for class II MHC molecules and, unlike myocardial cells, appear relatively resistant to induction of class II MHC molecule expression in the face of transplant rejection (Milton & Fabre, 1985). In fact, several characteristics of transplantation in rats suggest that endothelial cells do not play a major role in eliciting rejection (Fabre, 1982). In rats, passive enhancement of kidney allografts by administration of antibody against class II MHC antigens usually confers a significant improvement in graft outcome, and long-term graft survival can usually be achieved by administration of short courses of immunosuppression. In view of this it has been proposed that interstitial dendritic cells (passenger leukocytes) are the principal cells involved in eliciting a rejection response. These cells are short lived following transplantation and, unlike rodent endothelial cells, stain intensely for class II MHC antigens. Thus the immunogenicity of rat allografts would be predicted to decline as the graft becomes depleted of dendritic cells, whereas in species in which vascular endothelial cells express class II MHC molecules grafts would remain immunogenic. The importance of dendritic cells as participants in rodent allograft rejection is supported further by the observation that the immunogenicity of long-term surviving renal transplants can be restored by injection of donor dendritic cells, leading to allograft rejection (Lechler & Batchelor, 1982).

In contrast, in humans dendritic cells appear less important, perhaps because class II MHC molecule-bearing endothelial cells provide the major stimulus for initiating an immune response. Up-regulation of endothelial cell class II MHC molecules has been described on endothelial cells during acute rejection episodes in human renal transplants (Fuggle *et al.*, 1986). The increased class II molecule expression, which occurred on renal tubular cells in addition to large vessel endothelium, was associated with inflammatory cell infiltration of the graft and influenced by immunosuppressive therapy, being less marked in patients treated with cyclosporin A. Whether increased endothelial cell class II MHC molecule expression is also a feature of chronic rejection is less clear, although all patients with normal endothelial cell class II MHC molecule expression at 90 days maintained good renal function two years after transplantation.

A subsequent study confirmed the increase in large vessel endothelial cell class II MHC molecule expression during rejection episodes (Bishop *et al.*, 1989), but found that the expression of class II MHC molecules of capillary endothelium actually decreased in the presence of rejection. However, this apparent reduction in capillary endothelial cell class II molecule expression may, in fact, have reflected endothelial cell destruction by the rejection process (supporting the concept that endothelial cells may be a major target for acute rejection responses) as other endothelial cell surface molecules, including ICAM-1, were also decreased.

Whether increased endothelial cell class II MHC antigen expression contributes to acute human cardiac rejection is less clear, although immunocytochemical changes which suggest that endothelial cells may be involved in cell-mediated rejection have been described (Hengstenberg *et al.*, 1990).

Endothelial cells in transplant-associated arteriosclerosis

Several observations support the hypothesis that transplant associated arteriosclerosis may be an immune response to donor endothelium. The lesion itself differs histologically from that of atherosclerosis and involves both the arterial and venous systems (Oni, Ray & Hosenpund, 1992). In addition, there is no consistent correlation between the presence of traditional risk factors for atherosclerosis and the development of transplant arteriosclerosis. Other observations provide more direct evidence for an immune aetiology. Although the endothelium itself is usually preserved in transplant-associated arteriosclerosis, suggesting it is not the principal target for injury, the frequency of anti-endothelial cell antibodies is increased (Dunn *et al.*, 1992). In addition, coronary arterial endothelial cells from vessels which have undergone transplant-associated arteriosclerosis express high level of MHC class II molecules, whereas normal human coronary arteries or typical atherosclerotic lesions have few, if any, class II MHC molecule expressing cells. *In vitro* human arterial endothelial cells which have been induced to express class II MHC molecules are able to stimulate proliferation of allogenic CD4 lymphocytes, in addition to augmenting IL-2 secretion by PHA-activated CD4 cells (Salomon *et al.*, 1991). Immunohistochemical analysis of the inflammatory infiltrate within the expanded intima of transplanted coronary arteries reveals the presence of both CD4 and CD8

T lymphocytes (in approximately equal numbers) and macrophages, localized in a ring immediately subjacent to the luminal endothelium. Thus endothelial cells may play an important role in the development of transplant-associated coronary artery arteriosclerosis by promoting lymphocyte activation and sustaining an immune response.

Histologically, the predominant source of damage in transplant associated arteriosclerosis appears to be smooth muscle cell proliferation together with extracellular matrix deposition. Several mitogens may contribute to this smooth muscle cell proliferation including IL-1 (expressed on the surface of endothelial cells or secreted by macrophages recruited to the site of the lesion) and platelet-derived growth factor which may be secreted by several cells including platelets, macrophages, endothelial cells and smooth muscle cells. Platelet-derived growth factor is a potent mitogen of both smooth muscle cells and fibroblasts, which in its biologically active form is a dimeric molecule (Ross, Raines & Bowen Pope, 1986). Two distinct protein subunits (termed A and B) have been identified, and both A and B homodimers and the heterodimer can be mitogenic. Transcripts from both the *sis* gene (which encodes the PDGF B chain) and the PDGF A chain gene can be detected in cultured endothelial cells (Barrett *et al.*, 1984; Collins *et al.*, 1987). *Sis* gene transcript levels are increased in endothelial cells from human atherosclerotic lesions (Barrett & Benditt, 1987), and increased PDGF B receptors have been detected on smooth muscle cells in the arteriosclerotic lesions of chronically rejecting allograft kidneys (Rubin *et al.*, 1988).

Thus endothelial cells may contribute to chronic vascular rejection by promoting both leukocyte accumulation and activation and smooth muscle cell proliferation. Whether these proposed mechanisms have any relevance to the pathogenesis of classical atherosclerosis is unclear. Transplant associated coronary arteriosclerosis does not affect the recipient's own vessels supporting the view that immunological incompatibility is involved. Clearly, endothelial cells in usual atherosclerotic lesions do not bear alloantigens, and they typically do not express class II MHC molecules. Adherence of monocytes and lymphocytes to arterial endothelium is, however, one of the earliest detectable events in experimental and human atherosclerosis (Munro & Cotran, 1988), and an inducible endothelial–leukocyte adhesion molecule with high homology to human VCAM-1 has been identified early in the generation of atherosclerotic plaques in a rabbit model of atherosclerosis (Cybulsky & Gimbrone, 1991).

Endothelial cells in antibody-mediated rejection

Whilst MHC molecules play a major role in the development of allograft rejection (and have been identified as an important determinant of allograft survival), endothelial cells express many other antigens which may be recognized as foreign and contribute to allograft rejection. The expression of MHC molecules by endothelial cells endows them with the capacity to activate alloreactive T cells and thus contribute to both cell mediated and humoral rejection. Much of the evidence that other endothelial cell alloantigens may contribute to rejection responses come from studies of antibody mediated rejection. Endothelial cells constitutively express ABH blood group antigens, which are important histocompatibility antigens in transplantation, in addition to tissue specific antigens. Many endothelial cell antigens are also expressed on monocytes (Paul, Baldwin & van Es, 1985).

Antibodies against endothelial cell alloantigens may be preformed and contribute to hyperacute rejection or produced following transplantation by activated B lymphocytes, presumably with the help of CD4 cells which have also been activated by the allogenic endothelium. Virtually all patients with preformed anti-endothelial cell antibodies reject their grafts (Paul *et al.*, 1978; Paul *et al.*, 1979; Cerilli *et al.*, 1985). In such cases the presence of such preformed antibodies can usually be detected by the presence of a positive monocyte cross match, although hyperacute rejection can occur as a result of sensitization to endothelial cell antigens not present on monocytes (Jordan *et al.*, 1988).

Circulating anti-endothelial cell antibodies may also develop following transplantation and the presence of such antibodies correlates closely with the development of renal allograft rejection (Cerilli *et al.*, 1977). Furthermore, the frequency of antibodies reacting with endothelial cells is increased in eluates from rejected human renal allografts compared to eluates from normally functioning grafts or non-transplanted kidneys (Baldwin *et al.*, 1981).

The prevalence of anti-endothelial cell antibodies in transplant recipients is, however, likely to be underestimated as the identification of antibodies against endothelial cells is frequently masked by the presence of anti-HLA antibody (Cerilli *et al.*, 1985). Over 70% of recipients of HLA-identical living related renal transplants who reject their grafts exhibit cytotoxic antibody to antigens expressed on donor vascular endothelial cells and on corresponding peripheral blood monocytes. The antigens on endothelial cells and monocytes which are recognized by these antibodies are as yet largely uncharacterized, although several potential target antigens have been defined by monoclonal antibodies (Wood *et al.*, 1988).

It should be stressed that not all circulating antibodies that develop following transplantation necessarily participate in the development of graft rejection. The proposition that circulating anti-endothelial cell antibodies can induce vascular injury is, however, supported by the finding of antibodies that mediate complement-dependent endothelial cell lysis in various forms of systemic vasculitis. In Kawasaki disease, a paediatric vasculitis of unknown aetiology, IgM and IgG antibodies which selectively damage endothelial cells which have been stimulated by cytokines can be detected (Leung *et al.*, 1986*a*,*b*; see Chapter 9). Furthermore, the proliferative lesion which develops in Kawasaki syndrome is morphologically similar to the lesions of transplantation associated arteriosclerosis. In the haemolytic uraemic syndrome, another paediatric vasculitis which usually follows gastro-intestinal infection with Shiga or verotoxin positive bacteria, antibodies which lyse unstimulated but not interferon-γ treated endothelial cells circulate (Leung *et al.*, 1988; and see Chapter 10). Indeed, a possible association between an infectious agent and the development of anti-endothelial cell antibodies in paediatric transplant recipients who rejected their grafts has been reported (Harmer *et al.*, 1990).

In addition to acting as important mediators of the immunological response to foreign organs, vascular endothelial cells may also influence the development of tissue injury through other pro-inflammatory and procoagulant functions.

Endothelial cells as regulators of coagulation

Allograft rejection is commonly associated with intravascular fibrin deposition. Basally, the endothelial cell surface is anticoagulant in that it expresses thrombomodulin and secretes protein S (Esmon & Owen, 1981; Stern *et al.*, 1986), which catalyse the activated protein C pathway, and it also expresses heparin (Rosenberg & Rosenberg, 1984), which catalyses the anti-thrombin III pathway. As noted in Chapter 2, exposure of endothelial cells to tumour necrosis factor or IL-1 induces expression of tissue factor which binds factor VIIa, thereby initiating the extrinsic clotting pathway, and decreases the expression of thrombomodulin (Bevilacqua *et al.*, 1984; Nawroth *et al.*, 1986; Nawroth & Stern, 1986; Schorer *et al.*, 1986). In addition tumour necrosis factor and IL-1 increase endothelial cell synthesis of plasminogen activator inhibitor (Nachman *et al.*, 1986; Bevilacqua *et al.*, 1986). There is therefore both loss of basal endothelial cell surface anticoagulant activity, and induction of new procoagulant functions. Recent studies suggest that alterations in the coagulant properties of vascular endothelial cells may contribute to intragraft thrombin and fibrin deposition during rejection episodes. TNF production by infiltrating mononuclear cells in rat cardiac transplants is associated with widespread protein C and protein S deposition, resulting in low plasma concentrations of protein C and protein S. Human acute renal allograft rejection is associated with depression of plasma protein C and free protein S levels, decreased microvascular thrombomodulin expression, and widespread endothelial and interstitial deposition of protein C, protein S, thrombin, fibrin, and factors V and VII (Tsuchida *et al.*, 1992). Such changes are associated with increased plasma levels of tumour necrosis factor, suggesting that TNF may contribute to allograft rejection by promoting intragraft coagulation.

Expression of leukocyte endothelial cell adhesion molecules

Endothelial cells may also influence the development and progression of allograft rejection by expressing leukocyte adhesion molecules. Increased expression of E-selectin, ICAM-1 and VCAM-1 have all been reported on renal allograft vascular endothelium during rejection episodes (Briscoe *et al.*, 1992; Fuggle *et al.*, 1993). Furthermore, such increased expression appears to correlate with leukocytic infiltration of the graft. VCAM-1 and ICAM-1 expression are also increased on the endothelium of human hepatic allografts undergoing both acute and chronic rejection (Adams *et al.*, 1989; Bacchi *et al.*, 1993; Steinhoff *et al.*, 1993). Increased ICAM-1 expression is reduced in acute rejection by high dose corticosteroid treatment (Adams *et al.*, 1989). In human cardiac allografts, ICAM-1 and VCAM-1 expression are increased on endothelial cells in the presence of infiltrating lymphocytes (Briscoe *et al.*, 1991; Taylor *et al.*, 1992).

Endothelial cells as a target for therapeutic intervention

Support for a causal relationship between the expression of endothelial cell adhesion molecules and the development of an inflammatory response leading to allograft rejection is provided by antibody blocking studies. For example, antibodies against LFA-1, the ligand for ICAM-1 and ICAM-2 which is expressed on leukocytes, suppress migration of T lymphocytes through human umbilical vein endothelial cell monolayers (van Epps *et al.*, 1989). Such observations raise the possibility that therapy aimed at inhibiting endothelial cell–leukocyte interactions may be useful in preventing allograft rejection. In non-human primates, antibodies against ICAM-1 reduce T cell infiltration and prolong survival of renal and cardiac transplants (Cosimi *et al.*, 1990; Flavin *et al.*, 1991). Antibodies against VCAM-1 interfere with murine cardiac allograft rejection, although such treatment does not influence leukocytic infiltration into the graft, raising the possibility that the role of VCAM-1 in mediating transplant rejection may extend beyond that of an adhesion molecule (Pelletier *et al.*, 1992). Survival of murine cardiac allografts is also prolonged by treatment with a monoclonal antibody to ICAM-1 in combination with an antibody to the CD11a component of leukocyte function-associated antigen-1 (Isobe *et al.*, 1992).

Antibodies which block leukocyte receptors for endothelial adhesion molecules have been found to be effective in other animal models. For example, antibodies against CD-18 (the ligand for ICAM-1), and VLA-4 (the ligand for VCAM-1) are effective in reducing rabbit cardiac transplant rejection (Sadahiro *et al.* 1993).

Clinical trials in human subjects suggest that monoclonal antibodies against endothelial adhesion molecules may provide a safe and effective form of immunosuppression (Lehr *et al.*, 1993).

Conclusions

Endothelial cells may play a general role in regulating inflammatory responses by controlling local blood flow, recruiting leukocytes to sites of inflammation and facilitating extravasation of both inflammatory cells and macromolecules into the tissues. In addition, by providing conditions which facilitate lymphocyte accumulation and producing molecules which are important in lymphocyte activation, endothelial cells gain the ability to participate in the immune response to foreign antigens. Thus, endothelial cells can be induced to express class II MHC molecules by interferon-γ and can provide the necessary costimulatory signals to produce functional T cell activation. Whilst these properties may be shared by other antigen presenting cells, endothelial cells may be particularly important in the development of immune responses because of their unique anatomical position.

Although this capacity of endothelial cells to participate in immune mediated reactions has largely been defined *in vitro*, *in vivo* studies support the hypothesis that endothelial cells are involved in immune responses in several clinical settings, and particularly in the field of transplantation. The earliest histological studies of rejecting organs described evidence of endothelial cell injury, and more recent studies have shown increased expression of MHC class II molecules and adhesion molecules on vascular endothelium during rejection episodes. Furthermore, a proportion of patients have preformed, or develop, antibodies directed against foreign endothelial antigens. In cardiac transplantation the development of transplant associated arteriosclerosis, which may itself be an immune-mediated phenomenon, may also contribute to graft loss.

Thus vascular endothelial cells in organ transplants may present foreign antigens, together with the necessary costimulator signals, to host lymphocytes, thereby initiating an immune response against the graft. In turn, foreign endothelial cells may become a target for either cellular or antibody mediated immune reactions, in addition to contributing to allograft destruction by participating in the development of an inflammatory response. Current immunosuppressive regimes are directed predominantly against leukocytes. Defining the role of endothelial cells in the immunological response to foreign organs may not only increase understanding of the rejection process, but also open up new prospects for therapeutic intervention.

Acknowledgement

The author is a recipient of a National Kidney Research Fund Senior Fellowship.

References

Adams, D. H., Hubscher, S. G., Shaw, J., Rothlein, R. & Neuberger, J. M. (1989). Intercellular adhesion molecule 1 on liver allografts during rejection. *Lancet*, **ii**, 1122–5.

Bacchi, C. E., Marsh, C. L., Perkins, J. D., Carithers, R. L., McVicar, J. P., Hudkins, K. L., Benjamin, C. D., Harlan, J. M., Lobb, R. & Alpers, C. E. (1993). Expression of vascular cell adhesion molecule-1 (VCAM-1) in liver and pancreas allograft rejection. *American Journal of Pathology*, **142**, 579–91.

Bach, F. H., Bach, M. L., & Sondel, P. M. (1976). Differential function of major histocompatibility complex antigens in T-lymphocyte activation. *Nature*, **259**, 273–81.

Baldwin, W. M., Soulillou, J. P., Claas, F. H. J., Peyrat, M. A., van Es, L. A. & van Rood, J. J. (1981). Antibodies to endothelial antigens in eluates of 88 human kidneys: correlation with graft survival and presence of T- and B-cell antibodies. *Transplantation Proceedings*, **13**, 1547–50.

Barrett, T. B. & Benditt, E. P. (1987). *sis* (platelet derived growth factor B chain) gene transcript levels are elevated in human atherosclerotic lesions compared to normal artery. *Proceedings of the National Academy of Sciences USA*, **84**, 1099–1103.

Barrett, T. B., Gajduseck, C. M., Schwartz, S. M., McDougall, J. K. & Benditt, E. P. (1984). Expression of the *sis* gene by endothelial cells in culture and *in vivo*. *Proceedings of the National Academy of Sciences USA*, **81**, 6772–4.

Bevilacqua, M. P., Pober, J. S., Majeau, G. R., Cotran, R. S. & Gimbrone, M. A. Jr. (1984). Interleukin-1 (IL-1) induces biosynthesis and cell surface expression of procoagulant activity in human vascular endothelial cells. *Journal of Experimental Medicine*, **160**, 618–23.

Bevilacqua, M. P., Schleef, R. R., Gimbrone, M. A. Jr. & Loskutoff, D. J. (1986). Regulation of the fibrinolytic system of cultured human vascular endothelium by interleukin 1. *Journal of Clinical Investigation*, **78**, 587–91.

Bieber, C. P., Stinson, E. B., Shumway, N. E., Payne, R. & Kosek, (1970). Cardiac transplantation in man. VII. Cardiac allograft pathology. *Circulation*, **41**, 753–72.

Billingham, M. E. (1987). Cardiac transplant atherosclerosis. *Transplantation Proceedings*, **19**, 19–25.

Bishop, G. A., Waugh, J. A., Landers, D. V., Krensky, A. M. & Hall, B. M. (1989). Microvascular destruction in renal transplant rejection. *Transplantation*, **48**, 408–14.

Briscoe, D. M., Pober, J. S., Harmon, W. E. & Cotran, R. S. (1992). Expression of vascular cell adhesion molecule-1 in human renal allografts. *Journal of the American Society of Nephrology*, **3**, 1180–5.

Briscoe, D. M., Schoen, F. J., Rice, G. E., Bevilacqua, M. P., Ganz, P. & Pober, J. S. (1991). Induced expression of endothelial-leukocyte adhesion molecules in human cardiac allografts. *Transplantation*, **51**, 537–47.

Busch, G. J., Reynolds, E. S., Galvaneck, E. G., Braun, W. E. & Dammin, G. J. (1971). Human renal allografts: the role of vascular injury in early graft failure. *Medicine*, **50**, 29–79.

Cerilli, J. Brasile, L., Galouzis, T., Lempert, N. & Clarke, J. (1985). The vascular endothelial cell antigen system. *Transplantation*, **39**, 286–9.

Cerilli, J., Holliday, J. E., Fesperman, D. P. & Folger, M. R. (1977). Antivascular endothelial cell antibody—its role in transplantation. *Surgery*, **81**, 132–8.

Collins, T., Korman, A. J., Wake, C. T., Boss, J. M., Kappes, D. J., Fiers, W., Ault, K. A., Gimbrone, M. A., Strominger, J. L. & Pober, J. S. (1984). Immune interferon activates multiple class II major histocompatibility complex genes and the associated invariant chain gene in human endothelial cells and dermal fibroblasts. *Proceedings of the National Academy of Sciences USA*, **81**, 1878–84.

Collins, T., Pober, J. S., Gimbrone, M. A. Jr., Hammacher, A., Betsholtz, C., Westermark, B. & Heldin, C. H. (1987). Cultured human endothelial cells express platelet-derived growth factor A chain. *American Journal of Pathology*, **126**, 7–12.

Cosimi, A. B., Conti, D., Delmonicop, F. L., Preffer, F. I., Wee, S. L., Rothlein, R., Faanes, R. & Colvin, R. B. (1990). *In vivo* effects of monoclonal antibody to ICAM-1 (CD54) in nonhuman primates with renal allografts. *Journal of Immunology*, 144, 4604–12.

Cybulsky, M. I. & Gimbrone, M. A. (1991). Endothelial expression of a mononuclear leukocyte adhesion molecule during atherogenesis. *Science*, **251**, 788–91.

Dalmasso, A. P. (1992). The complement system in xenotransplantation. *Immunopharmacology*, **24**, 149–60.

Damle N. K. & Aruffo, A. (1991). Vascular cell adhesion molecule 1 induces T-cell antigen receptor-independent activation of CD4+ T lymphocytes. *Proceedings of the National Academy of Sciences USA*, **88**, 6403–7.

Darr, A. S., Fuggle, S. V., Fabre, J. W., Ting, A. & Morris, P. J. (1984). The detailed distribution of MHC class II antigens in normal human organs. *Transplantation*, **38**, 293–8.

Dunn, M. J., Crisp, S. J., Rose, M. L., Taylor, P. M. & Yacoub, M. H. (1992). Anti-endothelial cell antibodies and coronary artery disease after cardiac transplantation. *Lancet*, **339**, 1566–70.

van Epps, D. E., Potter, J., Vachula, M., Smith, C. W. & Anderson, D. C. (1989). Suppression of human lymphocyte chemotaxis and transendothelial migration by anti-LFA-1 antibody. *Journal of Immunology*, **143**, 3207–10.

Esmon, C. T. & Owen, W. G. (1981). Identification of an endothelial cofactor for thrombin-catalyzed activation of protein C. *Proceedings of the National Academy of Sciences USA*, **78**, 2249–52.

Fabre, J. W. (1982). Rat kidney allograft model: was it all too good to be true? *Transplantation*, **34**, 223–5.

Faull, R. J., Starr, R. J. & Russ, G. R. (1989). Vascular endothelial cell expression of adhesion molecules and HLA antigens in renal allografts. *Transplantation Proceedings*, **21**, 316–17.

Flavin, T., Ivens, K., Rothlein, R., Faanes, R., Clayberger, C., Billingham, M. & Starnes, V. A., (1991). Monoclonal antibodies against intercellular adhesion molecule-1 prolong cardiac allograft survival in cynomolgus monkeys. *Transplantation Proceedings*, **23**, 533–4.

Forbes, R. D. C. & Guttmann, R. D. (1982). Evidence for complement-induced endothelial injury *in vivo*: a comparative ultrastructural tracer study in a controlled model of hyperacute rat cardiac allograft rejection. *American Journal of Pathology*, **106**, 378–87.

Fuggle, S. V., McWhinnie, D. L., Chapman, J. R., Taylor, H. M. & Morris, P. J. (1986). Sequential analysis of HLA-class II antigen expression in human renal allografts: induction of tubular class II antigens and correlation with clinical parameters. *Transplantation*, **42**, 144–50.

Fuggle, S. V., Sanderson, J. B., Gray, D. W., Richardson, A. & Morris, P. J. (1993). Variation in expression of endothelial adhesion molecules in pretransplant and transplanted kidneys–correlation with intragraft events. *Transplantation*, **55**, 117–23.

Groenewegen, G. & Buurman, W. A. (1984). Vascular endothelial cells present alloantigens to unprimed lymphocytes. *Scandinavian Journal of Immunology*, **19**, 269–73.

Groenewegen, G., Buurman, W. A., Jeunhomme, M. A. A., van der Linden, C. J., Vegt, P. A. & Kootstra, G. (1984). *In vitro* stimulation of lymphocytes by vascular endothelial cells: a study with canine arterial and venous endothelial cells. *Transplantation*, 206–10.

Groenewegen, G., Buurman, W. A. & van der Linden, C. J. (1985). Lymphokine dependence of *in vivo* expression of MHC class II antigens by endothelium. *Nature*, **316**, 361–3.

Guinan, E. C., Smith, B. R., Doukas, J. T., Miller, R. A. & Pober, J. S. (1989). Vascular endothelial cells enhance T cell responses by markedly augmenting IL-2 concentrations. *Cellular Immunology*, **118**, 166–77.

Harmer, A. W., Rigden, S. P. A., Koffman, C. G. & Welsh, K. I. (1990). Preliminary report: dramatic rise in renal allograft failure rate. *Lancet*, **335**, 1184–5.

Hart, D. N. J., Fuggle, S. V., Williams, K. A., Fabre, J. W., Ting, A. & Morris, P. J. (1981). Localization of HLA-ABC and DR antigens in human kidney. *Transplantation*, **31**, 428–33.

Hayry, P., von Willebrand, E. & Andersson, L. C. (1980). Expression of HLA-ABC and -DR locus antigens on human kidney, endothelial, tubular and glomerular cells. *Scandinavian Journal of Immunology*, **11**, 303–10.

Hengstenberg, C., Rose, M. L., Page, C., Taylor, P. M. & Yacoub, M. H. (1990). Immunocytochemical changes suggestive of damage to endothelial cells during rejection of human cardiac allografts. *Transplantation*, **49**, 895–9.

Hirschberg, H., Bergh, O. J. & Thorsby, E. (1980). Antigen presenting properties of human vascular endothelial cells. *Journal of Experimental Medicine*, **152**, 249s–55s.

Hirschberg, H., Evenson, S. A., Henricksen, T. & Thorsby, E. (1975). The human mixed lymphocyte–endothelium culture interaction. *Transplantation*, **19**, 495–504.

Hughes, C. C. W., Savage, C. O. S. & Pober, J. S. (1990). Endothelial cells augment T cell interleukin 2 production by a contact-dependent mechanism involving CD2/LFA-3 interaction. *Journal of Experimental Medicine*, **171**, 1453–7.

Isobe, M., Yagita, H., Okumura, K. & Ihara, A. (1992). Specific acceptance of cardiac allograft after treatment with antibodies to ICAM-1 and LFA-1. *Science*, **255**, 1125–7.

Jirik, F. R., Podor, T.J., Hirano, T., Kishimoto, T., Loskutoff, D. J., Carson, D. A. & Lotz, M. (1989). Bacterial polysaccharide and inflammatory mediators augment IL-6 secretion by human endothelial cells. *Journal of Immunology*, **142**, 144–7.

Jordan, S. C., Yap, H. K., Sakai, R. S., Alfonso, P. & Fitchman, M. (1988). Hyperacute allograft rejection mediated by anti-vascular cell antibodies with a negative monocyte crossmatch. *Transplantation*, **46**, 585–602.

Koyama, K., Fukunishi, T., Barcos, M., Tanigaki, N. & Pressman, D. (1979). Human Ia-like antigens in non-lymphoid organs. *Immunology*, **38**, 333–41.

Kurt-Jones, E. A., Fiers, W. & Pober, J. S. (1987). Membrane interleukin 1 induction on human endothelial cells and dermal fibroblasts. *Journal of Immunology*, **139**, 2317–24.

Lechler, R. I. & Batchelor, J. R. (1982). Restoration of immunogenicity to passenger cell-depleted kidney allografts by the addition of donor strain dendritic cells. *Journal of Experimental Medicine*, **155**, 31–41.

Lechler, R. I., Giovanni, L., Batchelor, J. R., Reinsmoen, N. & Bach, F. H. (1990). The molecular basis of alloreactivity. *Immunology Today*, **11**, 83–8.

Lehr, H. A., Arfors, K. E., Hubner, C., Menger, M. D. & Messmer, K. (1993). Leukocyte-endothelium interaction as a target for anti-atherogenic strategies in allograft rejection. *Transplantation Proceedings*, **25**, 2067–9.

Leung, D. Y. M., Collins, T., Lapierre, L. A., Geha, R. S. & Pober, J. S. (1986*a*). IgM antibodies in the acute phase of Kawasaki syndrome lyse cultured vascular endothelial cells stimulated by gamma interferon. *Journal of Clinical Investigation*, **77**, 1428–35.

Leung, D. Y. M., Geha, R. S., Newburger, J. W., Burns, J. S., Fiers, W., Lapierre, L. A. & Pober, J. S. (1986*b*). Two monokines, interleukin 1 and tumor necrosis factor, render cultured vascular endothelial cells susceptible to lysis by antibodies circulating during Kawasaki syndrome. *Journal of Experimental Medicine*, **164**, 1958–72.

Leung, D. Y. M., Moake, J. L., Havens, P. L., Kim, J. M. & Pober, J. S. (1988). Lytic anti-endothelial cell antibodies are present in hemolytic uremic syndrome. *Lancet*, **i**, 183–6.

March, C. J., Mosley, B., Larsen, A., Cerretti, D. P., Braedt, G., Price, V., Gillis, S., Henney, C. S., Kronheim, S., Grabstein, K., Conlon, P. J., Hopp, T. P. & Cosman, D. (1985). Cloning, sequence and expression of two distinct human interleukin-1 complementary DNAs. *Nature*, **315**, 641–7.

Messadi, D. V., Pober, J. S. & Murphy, G. F. (1988). Effects of recombinant γ interferon on HLA-DR and DQ expression by skin cells in short term organ culture. *Laboratory Investigation*, **58**, 61–7.

Milton, A. D. & Fabre, J. W. (1985). Massive induction of donor-type class I and II major histocompatibility complex antigens in rejecting cardiac allografts in the rat. *Journal of Experimental Medicine*, **161**, 98–112.

Munro, J. M. & Cotran, R. S. (1988). The pathogenesis of atherosclerosis: atherogenesis and inflammation. *Laboratory Investigation*, **58**, 249–61.

Munro, J. M., Pober, J. S. & Cotran, R. S. (1989). Tumor necrosis factor and interferon-γ induce distinct patterns of endothelial activation and leukocyte accumulation in skin of *Papio anubis*. *American Journal of Pathology*, **135**, 121–33.

Nachman, R. L., Hajjar, K. A., Silverstein, R. L. & Dinarello, C. A. (1986). Interleukin 1 induces endothelial cell synthesis of plasminogen activator inhibitor. *Journal of Experimental Medicine*, **163**, 1595–600.

Natali, P. G., de Martino, C., Quaranta, V., Nicotra, M. R., Frezza, F., Pellegrino, M. A. & Ferrone (1981*a*). Expression of Ia-like antigens in normal human non-lymphoid tissues. *Transplantation*, **31**, 75–8.

Natali, P. G., Quaranta, V., Nicotra, M. R., Apolloni, C., Pellegrino, M. A. & Ferrone, S. (1981*b*). Tissue distribution of Ia-like antigens in different species: analysis with monoclonal antibodies. *Transplantation Proceedings*, **13**, 1026–9.

Nawroth, P. P., Handley, D. A., Esmon, C. T. & Stern, D. M. (1986). Interleukin-1 induces endothelial cell procoagulant while suppressing cell surface anticoagulant activity. *Proceedings of the National Academy of Sciences USA*, **83**, 3460–4.

Nawroth, P. P. & Stern, D. M. (1986). Modulation of endothelial cell haemostatic properties by tumor necrosis factor. *Journal of Experimental Medicine*, **163**, 740–5.

Oni, A. A., Ray, J. & Hosenpund, J. D. (1992). Coronary venous intimal thickening in explanted cardiac allografts. *Transplantation*, **53**, 1247–51.

O'Sullivan, D., Grey, H. & Shaw, S. (1991). Analysis of T cell stimulation by superantigen plus major histocompatibility complex class II molecules or by CD3 monoclonal antibody: costimulation by purified adhesion ligands VCAM-1, ICAM-1, but not ELAM-1. *Journal of Experimental Medicine*, **174**, 901–13.

Paul, L. C., Baldwin, III W. M. & van Es Leendert, A. (1985). Vascular endothelial alloantigens in renal transplantation. *Transplantation*, **40**, 117–23.

Paul, L. C., Claas, F. H. J., van Es L. A., Kalff, M. W. & de Graeff, J. (1979). Accelerated rejection of a renal allograft associated with pretransplantation antibodies directed against donor antigens on endothelium and monocytes. *New England Journal of Medicine*, **300**, 1258–60.

Paul, L. C., van Es, L. A., de la Riviere, G. B., Eernisse, G. & de Graeff, J. (1978). Blood group B antigen on renal endothelium as the target for rejection in an ABO-incompatible recipient. *Transplantation*, **26**, 268–71.

Pelletier, R. P., Ohye, R. G., Vanbuskirk, A., Sedmak, D. D., Kincade, P., Ferguson, R. M. & Orosz, C. G. (1992). Importance of endothelial VCAM-1 for inflammatory leukocytic infiltration *in vivo*. *Journal of Immunology*, **149**, 2473–81.

Pober, J. S. (1988). Cytokine mediated activation of vascular endothelium: physiology and pathology. *American Journal of Pathology*, **133**, 426–33.

Pober, J. S., Collins, T., Gimbrone, M. A., Cotran, R. S., Gitlin, J. D., Fiers, W., Clayberger, C., Krensky, A. M., Burakoff, S. J., Reiss, C. S. (1983*c*). Lymphocytes recognize human vascular endothelial and dermal fibroblast Ia antigens induced by recombinant immune interferon. *Nature*, **305**, 726–9.

Pober, J. S., Collins, T., Gimbrone, M. A., Libby, P. & Reiss, C. S. (1983*a*). Inducible expression of class II histocompatibility complex antigens and the immunogenicity of vascular endothelium. *Transplantation*, **41**, 141–6.

Pober, J. S., Gimbrone, M. A., Cotran, R. S., Reiss, C. S., Burakoff, S. J., Fiers, W. & Ault, K. A. (1983*b*). Ia expression by vascular endothelium is inducible by activated T cells and γ-interferon. *Journal of Experimental Medicine*, **157**, 1339–3.

Rosenberg, R. D. & Rosenberg, J. S. (1984). Natural anticoagulant mechanisms. *Journal of Clinical Investigation*, **74**, 1–5.

Ross, R., Raines, E. W. & Bowen Pope, D. F. (1986). The biology of platelet derived growth factor. *Cell*, **46**, 155–169.

Rowlands, D. T., Hill, G. S. & Zmijewski, C. M. (1976). The pathology of renal homograft rejection. *American Journal of Pathology*, **85**, 774–802.

Rubin, K., Tingstrom, A., Hansson, G. K. *et al.* (1988). Induction of B-type receptors for platelet-derived growth factor in vascular inflammation: possible implications for development of vascular proliferative lesions. *Lancet*, **i**, 1353–6.

Sadahiro, M., McDonald, T. O. & Allen, M. D. (1993). Reduction in cellular and vascular rejection by blocking leucocyte adhesion molecule receptors. *American Journal of Pathology*, **142**, 675–83.

Salomon, R. N., Hughes, C. C. W., Schoen, F. J., Payne, D. D., Pober, J. S. & Libby, P. (1991). Human coronary transplantation-associated arteriosclerosis: evidence of a chronic immune reaction to activated graft endothelial cells. *American Journal of Pathology*, **138**, 791–8.

Savage, C. O. S., Brooks, C., Picard, J., Harcourt, G. & Wilcox, N. (1993). Processing and presentation of peptides by vascular endothelial cells to CD4+ T cell lines. *Clinical and Experimental Immunology*, **16**(Suppl 1), 19.

Savage, C. O. S., Hughes, C. C. W., Pepinsky, R. B., Wallner, B. P., Freedman, A. S. & Pober, J. S. (1991). Endothelial cell lymphocyte function-associated antigen-3 and an unidentified ligand act in concert to provide costimulation to human peripheral blood CD4+ T cells. *Cellular Immunology*, **137**, 150–63.

Schorer, A. E., Kaplan, M. E., Rao, G. H. R. & Moldow, C. F. (1986). Interleukin-1 stimulates endothelial cell tissue factor production and expression by a prostaglandin independent mechanism. *Thrombosis and Haemostasis*, **56**, 256–9.

van Seventer, G. A., Newman, W., Shimizu, Y., Nutman, T. B., Tanaka, Y., Horgan, K. J., Gopal, T. V., Ennis, E., O'Sullivan, D., Grey, H. & Shaw, S. (1991). Analysis of T cell stimulation by superantigen plus major histocompatibility complex class II molecules or by CD3 monoclonal antibody: costimulation by purified adhesion ligand VCAM-1, ICAM-1 but not ELAM-1. *Journal of Experimental Medicine*, **174**, 901–13.

Sobel, R. A., Blanchette, B. W., Bhan, A. K. & Colvin, R. B. (1984). The immunopathology of experimental allergic encephalomyelitis. II. Endothelial cell Ia increases prior to inflammatory cell infiltrates. *Journal of Immunology*, **132**, 2402–7.

Steinhoff, G., Behrend, M., Schrader, B., Duijvestijn, A. M. & Wonigeit, K. (1993). Expression patterns of leukocyte adhesion ligand molecules on human liver endothelia. Lack of ELAM-1 and CD62 inducibility on sinusoidal endothelia and distinct distribution of VCAM-1, ICAM-1, ICAM-2, and LFA-3. *American Journal of Pathology*, **142**, 481–8.

Stern, D. M., Brett, J., Harris, K. & Nawroth, P. P. (1986). Participation of endothelial cells in the protein C-protein S anticoagulant pathway: the synthesis and release of protein S. *Journal of Cell Biology*, **102**, 1971–8.

Taylor, P. M., Rose, M. L. & Yacoub, M. (1989). Expression of class I and class II MHC antigens in normal and transplanted human lung. *Transplantation Proceedings*, **21**, 451–2.

Taylor, P. M., Rose, M. L., Yacoub, M. H. & Pigott, R. (1992). Induction of vascular adhesion molecules during rejection of human cardiac allografts. *Transplantation*, **54**, 451–7.

Terai, M., Kohno, Y., Namba, M. *et al.* (1990). Class II major histocompatibility antigen expression on coronary arterial endothelium in a patient with Kawasaki disease. *Human Pathology*, **21**, 231–4.

Tsuchida, A., Salem, H., Thomson, N. & Hancock, W. W. (1992). Tumor necrosis factor production during human renal allograft rejection is associated with depression of plasma protein C and free protein S levels and decreased intragraft thrombomodulin expression. *Journal of Experimental Medicine*, **175**, 81–90.

de Waal, R. M. W., Bogmann, M. J. J., Maass, C. N., Cornelissen, L. M. H., Tax, W. J. M. & Koene, R. A. P. (1983). Variable expression of Ia antigens on the vascular endothelium of mouse skin allografts. *Nature*, **303**, 426–9.

Wagner, C. R., Vetto, R. M. & Burger, D. R. (1984). The mechanisms of antigen presentation by endothelial cells. *Immunobiology*, **168**, 453–69.

Williams, G. M., ter Haar, A., Parks, L. C., & Krajewski, C. A. (1973). Endothelial changes associated with hyperacute, acute and chronic rejection in man. *Transplantation Proceedings*, **5**, 819–22.

Williams, G. M., Lee, D. M., Weymouth, R. F., Harlan, W. R. Jr., Holden, K. R., Stanley, C. M., Millington, G. A. & Hume, D. M. (1967). Studies in hyperacute and chronic renal homograft rejection in man. *Surgery*, **62**, 204–12.

Wood, N. L., Schook, L. B., Studer, E. J., Mohanakumar, T. (1988). Biochemical characterization of human vascular endothelial cell-monocyte antigens defined by monoclonal antibodies. *Transplantation*, **45**, 787–92.

Yousem, S. A., Burke, C. M. & Billingham, M. E. (1985). Pathological pulmonary alterations in long-term human heart–lung transplantation. *Human Pathology*, **16**, 911–23.

Index

Page numbers in italics refer to tables and figures.